RN Pediatric Nursing
REVIEW MODULE EDITION 12.0

Contributors

Alissa Althoff, Ed.D, MSN, RN

Honey C. Holman, MSN, RN

Norma Jean Henry, MSN/Ed., RN

Beth Cusatis Phillips, PhD,
RN, CNE, CHSE

Janean Johnson, DNP, RN, CNE

Pamela Roland, MSN, MBA, RN

LaKeisha Wheless, MSN, RN

Lori Grace, MSN, RN

Mendy Gearhart, DNP, MSN, CCCE

Michelle E. Cawley, MSN, RN

Shannon Davis, MSN, BSN, RN

Consultants

Jessica L. Johnson, DNP, MSN, RN

Judith Drumm, DNS, RN, CPN

Director of content review: Kristen Lawler

Director of development: Derek Prater

Project management: Meri Ann Mason

Coordination of content review: Alissa Althoff, Honey C. Holman

Copy editing: Kelly Von Lunen, Tricia Lunt, Bethany Robertson, Kya Rodgers, Rebecca Her, Sam Shiel, Alethea Surland, Graphic World

Layout: Bethany Robertson, Maureen Bradshaw, Haylee Hedge, scottie. o

Illustrations: Randi Hardy, Graphic World

Online media: Brant Stacy, Ron Hanson, Britney Fuller, Trevor Lund

Interior book design: Spring Lenox

IMPORTANT NOTICE TO THE READER

User's Guide

Welcome to the Assessment Technologies Institute® RN Pediatric Nursing Review Module Edition 12.0. The mission of ATI's Content Mastery Series® Review Modules is to provide user-friendly compendiums of nursing knowledge that will:

- Help you locate important information quickly.
- Assist in your learning efforts.
- Provide exercises for applying your nursing knowledge.
- Facilitate your entry into the nursing profession as a newly licensed nurse.

ORGANIZATION

This Review Module is organized into units covering the foundations of pediatric nursing, nursing care of children who have systems disorders, and nursing care of children who have other specific needs. Chapters within these units conform to one of four organizing principles for presenting the content.

- Nursing concepts
- Growth and development
- Procedures
- System disorders

Nursing concepts chapters begin with an overview describing the central concept and its relevance to nursing. Subordinate themes are covered in outline form to demonstrate relationships and present the information in a clear, succinct manner.

Growth and development chapters cover expected growth and development, including physical and psychosocial development, age-appropriate activities, and health promotion, including immunizations, health screenings, nutrition, and injury prevention.

Procedures chapters include an overview describing the procedure(s) covered in the chapter. These chapters provide nursing knowledge relevant to each procedure, including indications, nursing considerations, interpretation of findings, and complications.

System disorders chapters include an overview describing the disorder(s) and/or disease process. These chapters address assessments, including risk factors, expected findings, laboratory tests, and diagnostic procedures. Next, you will focus on patient-centered care, including nursing care, medications, therapeutic procedures, interprofessional care, and client education. Finally, you will find complications related to the disorder, along with nursing actions in response to those complications.

ACTIVE LEARNING SCENARIOS AND APPLICATION EXERCISES

Each chapter includes opportunities for you to test your knowledge and to practice applying that knowledge. Active Learning Scenario exercises pose a nursing scenario and then direct you to use an ATI Active Learning Template (included at the end of this book) to record the important knowledge a nurse should apply to the scenario. An example is then provided to which you can compare your completed Active Learning Template. Application exercises throughout the chapters include NCLEX-style questions, such as multiple-choice and multiple-select items, providing you with opportunities to practice answering the kinds of questions you might expect to see on ATI assessments or the NCLEX. Answers and rationales are provided to further your learning.

NCLEX® CONNECTIONS

To prepare for the NCLEX-RN, it is important to understand how the content in this Review Module is connected to the NCLEX-RN test plan. You can find information on the detailed test plan at the National Council of State Boards of Nursing's website, www.ncsbn.org. When reviewing content in this Review Module, regularly ask yourself, "How does this content fit into the test plan, and what types of questions related to this content should I expect?"

To help you in this process, we've included NCLEX Connections at the beginning of each unit and with each question in the Application Exercises Answer Keys. The NCLEX Connections at the beginning of each unit point out areas of the detailed test plan that relate to the content within that unit. The NCLEX Connections attached to the Application Exercises Answer Keys demonstrate how each exercise fits within the detailed content outline. These NCLEX Connections will help you understand how the detailed content outline is organized, starting with major client needs categories and subcategories and followed by related content areas and tasks. The major client needs categories are:

- Safe and Effective Care Environment
  - Management of Care
  - Safety and Infection Control
- Health Promotion and Maintenance
- Psychosocial Integrity
- Physiological Integrity
  - Basic Care and Comfort
  - Pharmacological and Parenteral Therapies
  - Reduction of Risk Potential
  - Physiological Adaptation

An NCLEX Connection might, for example, alert you that content within a unit is related to:

- Physiological Adaptation
  - Alterations in Body Systems

QSEN COMPETENCIES

As you use the Review Modules, you will note the integration of the Quality and Safety Education for Nurses (QSEN) competencies throughout the chapters. These competencies are integral components of the curriculum of many nursing programs in the United States and prepare you to provide safe, high-quality care as a newly licensed nurse. Icons appear to draw your attention to the six QSEN competencies.

Safety: The minimization of risk factors that could cause injury or harm while promoting quality care and maintaining a secure environment for clients, self, and others.

Patient-Centered Care: The provision of caring and compassionate, culturally sensitive care that addresses clients' physiological, psychological, sociological, spiritual, and cultural needs, preferences, and values.

Evidence-Based Practice: The use of current knowledge from research and other credible sources, on which to base clinical judgment and client care.

Informatics: The use of information technology as a communication and information-gathering tool that supports clinical decision-making and scientifically based nursing practice.

Quality Improvement: Care related and organizational processes that involve the development and implementation of a plan to improve health care services and better meet clients' needs.

Teamwork and Collaboration: The delivery of client care in partnership with multidisciplinary members of the health care team to achieve continuity of care and positive client outcomes.

ICONS

Icons are used throughout the Review Module to draw your attention to particular areas. Keep an eye out for these icons.

N This icon is used for NCLEX Connections.

G This icon indicates gerontological considerations, or knowledge specific to the care of older adult clients.

Qs This icon is used for content related to safety and is a QSEN competency. When you see this icon, take note of safety concerns or steps that nurses can take to ensure client safety and a safe environment.

QPCC This icon is a QSEN competency that indicates the importance of a holistic approach to providing care.

QEBP This icon, a QSEN competency, points out the integration of research into clinical practice.

QI This icon is a QSEN competency and highlights the use of information technology to support nursing practice.

QQI This icon is used to focus on the QSEN competency of integrating planning processes to meet clients' needs.

QTC This icon highlights the QSEN competency of care delivery using an interprofessional approach.

QSDoH This icon highlights content related to social determinants of health.

M This icon appears at the top-right of pages and indicates availability of an online media supplement, such as a graphic, animation, or video. If you have an electronic copy of the Review Module, this icon will appear alongside clickable links to media supplements. If you have a hard copy version of the Review Module, visit www.atitesting.com for details on how to access these features.

FEEDBACK

ATI welcomes your feedback. Please submit to comments@atitesting.com. Changes to the text are made for subsequent printings of the book and for subsequent releases of the electronic version. For the printed books, print runs are based on when existing stock is depleted. For the eBook, updates are made routinely depending on the volume of changes. As such, ATI encourages faculty and students to refer to the Review Module addendums for information on what updates have been made. These addendums, which are available in the Help/FAQs on the student site and the Resources/eBooks & Active Learning on the faculty site, are updated regularly and always include the most current information on updates to the Review Modules.

Table of Contents

NCLEX® Connections 1

UNIT 1   *Foundations of Pediatric Nursing*   3

SECTION: *Perspectives of Pediatric Nursing*   3

CHAPTER 1	Family-Centered Nursing Care	3
CHAPTER 2	Physical Assessment Findings	9
CHAPTER 3	Health Promotion of Infants (2 Days to 1 Year)	17
CHAPTER 4	Health Promotion of Toddlers (1 to 3 Years)	25
CHAPTER 5	Health Promotion of Preschoolers (3 to 6 Years)	31
CHAPTER 6	Health Promotion of School-Age Children (6 to 12 Years)	37
CHAPTER 7	Health Promotion of Adolescents (12 to 20 Years)	41

NCLEX® Connections 45

SECTION: *Specific Considerations of Pediatric Nursing*   47

CHAPTER 8	Safe Administration of Medication	47
CHAPTER 9	Pain Management	51
CHAPTER 10	Hospitalization, Illness, and Play	57
CHAPTER 11	Death and Dying	61

NCLEX® Connections   65

UNIT 2   *System Disorders*   67

SECTION: *Neurologic Disorders*   67

CHAPTER 12   Acute Neurologic Disorders   67

CHAPTER 13   Seizures   71

CHAPTER 14   Head Injury   77

CHAPTER 15   Cognitive and Sensory Impairments   83

NCLEX® Connections   89

SECTION: *Respiratory Disorders*   91

CHAPTER 16   Oxygen and Inhalation Therapy   91

CHAPTER 17   Acute and Infectious Respiratory Illnesses   99

CHAPTER 18   Asthma   109

CHAPTER 19   Cystic Fibrosis   115

NCLEX® Connections   119

SECTION: *Cardiovascular and Hematologic Disorders*   121

CHAPTER 20   Cardiovascular Disorders   121

CHAPTER 21   Hematologic Disorders   135

NCLEX® Connections   143

SECTION: *Gastrointestinal Disorders*   145

CHAPTER 22   Acute Infectious Gastrointestinal Disorders   145

CHAPTER 23   Gastrointestinal Structural and Inflammatory Disorders   151

NCLEX® Connections 159

SECTION: *Genitourinary and Reproductive Disorders* 161

CHAPTER 24   Enuresis and Urinary Tract Infections 161

CHAPTER 25   Structural Disorders of the Genitourinary Tract and Reproductive System 165

CHAPTER 26   Kidney Disorders 169

NCLEX® Connections 177

SECTION: *Musculoskeletal Disorders* 179

CHAPTER 27   Fractures 179

CHAPTER 28   Musculoskeletal Congenital Disorders 185

CHAPTER 29   Chronic Neuromusculoskeletal Disorders 193

NCLEX® Connections 205

SECTION: *Integumentary Disorders* 207

CHAPTER 30   Skin Infections and Infestations 207

CHAPTER 31   Dermatitis and Acne 213

NCLEX® Connections 219

SECTION: *Endocrine Disorders* 221

CHAPTER 32   Diabetes Mellitus 221

CHAPTER 33   Growth Hormone Deficiency 227

NCLEX® Connections 231

SECTION: *Immune and Infectious Disorders* 233

CHAPTER 34   Immunizations 233

CHAPTER 35   Communicable Diseases 241

CHAPTER 36   Acute Otitis Media 247

CHAPTER 37   HIV/AIDS 251

NCLEX® Connections   255

SECTION: *Neoplastic Disorders*   *257*

CHAPTER 38   Organ Neoplasms   257

CHAPTER 39   Blood Neoplasms   263

CHAPTER 40   Bone and Soft Tissue Cancers   267

NCLEX® Connections   273

Unit 3   *Other Specific Needs*   275

SECTION: *Integumentary Disorders*   275

CHAPTER 41   Burns   275

CHAPTER 42   Complications of Infants   281

CHAPTER 43   Pediatric Emergencies   297

CHAPTER 44   Psychosocial Issues of Infants, Children, and Adolescents   303

References   311

Active Learning Templates   *A1*

Basic Concept   A1

Diagnostic Procedure   A3

Growth and Development   A5

Medication   A7

Nursing Skill   A9

System Disorder   A11

Therapeutic Procedure   A13

Concept Analysis   A15

When reviewing the following chapters, keep in mind the relevant topics and tasks of the NCLEX outline, in particular:

Safety and Infection Control

ACCIDENT/ERROR/INJURY PREVENTION
Identify factors that influence accident/injury prevention.

Identify and facilitate correct use of infant and child car seats.

Health Promotion and Maintenance

AGING PROCESS
Provide care and education for the newborn, infant, and toddler client from birth through 2 years.

Provide care and education for the preschool, school-age, and adolescent client ages 3 through 17 years.

DEVELOPMENTAL STAGES AND TRANSITIONS
Provide education to clients/staff members about expected age-related changes and age-specific growth and development.

Identify family structures and roles of family members.

Modify approaches to care in accordance with client developmental stage.

HEALTH PROMOTION/DISEASE PREVENTION: Assess
and educate clients about health risks based on family, population, and/or community characteristics.

Basic Care and Comfort

NUTRITION AND ORAL HYDRATION: Monitor
the client's nutritional intake.

REST AND SLEEP: Assess client sleep/rest
pattern and intervene as needed.

Reduction of Risk

CHANGES/ABNORMALITIES IN VITAL SIGNS: Assess and
respond to changes and/or trends in client vital signs.

SYSTEM-SPECIFIC ASSESSMENTS: Perform focused assessments.

CHAPTER 1

CHAPTER 1 *Family-Centered Nursing Care*

Families are groups that should remain constant in children's lives. Family is defined as what an individual considers it to be. Families often include individuals with a biological, marital, or adoptive relationship, but in the absence of these characteristics, families also consist of individuals who have a strong emotional bond and commitment to one another. Due to the expanding concepts of family, the term household is sometimes used. Positive family relationships are characterized by parent-child interactions that show mutual warmth and respect.

COMPONENTS OF CARE

Family-centered nursing care includes the following. ⓆPCC
- Agreed-upon partnerships between families of children, nurses, and providers, in which the families and children benefit.
- Respecting cultural diversity, and incorporating cultural views in the plan of care.
- Understanding growth and developmental needs of children and their families.
- Treating children and their families as clients.
- Working with all types of families.
- Collaborating with families regarding hospitalization, home, and community resources.
- Allowing families to serve as experts regarding their children's health conditions, usual behaviors in different situations, and routine needs.

PROMOTING FAMILY-CENTERED CARE

Nurses should perform comprehensive family assessments to identify strengths and weaknesses.

Characteristics of healthy families

Members communicate well and listen to each other.
- There is affirmation and support for all members.
- There is a clear set of family rules, beliefs, and values.
- Members teach respect for others.
- There is a sense of trust.
- Members play and share humor together.
- Members interact with one another.

- There is a shared sense of responsibility.
- There are traditions and rituals.
- There is adaptability and flexibility in roles.
- Members seek help for their problems.

NURSING ACTIONS
- Nurses should pay close attention when family members state that a child "isn't acting right" or has other concerns.
- Children's opinions should be considered when providing care.

SOCIAL DETERMINANTS OF HEALTH (SDOH)

To promote the health and well-being of the pediatric population and adequately provide family centered nursing care, the nurse should assess the SDOH for each individual child and family. Children are born into conditions in the environment in which they live. These conditions affect their daily life and, eventually, their health. Nurses are in a unique position to screen children for SDOH factors and request referrals when needs are identified.

SDOH are divided into six categories: neighborhood and built environment, social and community context, economic stability, health care access and quality, and education access and quality.

Neighborhood and Built Environment

- Geographical layout of neighborhood
- Rate of crime
- Quality of air
- Living arrangements in the home
- Accessible outdoor spaces

IMPACT ON PEDIATRIC HEALTH AND WELL-BEING
- **Rate of crime:** High crime rates prevent caregivers from allowing children to play outside. Decreased activity levels place children at a greater risk for obesity and related co-morbidities.
- **Quality of air and water**: Poor air quality leads to a greater risk for respiratory illnesses such as asthma as well as higher hospitalization rates for those experiencing respiratory illness.

Social and Community Context

- Relationships and interactions with others
- Food insecurity

IMPACT ON PEDIATRIC HEALTH AND WELL-BEING
- **Relationships and interactions with others:** Impaired parent-child relationships due to parental incarceration increases the probability of behavioral problems, delays in speech and attention span development, and likelihood of the child spending time in jail later in life.
- **Food insecurities:** Food insecurities have a harmful impact on health and place children at risk for poor performance in school.

Economic Stability

- Ability to seek health care
- Employment status
- Child-care opportunities

IMPACT ON PEDIATRIC HEALTH AND WELL-BEING
- **Ability to seek health care:** Economic instability and poverty impact a parent's ability to access care for themselves and their children. This places the parent and child alike at greater risk for disease morbidity and mortality. (Hockenberry 2019)

Health care Access and Quality

- Availability of health care services
- Health insurance
- Availability of screening services

IMPACT ON PEDIATRIC HEALTH AND WELL-BEING
- **Health insurance:** Many children in the United States are either uninsured or underinsured. Most of these children live at or below the federal poverty level. These children are less likely to have a primary care provider and parents of these children report not having the finances needed to secure recommended cares and treatments. (Hockenberry 2019)

Education Access and Quality

- Level of education
- Quality of the educational system
- Presence of social discrimination

IMPACT ON PEDIATRIC HEALTH AND WELL-BEING
- **Level of education:** Parental level of education can influence earnings and household income which in turn impact the ability to provide housing, nourishment, and safe environmental conditions for the child. Lower educational levels also have a negative impact on health literacy and the parent's ability to understand and follow through with health care recommendations. (Stanhope 2020)
- **Quality of the educational system:** Children who receive higher quality education have a greater likelihood of graduating from high school and attending college. Those who receive a higher-quality education have been found to be better candidates for higher paying jobs, less likely to live in poverty, and have a decreased risk for chronic health conditions.

FAMILY THEORIES

FAMILY SYSTEMS

The family is viewed as a whole system, instead of the individual members.
- A change to one member affects the entire system.
- The system can both initiate and react to change.
- Too much and too little change can lead to dysfunction.

FAMILY STRESS

Describes stress as inevitable.
- Stressors can be expected or unexpected.
- Explains the reaction of a family to stressful events.
- Offers guidance for adapting to stress.

DEVELOPMENTAL

Views families as small groups that interact with the larger social system.
- Emphasizes similarities and consistencies in how families develop and change.
- Uses Duvall's family life cycle stages to describe the changes a family goes through over time.
- How the family functions in one stage have a direct effect on how the family will function in the next stage.

FAMILY COMPOSITION

Traditional nuclear family: Married couple and their biologic children (only full brothers and sisters)

Nuclear family: Two parents (married/unmarried) and their children (biologic, adoptive, step, foster)

Single-parent family: One parent and one or more children

Blended family (also called reconstituted): At least one stepparent, stepsibling, or half-sibling

Extended family: At least one parent, one or more children, and other individuals (related/unrelated)

LGBTQIA families: Two people, who identify as parents/ partners, to children in which there could be legal or common-law tie

Foster family: A child or children who have been placed in an approved living environment away from the family of origin, usually with one or two parents

Binuclear family: Parents who have terminated spousal roles but continue their parenting roles

Communal family: Individuals who share common ownership of property and goods, and exchange services without monetary consideration

Polygamous family: Spouse with polygamous partner and children in which all may/may not reside in the same household

OTHER FAMILY SITUATIONS

Adoption of a child
- Legal bond of child and parents (nonbiological)
- Attachment concerns with older children
- Older child should be included in decision making process
- May encounter behavioral concerns

Divorce
- Separation of parents
- Impacts a child socially, emotionally, and physically

Single parenting
- Result of death, divorce, separation
- Risk of financial instability
- Provide support and referral to resources as indicated

Birth of new child
- Parents' sense of self as they transition to the new parental role
- Increased financial responsibilities and possible loss of income
- Sleep habit changes
- Relationships with grandparents
- Work relationships

Foster parenting
- Guidelines are regulated on local/state level
- Can include placement with relative and non–relatives

PARENTING STYLES

TYPES OF PARENTING

Authoritarian

Parents try to control the child's behaviors and attitudes through unquestioned rules and expectations.

> The child is never allowed to watch television on school nights.

Permissive

Parents exert little or no control over the child's behaviors and consult the child when making decisions.

> The child assists with deciding whether they will watch television.

Authoritative

Parents direct the child's behavior by setting rules and explaining the reason for each rule setting.

> The child can watch television for 1 hr on school nights after completing all homework and chores.

Parents negatively reinforce deviations from the rules.

> The privilege is taken away but later reinstated based on new guidelines.

Uninvolved

Parents are indifferent and emotionally removed.

> The child may watch television whenever they want.

GUIDELINES FOR PROMOTING ACCEPTABLE BEHAVIOR IN CHILDREN

- Set clear and realistic limits and expectations based on the developmental level of the child.
- Validate the child's feelings, and offer sympathetic explanations.
- Provide role modeling and reinforcement for appropriate behavior.
- Focus on the child's behavior when disciplining the child.

FAMILY ASSESSMENT

History: Medical history for parents, siblings, and grandparents

Structure: Family members (mother, father, son)

Developmental tasks: Tasks a family works on as the child grows (parents helping a school–age child develop peer relations)

Family characteristics: Cultural, religious, and economic influences on behavior, attitudes, and actions

Family stressors: Expected (birth of a child) and unexpected (illness, divorce, disability, or death of a family member) events that cause stress

Environment: Availability of and family interactions with community resources

Family support system: Availability of extended family, work and peer relationships, as well as social systems and community resources to assist the family in meeting needs or adapting to a stressor.

Active Learning Scenario

A nurse is providing anticipatory guidance to the mother of a toddler. The nurse learns that the household includes the mother, toddler, an older brother, and a grandmother. Use the ATI Active Learning Template: Basic Concept to complete this item.

RELATED CONTENT: Describe the composition of this family.

UNDERLYING PRINCIPLES

- Describe two methods the parent can use to positively influence the child.
- Describe two ways the parent can promote acceptable behavior in the child.

NURSING INTERVENTIONS: Include two additional family assessments the nurse should perform.

Active Learning Scenario Key

Using the ATI Active Learning Template: Basic Concept

RELATED CONTENT: This is an extended family, which includes at least one parent, one or more children, and other individuals who are either related or not related.

UNDERLYING PRINCIPLES

- Positive parental influences
  - Have good mental health.
  - Maintain structure and routine in the household.
  - Engage in activities with the child.
  - Validate the child's feelings when communicating.
  - Monitor for safety concerns with special consideration for the child's developmental needs.
- Promoting acceptable behavior
  - Validate the child's feelings, and offer sympathetic explanations.
  - Provide role modeling and reinforcement for acceptable behavior.
  - Set clear and realistic limits and expectations based on the child's developmental level.
  - Focus on the behavior when implementing discipline.

NURSING INTERVENTIONS: Family assessments

- Medical history on parents, siblings, and grandparents
- Family structure for roles/position within the family, as well as occupation and education of family members
- Developmental tasks a family works on as the child grows
- Family characteristics (cultural, religious, and economic influences on behavior, attitudes, and actions)
- Family stressors, (expected [birth of a child] and unexpected [illness of a child, divorce, disability or death of a family member] events that cause stress)
- Availability of and family interactions with community resources
- Family support systems (availability of extended family; work and peer relationships; and social systems and community resources to assist the family in meeting needs or adapting to a stressor)

Ⓝ *NCLEX® Connection: Health Promotion and Maintenance, Aging Process*

Application Exercises

1. A nurse manager on a pediatric unit is preparing an education program on working with families for a group of newly hired nurses. Which of the following should the nurse include when discussing the developmental theory?

A. Describes that stress is inevitable

B. Emphasizes that change with one member affects the entire family

C. Provides guidance to assist families adapting to stress

D. Defines consistencies in how families change

2. Match the family type to the correct definition.

A. Nuclear family

B. Blended family

C. Binuclear family

D. Extended family

E. Communal family

1. Parents who have terminated spousal roles but continue their parenting roles

2. At least one stepparent, stepsibling, or half-sibling

3. Two parents and their children

4. Individuals who share common ownership of property and goods, and exchange services without monetary consideration

5. At least one parent, one or more children, and other individuals

3. A nurse is assisting a group of guardians of adolescents to develop skills that will improve communication within the family. The nurse hears one guardian state, "My son knows he better do what I say." Which of the following parenting styles is the parent exhibiting?

A. Authoritarian

B. Permissive

C. Authoritative

D. Passive

4. You are caring for a child in a pediatric setting when a parent asks you to provide information that will help them foster positive behavior in their child. Compose a statement that you would use when faced with this type of question.

5. A nurse is performing family assessment. Which of the following should the nurse include? (Select all that apply.)

A. Medical history

B. Parents' education level

C. Child's physical growth

D. Support systems

E. Stressors

Application Exercises Key

1. A. The family stress theory describes that stress is inevitable; therefore, the nurse should not include this information when discussing the developmental theory.
   B. The family systems theory emphasizes that change with one member affects the entire family; therefore, the nurse should not include this information when discussing the developmental theory.
   C. The family stress theory provides guidance to assist families adapting to stress; therefore, the nurse should not include this information when discussing the developmental theory.
   D. **CORRECT:** When discussing the developmental theory, the nurse should include that the developmental theory defines consistencies in how families change.

   Ⓝ *NCLEX® Connection: Health Promotion and Maintenance, Developmental Stages and Transitions*

2. A, 3; B, 2; C, 1; D, 5; E, 4

   A nuclear family consists of two parents and their children regardless of whether the children are biologic, step, adopted, or foster children. A blended family consists of at least one stepparent, stepsibling, or half sibling. A binuclear family consists of two parents who have terminated their spousal roles but continue their roles as parents for the children in the family. An extended family consists of at least one parent, one or more children, as well as other individuals who may or may not be related. A communal family consists of individuals who share common ownership of property and goods, and exchange services without monetary consideration.

   Ⓝ *NCLEX® Connection: Health Promotion and Maintenance, Developmental Stages and Transitions*

3. A. **CORRECT:** The nurse should identify that this parent is exhibiting an authoritarian parenting style. The parent controls the adolescent's behaviors and attitudes through unquestioned rules and expectations.
   B. This parent is not exhibiting a permissive parenting style. Using this style, the parent exerts little or no control over the adolescent's behaviors and consults the adolescent when making decisions.
   C. This parent is not exhibiting an authoritative parenting style. Using this style, the parent directs the adolescent's behavior by setting rules and explaining the reason for each rule setting.
   D. This parent is not exhibiting an uninvolved parenting style. Using this style, the parent is indifferent and emotionally removed.

   Ⓝ *NCLEX® Connection: Health Promotion and Maintenance, Developmental Stages and Transitions*

4. There are several factors to consider when fostering positive behavior. When a child misbehaves, focus your attention on the behavior that the child is exhibiting and not the child themself. An example of focusing on the behavior may sound like this, "Throwing rocks at cars is not an ok thing to do" instead of "You know you should not throw rocks at cars." When interacting with your child, let them know that you care about their feelings while maintaining that the behavior is unacceptable. Children also need clear, consistent boundaries that are appropriate for their developmental age. Also, remember when interacting with your child to behave in the way that you wish for your child to behave in difficult situations.

   Ⓝ *NCLEX® Connection: Psychosicial Integrity, Behavioral Interventions*

5. When performing family data collection, the nurse should include a medical history on the parents, siblings, and grandparents. The nurse should also collect data about the family's structure, which includes family members, family size, roles and positions within the family, and occupation and education of family members. Support systems should be included with family data collection to determine the availability of extended family, work and peer relationships, social systems, and access to community resources. Lastly, stressors, both expected and unexpected, should be included when performing family data collection. The child's physical growth should be determined when performing individual data collection on the child, not when conducting family data collection.

   Ⓝ *NCLEX® Connection: Health Promotion and Maintenance, Health Promotion/Disease Prevention*

CHAPTER 2 Physical Assessment Findings

Alter exams to accommodate chronological age and developmental needs. Involve children and family members in examinations. Praise children for cooperation during exams. Qpcc

Observe for behaviors (interacting with nurse, making eye contact, permitting physical touch, and willingly sitting on the examination table) to determine the child's readiness to cooperate.

Language, cognition, and fine and gross motor development can be screened using a standardized tool (the Denver Developmental Screening Test – Revised [Denver II]). A combination of data collected from psychosocial and medical histories and a physical examination is used to determine need and make a referral for further evaluation.

NURSING ACTIONS

- Keep the room warm and well lit.
- Perform examinations in nonthreatening environments. Keep medical equipment out of sight.
- Provide privacy. Determine whether older school-age children and adolescents prefer a caregiver to remain during examination.
- Take time to play and develop rapport prior to beginning an examination.
- Observe for behaviors that demonstrate child's readiness to cooperate (interacting with nurse, making eye contact permitting physical touch, and willingly sitting on the examination table).
- Explain each step of the examination to the child.
  - Use age-appropriate language.
  - Demonstrate what will happen using dolls, puppets, or paper drawings.
  - Allow the child to manipulate and handle equipment.
  - Encourage the child to use equipment on others.
- Examine the child in a secure, comfortable position. For example, a toddler may sit on a parent's lap if desired.

- Proceed to examine the child in an organized sequence when possible.
- If the child is uncooperative, assess reasons, be firm and direct about expected behavior, complete the assessment quickly, and use a calm voice.
- Encourage the child and family to ask questions during physical exams. Discuss findings with family after the examination.

PHYSIOLOGIC AND GROWTH MEASUREMENTS

TEMPERATURE

2.1 Temperature by age

	EXPECTED LEVEL	RECOMMENDED ROUTES
3 months	37.5° C (99.5° F)	Axillary
6 months		Rectal (if exact measurement necessary)
1 year	37.7° C (99.9° F)	
3 years	37.2° C (99.0° F)	Axillary Tympanic Oral (if child cooperative)
5 years	37.0° C (98.6° F)	Rectal (if exact measurement necessary)
7 years	36.8° C (98.2° F)	Oral
9 years	36.7° C (98.1° F)	
11 years		Axillary
13 years	36.6° C (97.9° F)	Tympanic

PULSE RATE

Values listed are general guidelines and may vary according to reference, as well as the child's specific age and activity level.

Newborn (birth to 4 weeks): 110 to 160/min

Infant (1 to 12 months): 90 to 160/min

Toddler (1 to 2 years): 80 to 140/min

Preschooler (3 to 5 years): 70 to 120/min

School aged (6 to 12 years): 60 to 110/min

Adolescent (13 to 18 years): 50 to 100/min

RESPIRATIONS

Values listed are general guidelines and may vary according to reference, as well as the child's specific age and activity level.

Newborn (birth to 4 weeks): 30 to 60/min

Infant (1 to 12 months): 25 to 30/min

Toddler (1 to 2 years): 25 to 30/min

Preschooler (3 to 5 years): 20 to 25/min

School aged (6 to 12 years): 20 to 25/min

Adolescent (13 to 18 years): 16 to 20/min

BLOOD PRESSURE

- Readings should be compared with standard measurements (National High Blood Pressure Education Program Working Group on High Blood Pressure in Children and Adolescents). Q EBP
- Age, height, and sex all influence blood pressure readings. (2.2)

GROWTH

Growth can be evaluated using weight, length/height, body mass index (BMI), and head circumference. Growth charts are tools that can be used to assess the overall health of a child.

- It is recommended to use the World Health Organizations (WHO) growth standards for infants and children ages 0 to 2 in the United States and CDC growth charts for children 2 years and older.
- To see growth charts by age and sex, visit the website for the Centers for Disease Control and Prevention. Q EBP

EXPECTED PHYSICAL FINDINGS

GENERAL APPEARANCE

- Appears undistressed, clean, well-kept, and without body odors.
- Muscle tone: Erect head posture is expected in infants after 4 months of age.
- Makes eye contact when addressed (except infants).
- Follows simple commands as age-appropriate.
- Uses speech, language, and motor skills spontaneously.

SKIN, HAIR, AND NAILS

Skin

- Variations in skin color are expected.
- Temperature should be warm or slightly cool to the touch.
- Skin texture should be smooth and slightly dry, not oily.

- Skin turgor exhibits brisk elasticity with adequate hydration.
- Lesions are unexpected findings.
- Skin folds should be symmetric.

Hair and Scalp

- Hair should be evenly distributed, smooth, and strong.
  - Hair that is dull, brittle, or dry could possibly indicate potential nutritional deficiencies.
  - Hair loss or balding spots on infants can indicate the child is spending too much time in the same position.
- Scalp should be clean and absent from any scaliness, infestations, and trauma.
- Assess children approaching adolescence for the presence of secondary hair growth.

Nails

- Nailbeds can be pink or more pigmented in coloration; the tip of the nails are white.
- Smooth and firm (but slightly flexible in infants).

LYMPH NODES

Lymph nodes should be nonpalpable. Lymph nodes that are small, palpable, nontender, and mobile can be an expected finding in children.

HEAD AND NECK

Head

- The shape of the head should be symmetric.
- Fontanels should be flat. The posterior fontanel usually closes by 8 weeks of age, and the anterior fontanel usually closes between 12 and 18 months of age.

Face

- Symmetric appearance and movement
- Proportional features

2.2 Expected blood pressure ranges by age and sex

		Average (50th Percentile)		Hypertension (95th Percentile)	
		SYSTOLIC (mm Hg)	DIASTOLIC (mm Hg)	SYSTOLIC GREATER THAN (mm Hg)	DIASTOLIC GREATER THAN (mm Hg)
Newborn (full term: birth to 4 weeks)		64	41	n/a	
Infant (1 month to 12 months)		85	50	n/a	
Toddler (1 year to 2 years)	Male	85 to 91	37 to 46	103 to 109	56 to 65
	Female	86 to 89	40 to 49	104 to 107	58 to 67
Preschooler (3 to 5 years)	Male	91 to 98	46 to 53	109 to 112	65 to 72
	Female	89 to 93	49 to 52	107 to 110	67 to 72
School aged (6 to 12 years)	Male	96 to 106	55 to 62	114 to 123	74 to 81
	Female	94 to 105	56 to 62	111 to 123	74 to 80
Adolescent (13 to 18 years)		less than 120	less than 80	n/a	

Neck

- Short in infants
- No palpable masses
- Midline trachea
- Full range of motion present whether assessed actively or passively

EYES

Eyebrows should be symmetric and evenly distributed from the inner to the outer canthus.

Eyelids should close completely and open to allow the lower border and most of the upper portion of the iris to be seen.

Eyelashes should curve outward and be evenly distributed with no inflammation around any of the hair follicles.

Conjunctiva

- Palpebral fissures and conjunctiva are pink.
- Bulbar conjunctiva are transparent.

Lacrimal apparatus is without excessive tearing, redness, or discharge.

Sclera should be white.

Corneas should be clear.

Pupils should be:
- Round
- Equal in size
- Reactive to light
- Accommodating

Irises should be round with the permanent color manifesting around 6 to 12 months of age.

Visual acuity

- Can be difficult to determine in children younger than 3 years of age.
- Visual acuity in infants can be assessed by holding an object in front of the eyes and checking to see whether the infant is able to fix on the object and follow it.
- Use the tumbling E or HOTV test to check visual acuity of children who are unable to read letters and numbers.
- Older children should be tested using a Snellen chart or symbol chart.

Peripheral visual fields should be:
- Upward 50°
- Downward 70°
- Nasally 60°
- Temporally 90°

Extraocular movements

- Might not be symmetric in newborns.
- Corneal light reflex should be symmetric.
- Cover/uncover test should demonstrate equal movement of the eyes.
- Six cardinal fields of gaze should demonstrate no nystagmus.

Color vision

- Should be determined using the Ishihara color test or the Hardy-Rand-Rittler test.
- The child should be able to correctly identify shapes, symbols, or numbers.

Internal exam

- Red reflex should be present.
- Arteries, veins, optic discs, and maculae can be visualized in older children and adolescents.

EARS

Alignment: The top of the auricles should meet in an imaginary horizontal line that extends from the outer canthus of the eye.

External ear

- The external ear should be free of lesions and nontender.
- The ear canal should be free of foreign bodies or discharge.
- Cerumen is an expected finding.

Internal ear

- In infants and toddlers, pull the pinna down and back to visualize the tympanic membrane. Qpcc
- In children older than 3 years of age, pull the pinna up and back to visualize.
- The ear canal should be pink with fine hairs.
- The tympanic membrane should be pearly pink, or gray.
- The light reflex should be visible.

Hearing

- Newborns should have intact acoustic blink reflexes to sudden sounds.
- Infants should turn toward sounds.
- Older children can be screened by whispering a word from behind to see whether they can identify the word.

NOSE

- The position should be midline.
- Patency should be present for each nostril without excessive flaring.
- Sense of smell can be assessed in older children.

Internal structures

- The septum is midline and intact.
- The mucosa is deep pink in light-skinned clients and various shades of brown or gray in dark-skinned clients. The mucosa should be moist without evidence of discharge.

MOUTH AND THROAT

Lips

- Darker pigmented than facial skin
- Smooth, soft, moist, and symmetric

Gums

- Coral pink in light-skinned clients, and various shades of brown or gray in dark-skinned clients
- Tight against the teeth

Mucous membranes

- Without lesions
- Moist, smooth, and glistening. Pink in light-skinned clients and various shades of brown or gray in dark-skinned clients

Tongue

- Infants can have white coatings on their tongues from milk that can be easily removed. Oral candidiasis coating is not easily removed.
- Children and adolescents should have pink, symmetric tongues that they are able to move beyond their lips.

Teeth

- Infants should have six to eight teeth by 1 year of age.
- Children and adolescents should have teeth that are white and smooth, and begin replacing the 20 deciduous teeth with 32 permanent teeth.

Hard and soft palates: Intact, firm, and concave

Uvula: Intact and moves with vocalization

Tonsils

- Infants: Might not be able to visualize
- Children: Barely visible to prominent, same color as surrounding mucosa

Voice

- Infants: Strong cry
- Children and adolescents: Clear and articulate

THORAX AND LUNGS

Chest shape

- Infants: Shape is almost circular with anteroposterior diameter equaling the transverse or lateral diameter.
- Children and adolescents: The transverse diameter to anteroposterior diameter changes to 2:1.

Ribs and sternum: More soft and flexible in infants; symmetric and smooth, with no protrusions or bulges

Movement

- Symmetric, no retractions.
- Infants: Irregular rhythms are common.
- Children younger than 7 years: More abdominal movement is seen during respirations.

Breath sounds

- Inspiration is longer and louder than expiration.
- Vesicular, or soft, swishing sounds, are heard over most of the lungs.

Breasts

- Newborns: Breasts can be enlarged during the first few days.
- Children and adolescents: Nipples and areolas are darker pigmented and symmetric.
  - Females: Breasts typically develop between 10 to 14 years of age. The breasts should appear asymmetric, have no masses, and be palpable.
  - Males can develop gynecomastia, which is unilateral or bilateral breast enlargement that occurs during puberty.

2.3 Infant reflexes

	EXPECTED FINDING	EXPECTED AGE
SUCKING AND ROOTING REFLEXES	Elicited by stroking an infant's cheek or the edge of an infant's mouth	Birth to 4 months
	The infant turns their head toward the side that is touched and starts to suck.	
PALMAR GRASP	Elicited by placing an object in an infant's palm	Birth to 4 months
	The infant grasps the object.	
PLANTAR GRASP	Elicited by touching the sole of an infant's foot	Birth to 8 months
	The infant's toes curl downward.	
MORO REFLEX	Elicited by allowing the head and trunk of an infant in a semi-sitting position to fall backward to an angle of at least 30°	Birth to 4 months
	The infant's arms and legs symmetrically extend, then abduct while fingers spread to form C shape.	
TONIC NECK REFLEX (FENCER POSITION)	Elicited by turning an infant's head to one side	Birth to 3 to 4 months
	The infant extends the arm and leg on that side and flexes the arm and leg on the opposite side.	
BABINSKI REFLEX	Elicited by stroking the outer edge of the sole of an infant's foot up toward the toes	Birth to 1 year
	The infant's toes fan upward and out.	
STEPPING	Elicited by holding an infant upright with his feet touching a flat surface	Birth to 4 weeks
	The infant makes stepping movements.	

CIRCULATORY SYSTEM

A comprehensive assessment of the circulatory system includes assessment of the pulses, capillary refill time, neck veins, clubbing of fingers, peripheral cyanosis, edema, blood pressure, and respiratory status.

Heart sounds

- Auscultation should be done in both a sitting and reclining position. QEBP
- S1 and S2 heart sounds should be clear and crisp. S1 is louder at the apex of the heart. S2 is louder near the base of the heart. Physiologic splitting of S2 and S3 heart sounds are expected findings in some children. Sinus arrhythmias that are associated with respirations are common.

Pulses

- Infants: Brachial, temporal, and femoral pulses should be palpable, full, and localized.
- Children and adolescents: Pulse locations and expected findings are the same as those in adults.

Abdomen

- Without tenderness, no guarding. Peristaltic waves can be visible in thinner children.
- Shape: Symmetric and without protrusions around the umbilicus.
  - Infants and toddlers have rounded abdomens.
  - Children and adolescents should have flat abdomens.
- Bowel sounds should be heard every 5 to 30 seconds.

GENITALIA

Anus: Surrounding skin should be intact with sphincter tightening noted if the anus is touched. Routine rectal exams are not done with the pediatric population.

Male

Hair distribution is diamond shaped after puberty in adolescent males. No pubic hair is noted in infants and small children.

Penis
- Penis should appear straight.
- Urethral meatus should be at the tip of the penis.
- Foreskin might not be retractable in infants and small children.
- Enlargement of the penis occurs during adolescence.
- The penis can look disproportionately small in males who are obese because of skin folds partially covering the base.

Scrotum
- The scrotum hangs separately from the penis.
- The skin on the scrotum has a rugose appearance and is loose.
- The left testicle hangs slightly lower than the right.
- The inguinal canal should be absent of swelling.
- During puberty, the testes and scrotum enlarge with darker scrotal skin.

2.4 Cranial nerves: Expected findings

NERVES	INFANTS	CHILDREN AND ADOLESCENTS
I Olfactory	Difficult to test	Identifies smells through each nostril individually
II Optic	Looks at face and tracks with eyes	Has intact visual acuity, peripheral vision, and color vision
III Oculomotor	Blinks in response to light. Has pupils that are reactive to light	Has no nystagmus and PERRLA is intact
IV Trochlear	Looks at face and tracks with eyes	Has the ability to look down and in with eyes
V Trigeminal	Has rooting and sucking reflexes	Is able to clench teeth together. Detects touch on face with eyes closed
VI Abducens	Looks at face and tracks with eyes	Is able to move eyes laterally toward temples
VII Facial	Has symmetric facial movements	Has the ability to differentiate between salty and sweet on tongue. Has symmetric facial movements
VIII Acoustic	Tracks a sound. Blinks in response to a loud noise	Does not experience vertigo. Has intact hearing
IX Glossopharyngeal	Has an intact gag reflex	Has an intact gag reflex. Is able to taste sour sensations on back of tongue
X Vagus	Has no difficulties swallowing	Speech clear, no difficulties swallowing. Uvula is midline
XI Spinal Accessory	Moves shoulders symmetrically	Has equal strength of shoulder shrug against examiner's hands
XII Hypoglossal	Has no difficulties swallowing. Opens mouth when nares are occluded	Has a tongue that is midline. Is able to move tongue in all directions with equal strength against tongue blade resistance

Female

Hair distribution over the mons pubis should be documented in terms of amount and location during puberty. Hair should appear in an inverted triangle. No pubic hair should be noted in infants or small children.

- **Labia:** Symmetric, without lesions, moist on the inner aspects
- **Clitoris:** Small, without bruising or edema
- **Urethral meatus:** Slit-like in appearance with no discharge
- **Vaginal orifice:** Hymen can be absent or completely or partially cover the vaginal opening prior to sexual intercourse.

MUSCULOSKELETAL SYSTEM

Length, position, and size of extremities are symmetric.

Joints

Stable and symmetric with full range of motion and no crepitus or redness

Spine

Infants: Spines should be without dimples or tufts of hair. They should be midline with an overall C-shaped lateral curve.

Toddlers appear squat with short legs and protuberant abdomens.

Preschoolers appear more erect than toddlers.

Children should develop the cervical, thoracic, and lumbar curvatures like that of adults.

Adolescents should remain midline (no scoliosis noted).

Gait

Toddlers and young children: A bowlegged or knock-knee appearance is a common finding. Feet should face forward while walking.

Older children and adolescents: A steady gait should be noted with even wear on the soles of shoes.

NEUROLOGIC SYSTEM

Infant reflexes (2.3)

Cranial nerves (2.4)

Deep tendon reflexes

Deep tendon reflexes should demonstrate the following.
- Partial flexion of the lower arm at the biceps tendon
- Partial extension of the lower arm at the triceps tendon
- Partial extension of the lower leg at the patellar tendon
- Plantar flexion of the foot at the Achilles tendon

Cerebellar function (children and adolescents)

Finger to nose test: Rapid coordinated movements

Heel to shin test: Able to run the heel of one foot down the shin of the other leg while standing

Romberg test: Able to stand with slight swaying while eyes are closed

---

Active Learning Scenario

A nurse is preparing to examine a preschool-age child. Use the ATI Active Learning Template: Basic Concept to complete this item.

UNDERLYING PRINCIPLES: Describe two behaviors that indicate the child is ready to cooperate.

NURSING INTERVENTIONS

- Describe two actions to take if child is uncooperative.

- Include three actions to promote the child's comfort during the examination.

Active Learning Scenario Key

Using the ATI Active Learning Template: Basic Concept

UNDERLYING PRINCIPLES
- Child is ready to cooperate.
- Interacting with nurse.
- Making eye contact.
- Permitting physical touch.
- Willingly sitting on examination table.
- Accepting and handling equipment.

NURSING INTERVENTIONS
- Actions to take if child is uncooperative
  - Engage both the child and parent.
  - Be firm and direct about expected behavior.
  - Complete the assessment as quickly as possible.
  - Use a calm voice.
  - Reduce environmental stimuli.
  - Limit the people in the room.
- Actions to enhance child's comfort
  - Perform examination in nonthreatening environment.
  - Take time to play and develop rapport prior to beginning the examination.
  - Keep the room warm and well lit.
  - Keep medical equipment out of sight until needed.
  - Provide privacy.
  - Explain each step of the examination to the child.
  - Examine the child in a secure, comfortable position.
  - Examine the child in an organized sequence when possible.
  - Encourage the child and family to ask questions during the examination.

Ⓝ *NCLEX® Connection: Health Promotion and Maintenance, Developmental Stages and Transitions*

Application Exercises

1. A nurse is preparing to assess a preschooler. Which of the following actions should the nurse take to prepare the child?

   A. Allow the child to role-play using miniature equipment.

   B. Use medical terminology to describe what will happen.

   C. Separate the child from the caregiver during the examination.

   D. Keep medical equipment visible to the child.

2. A nurse is checking the vital signs of a 3-year-old child during a well-child visit. Which of the following findings should the nurse report to the provider?

   A. Temperature 37.2° C (99.0° F)

   B. Heart rate 106/min

   C. Respirations 30/min

   D. Blood pressure 88/54 mm Hg

3. A nurse is assessing a child's ears. Which of the following findings should the nurse expect?

   A. Light reflex is located at the 2 o'clock position.

   B. Tympanic membrane is red in color.

   C. Bony landmarks are not visible.

   D. Cerumen is present bilaterally.

4. A nurse is performing a physical assessment on a 16-month-old toddler. Sort the following findings into the following categories: Expected or Unexpected.

   A. Concave soft palate

   B. Heart rate of 70/min

   C. Open anterior fontanel

   D. Positive Babinski reflex

   E. Schaphoid abdomen

   F. Variations in skin color

5. A nurse is assessing a 6-month-old infant. Which of the following reflexes should the infant exhibit?

   A. Moro

   B. Plantar grasp

   C. Stepping

   D. Tonic neck

6. A nurse is performing a neurologic assessment on an adolescent. Which of the following responses should the nurse expect the adolescent to exhibit when assessing the trigeminal nerve? (Select all that apply.)

   A. Clenching teeth together tightly

   B. Recognizing sour tastes on the back of the tongue

   C. Identifying smells through each nostril

   D. Detecting facial touches with eyes closed

   E. Looking down and in with the eyes

Application Exercises Key

1. A. **CORRECT:** When generating solutions to prepare a preschool aged child for an assessment, the nurse should allow the child to role-play or manipulate actual or miniature equipment that will be used during the assessment. This action helps reduce anxiety and fear related to the examination.
   B. The nurse should use neutral words, not medical terminology, when describing to the child what will happen during the assessment.
   C. The nurse should encourage caregiver presence and not separate the child from the caregiver during the examination.
   D. The nurse should keep medical equipment out of sight unless showing or using it on the child.

   Ⓝ *NCLEX® Connection: Health Promotion and Maintenance, Developmental Stages and Transitions*

2. A. A temperature of 37.2° C (99.0° F) is within the expected reference range for a 3-year-old child and should not be reported to the provider.
   B. A heart rate of 106/min is within the expected reference range for a 3-year-old child and should not be reported to the provider.
   C. **CORRECT:** When analyzing cues while checking the vital signs of a 3 year old during a well child visit, the nurse should recognize that respirations of 30/min are above the expected reference range for a 3 year old and should be reported to the provider.
   D. A blood pressure of 90/52 mm Hg is within the expected reference range for a 3-year-old child and should not be reported to the provider.

   Ⓝ *NCLEX® Connection: Management of Care, Collaboration with Multidisciplinary Team*

3. A. The light reflex should be located around the 5 or 7 o'clock position; therefore, a light reflex located at the 2 o'clock position is not a finding the nurse should expect.
   B. The tympanic membrane should be a pearly pink, or gray color; therefore, a tympanic membrane that is red in color is not a finding the nurse should expect.
   C. Bony landmarks should be visible; therefore, bony landmarks that are not visible is not a finding the nurse should expect.
   D. **CORRECT:** The presence of cerumen bilaterally is an expected finding.

   Ⓝ *NCLEX® Connection: Reduction of Risk Potential, Potential for Alterations in Body Systems*

4. **EXPECTED:** A, B, F; **UNEXPECTED:** C, D, E

   A heart rate of 80 to 140/min is within the expected reference range for a toddler; therefore, a heart rate of 70 is an unexpected finding. Variations in skin color is an expected finding in the toddler. For example, the skin on the front of the arms of a light skinned toddler may be darker than the skin on the back of the arms due to differences in sun exposure times. Open anterior fontanel is an expected finding in a 16-month-old toddler. The anterior fontanel usually closes between 12 and 18 months of age. A concave soft palate is an expected finding for the toddler. Both the hard and soft palate should be intact, firm, and concave. The Babinski reflex usually disappears by one year of age; therefore, a positive Babinski reflex is an unexpected finding for the 16-month-old toddler. A protuberant or rounded abdomen, not a scaphoid abdomen, is an expected finding in the toddler. The abdomen appears rounded due to the increased curvature of the lumbar spine during the toddler years.

   Ⓝ *NCLEX® Connection: Health Promotion and Maintenance, Techniques of Physical Assessment*

5. A. The Moro reflex is exhibited by infants from birth to the age of 4 months. The 6-month-old infant should no longer exhibit the Moro reflex.
   B. **CORRECT:** When recognizing cues during the assessment of a 6-month-old infant, the nurse should recognize that the plantar grasp is exhibited by infants from birth to the age of 8 months; therefore, a 6-month-old infant should still be exhibiting the plantar grasp reflex.
   C. The stepping reflex is exhibited by infants from birth to the age of 4 weeks. The 6-month-old infant should no longer exhibit the stepping reflex.
   D. The tonic neck reflex is exhibited by infants from birth to the age of 3 to 4 months. The 6-month-old infant should no longer exhibit the tonic neck reflex.

   Ⓝ *NCLEX® Connection: Health Promotion and Maintenance, Developmental Stages and Transitions*

6. A, D. **CORRECT:** When recognizing cues during the assessment of the trigeminal nerve, the nurse should expect the adolescent to clench the teeth together tightly and to detect facial touches when the eyes are closed.
   B. Recognizing sour tastes on the back of the tongue is an expected response by the adolescent when checking the glossopharyngeal cranial nerve.
   C. Identifying smells through each nostril is an expected response by the adolescent when checking the olfactory cranial nerve.
   E. Looking down and in with the eyes is an expected response by the adolescent when checking the trochlear cranial nerve.

   Ⓝ *NCLEX® Connection: Reduction of Risk Potential, System-Specific Assessments*

UNIT 1   FOUNDATIONS OF PEDIATRIC NURSING
SECTION: PERSPECTIVES OF PEDIATRIC NURSING

CHAPTER 3   *Health Promotion of Infants (2 Days to 1 Year)*

EXPECTED GROWTH AND DEVELOPMENT

GENERAL MEASUREMENTS OF FULL-TERM NEWBORN

Head circumference: The head circumference averages between 33 and 35 cm (13 and 14 in).

Crown to rump length: The crown to rump length is 31 to 35 cm (12.5 to 14 in), approximately equal to head circumference.

Length: Head to heel length averages 48 to 53 cm (19 to 21 in).

Weight: Newborn weight averages 2,700 to 4,000 g (6 to 9 lb).

Newborns will lose up to 10% of their birth weight by 3 to 4 days of age. This is due to fluid shifts, loss of meconium, and limited intake, especially in infants who are breastfed. The birth weight is usually regained by the tenth to fourteenth day of life, depending on the feeding method used. Q EBP

PHYSICAL DEVELOPMENT

Fontanel
- Posterior fontanel closes by 2 months of age.
- Anterior fontanel closes by 12 to 18 months of age.

Infant size is tracked using weight, height, and head circumference measurements.
- **Weight**: Infants gain approximately 680 g (1.5 lb) per month during the first 5 months of life. The average weight of a 6 month old infant is 7.26 kg (16 lb). Birth weight is at least doubled by the age of 5 months, and tripled by the age of 12 months to an average of 9.75 kg (21.5 lb).
- **Height**: Infants grow approximately 2.5 cm (1 in) per month the first 6 months of life. Growth occurs in spurts after the age of 6 months, and the birth length increases by 50% by the age of 12 months.
- **Head circumference**: The circumference of infants' heads increases approximately 2 cm (0.75 in) per month during the first 3 months, 1 cm (0.4 in) per month from 4 to 6 months, and then approximately 0.5 cm (0.2 in) per month during the second 6 months.

Dentition
- Six to eight teeth should erupt in infants' mouths by the end of the first year of age. The first teeth typically erupt between the ages of 6 and 10 months (average age 8 months).
- Some children show minimal indications of teething (sucking or biting on their fingers or hard objects and drooling). Others are irritable, have difficulty sleeping, have a mild fever, rub their ears, and have decreased appetite for solid foods.
- Teething pain can be eased using frozen teething rings or an ice cube wrapped in a washcloth and over-the-counter teething gels. Topical anesthetic ointments are available but should be used under the direction of a health care provider. Acetaminophen and/or ibuprofen are appropriate if irritability interferes with sleeping and feeding but should not be used for more than 3 days. Ibuprofen should be used only in infants over the age of 6 months. Qs
- Clean infants' teeth using cool, wet washcloths.
- Bottles should not be given to infants when they are falling asleep because prolonged exposure to milk or juice can cause early childhood dental caries.

COGNITIVE DEVELOPMENT

Piaget: Sensorimotor stage (birth to 24 months) Q EBP
- Infants progress from reflexive to simple repetitive to imitative activities.
- Separation, object permanence, and mental representation are the three important tasks accomplished in this stage.
  - **Separation**: Infants learn to separate themselves from other objects in the environment.
  - **Object permanence**: The process by which infants learn that an object still exists when it is out of view. This occurs at approximately 9 to 10 months of age.
  - **Mental representation**: The ability to recognize and use symbols.

Language development
- Crying is the first form of verbal communication.
- Infants cry for 1 to 1 ½ hr each day up to 3 weeks of age and build up to 2 to 4 hr by 6 weeks.
- Crying decreases by 12 weeks of age.

PSYCHOSOCIAL DEVELOPMENT

Erikson: trust vs. mistrust (birth to 1 year) Q EBP
- Achieving this task is based on the quality of the caregiver–infant relationship and the care received by the infant.
- The infant begins to learn delayed gratification. Failure to learn delayed gratification leads to mistrust.
- Trust is developed by meeting comfort, feeding, stimulation, and caring needs.
- Mistrust develops if needs are inadequately or inconsistently met, or if needs are continuously met before being vocalized by the infant.

3.1 Motor Skill Development

1 to 2 months

Infant in prone position lifting head from mattress

3 to 4 months

Infant lying on back holding object with both hands

5 to 6 months

Infant rolling from front to back

5 to 6 months

Infant holding a bottle with both hands

7 to 8 months

Infant sitting up leaning forward onto both hands

9 to 10 months

Infant crawling on hands and knees

9 to 10 months

Infant holding a rattle by the handle

11 to 12 months

Infant walking with hand being held

11 to 12 months

Infant placing objects into a container

Social development

- Social development is initially influenced by infants' reflexive behaviors and includes attachment, separation, recognition/anxiety, and stranger fear.
- Attachment is seen when infants begin to bond with their parents. This development is seen within the first month, but it actually begins before birth. The process is enhanced when infants and parents are in good health, have positive feeding experiences, and receive adequate rest.
- Separation–individuation occurs during the first year of life as infants first distinguish themselves and their primary caregiver as separate individuals at the same time that object permanence is developing.
- Separation anxiety begins around 4 to 8 months of age. Infants will protest when separated from parents, which can cause considerable anxiety for parents. By 11 to 12 months, infants are able to anticipate the mother's imminent departure by watching the behaviors.
- Stranger fear becomes evident between 6 and 8 months of age, when infants have the ability to discriminate between familiar and unfamiliar people.
- Reactive attachment disorder results from maladaptive or absent attachment between the infant and primary caregiver and continues through childhood and adulthood. Q SDoH

Body-image changes

- Infants discover that mouths are pleasure producers.
- Hands and feet are seen as objects of play.
- Infants discover that smiling causes others to react.

AGE-APPROPRIATE ACTIVITIES Q PCC

- Play should provide interpersonal contact and educational stimulation.
- Infants have short attention spans and will not interact with other children during play (solitary play). Appropriate toys and activities that stimulate the senses and encourage development include the following.
  - Rattles
  - Soft stuffed toys
  - Teething toys
  - Nesting toys
  - Playing pat-a-cake
  - Playing with balls
  - Reading books
  - Mirrors
  - Brightly colored toys
  - Playing with blocks

3.2 Development Milestones

	MOTOR (FINE AND GROSS)	COGNITIVE	LANGUAGE	SOCIAL	CLIENT EDUCATION
2 MONTHS	• Demonstrates head lag (1 month) • Strong grasp reflex (1 month) • Holds head up when in a prone position • Moves bilateral extremities • Opens hands briefly • Grasp reflex fading	• Observes movement • Gazes at an object for several seconds	• Cries and makes other sounds • Startled from loud noises	• Calms down when picked up • Makes facial contact Smiles when spoken to	• Talk, read, or sing to infant • Cuddle and hold infant • Position infant on their tummy when awake periodically while providing supervision
4 MONTHS	• Pushes up onto elbows when in prone position • Holds head unsupported when being held • Hold object/toy when placed in hand • Brings hand to mouth • Grasp objects with both hands • Uses palmar grasp dominantly	• Opens mouth when notices breast or bottle when hungry • Shows interest in hands by observation	• Makes cooing sounds • Makes constant sounds • Makes sound back when you talk to them • Turns head towards familiar voice or sound of a rattle	• Smiles, moves, make sounds to get attention • Slight chuckling noted • Shows interest in environment	• Talk with infant in positive manner when infant makes sounds • Allow infant to reach for objects • Talk, read, or sing to infant • Provide routine for feeding and sleeping • Allow infant to put a safe clean object in their mouth
6 MONTHS	• Rolls from front to back position (prone to supine) • Sits leaning forward on both hands (7 months) • Pushes up with arms straight when in prone position • Holds bottle • Moves objects from hand to hand (7 months) • Begin using pincer grasp (8 months)	• Put objects in their mouth • Grabs toy	• Makes high pitched squealing sounds • Stick out tongue and blows • Alternates make sounds with another person	• Laughs • Enjoys looking at self in mirror • Recognizes familiar people	• Allow for reciprocal play with infant • Read, sing, or play music • Point to items infant looks at • Discuss with provider about initiation of complementary/solid foods
9 MONTHS	• Able to get into a sitting position independently • Sits unsupported • Uses fingers to move food towards themselves • Moves objects from one hand to another • Has a crude pincer grasp at 9 months by 11 months has neat pincer grasp • Changes from prone to sitting position (10 months) • Grasp rattle by its handle (10 months)	• Bang 2 objects together • Looks for objects when dropped or hidden	• Makes lots of various sounds with longer syllables • Lift arms to be picked up • Begins to comprehend simple commands accompanied by gestures	• Shy among strangers • Makes various facial expressions • Looks when name is called • Reacts when familiar face leaves room (parent, guardian) • Smiles or laugh when playing games	• Repeat sounds infant makes use simple words • Show infant how to wave "bye-bye" and shake their head "no" • Play games such as peek-a-boo, blocks in containers • Allow your infant to consume various foods • Schedule child's developmental screening assessment with their provider

Information adopted from the Centers for Disease Control and Prevention, CDC's Developmental Milestones 2022 Update

HEALTH PROMOTION

CARE OF THE NEWBORN AFTER DISCHARGE

- Newborn infants should be placed in a federally approved car seat at a 45-degree angle to prevent slumping and airway obstruction. The car seat is placed rear facing in the rear seat of the vehicle and secured using the safety belt. The shoulder harnesses are placed in the slots at or below the level of the infant's shoulders. The harness should be snug and the retainer clip placed at the level of the infant's armpits.
- Instruct parents that their newborn will require a checkup by a provider. Infants discharged sooner than 48 hours after birth should be examined within 48 hours after discharge from the hospital. Qpcc

IMMUNIZATIONS Qebp

The Centers for Disease Control and Prevention (CDC) immunization recommendations for healthy infants less than 12 months of age include:

- Birth: hepatitis B (Hep B)
- 2 months: diphtheria and tetanus toxoids and pertussis (DTaP), rotavirus vaccine (RV), inactivated poliovirus (IPV), Haemophilus influenzae type B (Hib), pneumococcal vaccine (PCV), and Hep B
- 4 months: DTaP, RV, IPV, Hib, PCV
- 6 months: DTaP, IPV (6 to 18 months), PCV, and Hep B (6 to 18 months); RV; Hib
- 6 to 12 months: seasonal influenza vaccination yearly (the inactivated influenza vaccine is available as an intramuscular injection)

NUTRITION

- Feeding alternatives
  - The Centers for Disease Control and Prevention (CDC), World Health Organization (WHO), and the American Academy of Pediatrics (AAP) recommend that infants receive breast milk solely until 6 months of age and breastfeeding should be continued while introducing complementary foods up to 2 years of age, or longer.
  - Iron-fortified formula is an acceptable alternative to breast milk. Cow's milk is not recommended.
  - It is recommended to begin vitamin D supplements within the first few days of life to prevent rickets and vitamin D deficiency (if consuming less than 28 ounces of formula or breastmilk per day. Qebp
  - Iron supplements could be prescribed for the infant if indicated.
  - Alternative sources of fluids (juice or water) are not needed during the first 4 months of life. Excessive intake of water could result in hyponatremia and water intoxication.
  - After the age of 6 months, 100% fruit juice should be limited to 4 to 6 oz per day.

- Solids (complementary foods) are introduced around 6 months of age.
  - Indicators for readiness include interest in solid foods, voluntary control of the head and trunk, and disappearance of the extrusion reflex.
  - Iron-fortified cereal is typically introduced first due to its high iron content.
  - Solid food choices may be introduced in any order. Introduce one single-ingredient new food from any food group every 3 to 5 days and monitor for allergy or intolerance, which can include fussiness, rash, upper respiratory distress, vomiting, diarrhea, or constipation.
  - Breast milk/formula should be decreased as intake of solid/complementary foods increases but should remain the primary source of nutrition through the first year or longer if breastfeeding.
  - Table foods that are well-cooked, chopped, and unseasoned are appropriate by 1 year of age.
  - Appropriate finger foods include ripe bananas, toast strips, graham crackers, cheese cubes, noodles, firmly-cooked vegetables, and raw pieces of fruit (except grapes).
- Weaning can be accomplished when infants show signs of readiness and are able to drink from a cup (sometime in the second 6 months).
  - Gradually replace one bottle or breastfeeding at a time with breast milk or formula in a cup with handles.
  - Bedtime feedings are the last to be stopped.

SLEEP AND REST

- Nocturnal sleep pattern is established by 3 to 4 months of age.
- Infants sleep 14 to 15 hr daily and 9 to 11 hr at night around the age of 4 months.
- Infants sleep through the night and take one to two naps during the day by the age of 12 months.

INJURY PREVENTION Qs

Aspiration of foreign objects
- Hold the infant for feedings; do not prop bottles.
- Small objects that can become lodged in the throat (grapes, coins, candy) should be avoided.
- Age-appropriate toys should be provided.
- Clothing should be checked for safety hazards (loose buttons).

Bodily harm
- Sharp objects should be kept out of reach.
- Anchor heavy objects and furniture so they cannot be overturned on top of the infant.
- Infants should not be left unattended with any animals present.

Burns

- Avoid warming formula in a microwave; check temperature of liquid before feeding.
- The temperature of bath water should be checked.
- Hot water thermostats should be set at or below 49° C (120° F).
- Working smoke detectors should be kept in the home.
- Handles of pots and pans should be kept turned to the back of stoves.
- Sunscreen should be used when infants are exposed to the sun.
- Electrical outlets should be covered.

Drowning

- Infants should not be left unattended in bathtubs or around water sources (toilets, cleaning buckets, or drainage areas).
- Secure fencing around swimming pools.
- Close bathroom doors.

Falls

- Crib mattresses should be kept in the lowest position possible with the rails all the way up.
- Restraints should be used in infant seats.
- Infant seats should be placed on the ground or floor if used outside of the car, and they should not be left unattended or on elevated surfaces.
- Place safety gates at the top and bottom of stairs.

Poisoning

- Exposure to lead paint should be avoided. Ⓠ SDoH
- Toxins and plants should be kept out of reach.
- Safety locks should be kept on cabinets that contain cleaners and other household chemicals.
- The phone number for a poison control center should be kept near the phone.
- Medications should be kept in childproof containers, away from the reach of infants.
- A working carbon monoxide detector should be kept in the home.

Motor-vehicle injuries

- Infant-only and convertible infant–toddler car seats are available.
- Infants and toddlers remain in a rear-facing car seat until the age of 2 years or the height recommended by the manufacturer.
- The safest area for infants and children is the backseat of the car.
- Do not place rear-facing car seats in the front seat of vehicles with passenger airbags.
- Infants should not be left in parked cars.

Suffocation

- Plastic bags should be avoided.
- Balloons should be kept away from infants.
- Crib mattresses should fit snugly.
- Crib slats should be no farther apart than 6 cm (2.375 in).
- Crib mobiles and/or crib gyms should be removed by 4 to 5 months of age.
- Pillows should be kept out of the crib.
- Infants should be placed on their backs for sleep.
- Toys with small parts should be kept out of reach.

Active Learning Scenario

A nurse is preparing an educational program for a group of caregivers of infants. Use the ATI Active Learning Template: Growth and Development to complete this item.

DEVELOPMENTAL STAGE: Identify the infant's developmental stage according to Piaget and Erikson.

COGNITIVE DEVELOPMENT: List two cognitive developmental tasks the infant should accomplish in the first year of life.

AGE-APPROPRIATE ACTIVITIES: List five activities appropriate for infants.

INJURY PREVENTION: Identify two injury prevention methods in each of the following categories.

- Aspiration
- Poisoning
- Drowning
- Suffocation

Active Learning Scenario Key

Using the ATI Active Learning Template: Growth and Development

DEVELOPMENTAL STAGE
- Piaget: Sensorimotor stage
- Erikson: Trust vs. mistrust

COGNITIVE DEVELOPMENT
- Infants progress from reflexive to simple repetitive to imitative activities.
- Separation: Learning to separate themselves from other objects in the environment.
- Object permanence: Understanding that an object still exists when it is out of view.
- Mental representation: Ability to recognize and use symbols.

AGE-APPROPRIATE ACTIVITIES
- Rattles
- Soft stuffed toys
- Teething toys
- Nesting toys
- Playing pat-a-cake
- Playing with balls
- Reading books
- Mirrors
- Brightly colored toys
- Playing with blocks

INJURY PREVENTION
- Aspiration
  - Avoid small objects.
  - Hold infant for feedings; do not prop bottles.
  - Provide age-appropriate toys.
  - Check clothing for hazards (loose buttons).
- Poisoning
  - Keep toxins and plants out of reach.
  - Place safety locks on cabinets where cleaners/chemicals are stored.
  - Use a carbon monoxide detector in the home.
  - Keep medications in childproof containers and out of reach.
- Drowning
  - Do not leave unattended around any water source.
  - Secure fencing around swimming pool.
  - Keep bathroom door closed.
- Suffocation
  - Avoid plastic bags.
  - Ensure crib mattress fits snugly.
  - Remove crib mobiles by 4 to 5 months of age.
  - Keep pillows out of the crib.
  - Place on back to sleep.

Ⓝ *NCLEX® Connection: Health Promotion and Maintenance, Health Promotion/Disease Prevention*

Application Exercises

1. A nurse is assessing a 12-month-old infant during a well-child visit. Which of the following findings should the nurse report to the provider?

   A. Closed anterior fontanel

   B. Eruption of six teeth

   C. Birth weight doubled

   D. Birth length increased by 50%

2. A nurse is providing teaching about dental care and teething to the caregiver of a 9-month-old infant. Which of the following statements by the caregiver indicates an understanding of the teaching?

   A. "I can give my baby a warm teething ring to relieve discomfort."

   B. "I should clean my baby's teeth with a cool, wet wash cloth."

   C. "I can give ibuprofen for up to 5 days while my baby is teething."

   D. "I should place diluted juice in the bottle my baby drinks while falling asleep."

3. A nurse is performing a developmental screening on a 9-month-old infant. Which of the following fine motor skills should the nurse expect the infant to perform? (Select all that apply.)

   A. Grasp a rattle by the handle

   B. Try building a two-block tower

   C. Use a crude pincer grasp

   D. Place objects into a container

   E. Sit unsupported

4. A nurse is conducting a well-baby visit with a 4-month-old infant. Which of the following immunizations should the nurse plan to administer to the infant? (Select all that apply.)

   A. Measles, mumps, rubella (MMR)

   B. Polio (IPV)

   C. Pneumococcal vaccine (PCV)

   D. Varicella

   E. Rotavirus vaccine (RV)

5. A nurse is providing education to the guardian of a 3-month-old infant about care of the infant during the first year of life. Which of the following statements by the guardian indicates an understanding of the teaching?

   A. "My baby can have up to 6 ounces of fruit juice a day after they are 6 months old."

   B. "I should expect my baby to begin showing signs of separation anxiety around 10 months of age."

   C. "I should consider starting my baby on vitamin D when they are 4 months old."

   D. "My baby should be able to say 6 to 8 words by the time they are 1-year-old."

6. A nurse is visiting the home of a 9-month-old infant who is receiving home health services. The nurse is conducting a safety assessment of the home environment shown in the image below. Sort the findings into the following categories: Hazards or Non-hazards.

   A. Cabinet with lock

   B. Fire in the fireplace with fireplace cover present

   C. Infant on the floor with dog, no adult present

   D. Jacks on the floor

   E. Plate with a fork on the coffee table

   F. Pool with locked gate

   G. Potted plant sitting on floor

   H. Smoke alarm on wall

   I. Stairs with safety gate at top but not bottom

   J. Steaming cup of coffee by the plate

   K. Uncovered electrical outlets

1. C. **CORRECT:** When analyzing data during the assessment of a 12-month-old infant, the nurse should report to the provider that the infants birth weight has doubled. By the age of 12 months, the infant's birth weight should have tripled.

   A, B, D. By the age of 12 to 18 months, the infant's anterior fontanel should close; therefore, this is not a finding that the nurse should report to the provider.

   Ⓝ *NCLEX® Connection: Management of Care, Collaboration with Multidisciplinary Team*

2. A. Teething pain can be relieved using frozen teething rings or an ice cube wrapped in a wash cloth.

   B. **CORRECT:** When evaluating the outcomes of teaching about dental care to the caregiver of a 9-month-old infant, the nurse should recognize that, "I should clean my baby's teeth with a cool, wet wash cloth" indicates understanding of the teaching.

   C. Ibuprofen (Advil) should not be used for more than 3 days.

   D. To prevent early childhood caries, infants should not be given bottles while falling asleep.

   Ⓝ *NCLEX® Connection: Health Promotion and Maintenance, Health Promotion/Disease Prevention*

3. A, C. **CORRECT:** When recognizing cues while performing a developmental screening on a 9-month-old infant, the nurse should recognize that by the age of 9 months the infant should be able to grasp a rattle by the handle, have a crude pincer grasp, and sit unsupported.

   B, D, E. An infant who is at least 12 months of age should be able to build a two-block tower and place objects in a container.

   Ⓝ *NCLEX® Connection: Health Promotion and Maintenance, Developmental Stages and Transitions*

4. B, C, E. **CORRECT:** When generating solutions during a well-baby visit for a 4-month-old infant, the nurse should plan to administer the IPV, PCV, and RV vaccine to the 4-month-old infant.

   A. The first MMR vaccine is given between the ages of 12 and 15 months; therefore, the nurse should not plan to administer the MMR vaccine to the 4-month-old infant.

   D. The first varicella vaccine is given at a minimum age of 12 months; therefore, the nurse should not plan to administer the varicella vaccine to the 4-month-old infant.

   Ⓝ *NCLEX® Connection: Health Promotion and Maintenance, Health Promotion/Disease Prevention*

5. A. **CORRECT:** When evaluating the client's response to the education provided, the nurse should identify that the following statement by the client indicates an understanding of the teaching, "My baby can have up to 6 ounces of fruit juice a day after they are 6 months old."

   B. "I should expect my baby to begin showing signs of separation anxiety around 10 months of age" does not indicate understanding of the teaching. The nurse should reinforce to the guardian that separation anxiety usually begins around 4 to 8 months of age.

   C. "I should consider starting my baby on vitamin D when they are 4 months old" does not indicate understanding of the teaching. The nurse should reinforce to the guardian that vitamin D supplementation is recommended to begin within the first few days of life to help prevent vitamin D deficiency if the infant is consuming less than 28 ounces of formula per day.

   D. "My baby should be able to say 6 to 8 words by the time they are 1-year-old" does not indicate understanding of the teaching. The nurse should reinforce to the guardian that most infants have a vocabulary of 3 to 5 words by one year of age.

   Ⓝ *NCLEX® Connection: Basic Care and Comfort, Nutrition and Oral Hydration*

6. **HAZARDS:** C, D, E, G, I, J, K; **NON-HAZARDS:** A, B, F, H

   When performing a safety assessment on the home of an infant the nurse should identify the following findings as hazardous to the safety of the infant: small toys in the floor, a fork on the coffee table, a cup of hot liquid on the coffee table, the infant is unsupervised with an animal, there are no covers on the electrical outlets, the stairs to not have a gate at the bottom, and a potted plant is sitting in the floor. The fireplace with a screen present, smoke alarm on the wall, locked gate on the pool, and lock on the cabinet all serve to protect the infant from harm.

CHAPTER 4

Health Promotion of Toddlers (1 to 3 Years)

EXPECTED GROWTH AND DEVELOPMENT

PHYSICAL DEVELOPMENT

- Anterior fontanels close by 18 months of age.
- **Weight**: At 30 months of age, toddlers should weigh four times their birth weight. Toddlers gain approximately 1.8 to 2.7 kg (4 to 6 lb) per year.
- **Height**: Toddlers grow about 7.5 cm (3 in) per year.
- **Head circumference** and chest circumference are usually equal by 1 to 2 years of age.

COGNITIVE DEVELOPMENT

Piaget: Sensorimotor stage transitions to the preoperational stage around 2 years of age. Q EBP
- The concept of object permanence increases.
- Toddlers have and demonstrate memories of events that relate to them.
- Domestic mimicry (playing house) is evident.
- Preoperational thought does not allow for toddlers to understand other viewpoints, but it does allow them to symbolize objects and people to imitate previously seen activities.

PSYCHOSOCIAL DEVELOPMENT

Erikson: autonomy versus shame and doubt Q EBP
- Independence is paramount for toddlers, who are attempting to do everything for themselves.
- Toddlers often use negativism, or negative responses, as they begin to express their independence.
- Ritualism, or maintaining routines and reliability, provides a sense of comfort for toddlers as they begin to explore the environment beyond those most familiar to them.

Moral development

- Moral development is closely associated with cognitive development.
- Egocentric: Toddlers are unable to see things from the perspectives of others; they can only view things from their personal points of view.
- Punishment and obedience orientation begin with a sense that good behavior is rewarded, and bad behavior is punished.

Self-concept development

Toddlers progressively see themselves as separate from their parents and increase their explorations away from them.

Body-image changes

- Toddlers appreciate the usefulness of various body parts.
- Toddlers develop gender identity by 3 years of age.

AGE-APPROPRIATE ACTIVITIES Q PCC

- Solitary play evolves into parallel play, in which toddlers observe other children and then might engage in activities nearby.
- Appropriate activities
  - Filling and emptying containers
  - Water toys and clay
  - Playing with blocks
  - Looking at books
  - Push-pull toys
  - Tossing balls
  - Finger paints
  - Large-piece puzzles
  - Thick crayons
- Temper tantrums result when toddlers are frustrated with restrictions on independence. Providing consistent, age-appropriate expectations helps toddlers to work through frustration.
- Toilet training can begin when toddlers have the sensation of needing to urinate or defecate. Parents should demonstrate patience and consistency in toilet training. Nighttime control might develop last.
- Discipline should be consistent with well-defined boundaries that are established to develop appropriate social behavior.

HEALTH PROMOTION

IMMUNIZATIONS

The Centers for Disease Control and Prevention immunization recommendations for healthy toddlers 12 months to 3 years of age include: Q EBP
- 12 to 15 months: inactivated poliovirus (third dose between 6 to 18 months); Haemophilus influenzae type B; pneumococcal conjugate vaccine; measles, mumps, and rubella; and varicella
- 12 to 23 months: hepatitis A (Hep A), given in two doses at least 6 months apart
- 15 to 18 months: diphtheria, tetanus, and acellular pertussis
- 12 to 36 months: yearly seasonal inactivated influenza vaccine; live, attenuated influenza vaccine by nasal spray (must be 2 years or older)
- Follow the current CDC recommendations for administration of the COVID-19 vaccine to children 12 months to 3 years of age.

4.1 Developmental Milestones According to Age

	MOTOR (FINE AND GROSS)	COGNITIVE	LANGUAGE	SOCIAL	CLIENT EDUCATION
12 MONTHS (1 YEAR)	• Pulls up to a standing position • Drinks from a cup without a lid • Picks things up between thumb and pointer finger • Walks holding onto furniture • Attempts to build a 2-block tower	• Able to place a block in a container • Looks for hidden object/toys	• Waves "bye-bye" • Calls parent/guardian by their special name • Comprehends the word "no"	• Plays games with others	• Ensure environment is safe • Limit screen time • Encourage baby to make noises • Teach baby positive behaviors
15 MONTHS	• Takes a few steps independently • Uses fingers to feed themselves food	• Stacks 2 small objects (blocks) • Attempts to use things in a correct manner (phone, book, cup)	• Tries to speak one or two words other than "mama" or "dada" • Follows simple directions given with both a gesture and words • Ask for things by pointing	• Mimics other children while playing • Claps hands together when excited • Shows affection (hugging, kissing, cuddling)	• Assist child with learning to speak by repeating and adding to what they say • Allow child to assist with daily activities • Encourage child play with blocks—stack them and allow child to knock over
18 MONTHS	• Walks independently without holding on to anyone or furniture • Climbs on and off furniture independently • Scribbles • Drinks from a lidless cup • Uses fingers to feed themselves • Attempts using a spoon	• Mimics someone performing household chores • Plays with toys in a simple manner	• Tries to say three or more different words • Follows one-step directions	• Points to something of interest • Assists with putting on clothes (pushing leg through pants or arms through sleeve) • Looks at pages in book with others	• Schedule child's developmental screening assessment with their provider • Inquire about toilet training with provider • Allow child to play, talk, and interact with others • Give child simple choices to make • Read a book with child and discuss pictures
24 MONTHS (2 YEARS)	• Kicks a ball • Runs • Walks up a few stairs with or without help • Uses a spoon when eating	• Plays with several toys simultaneously • Attempts to use knobs, buttons, or switches on toys • Holds something in one hand while using the other hand	• Uses more gestures such as blowing a kiss or affirmative nodding • Points to things in a book when asked • Says at least two words together • Points to two or more body parts when asked	• Notices emotions of others (looks sad when someone is crying) • Looks for the reaction of others	• Schedule child's developmental screening assessment with their provider • Allow child to throw, roll, or kick a ball • Provide consistent routines for sleeping and eating • Allow child to explore and learn new things
30 MONTHS	• Uses hands to twist items (doorknob) • Takes some clothes off independently • Jumps off the ground with both feet • Turns book pages, one at a time (while book is being read)	• Uses pretend play Demonstrates simple problem-solving skills Follows two-step instructions • Knows at least one color when asked	• Speaks about 50 words Speaks with 2 or more words and verb • Identifies pointed items in a book when asked	• Uses parallel play and/or plays with others • Follows simple routines when asked	• Schedule child's developmental screening assessment with their provider • Encourage child to name pictures in a book, colors, body parts • Allow child to draw with crayons or chalk • Demonstrate with child how to play with others

Table is based on the Centers for Disease Control and Prevention, CDC's Developmental Milestones 2022 Update

NUTRITION

- Children might establish lifetime eating habits during early childhood. **Q**sDoH
- Toddlers begin developing taste preferences and are generally picky eaters who repeatedly request their favorite foods.
- Physiologic anorexia occurs, resulting in toddlers becoming fussy eaters because of a decreased appetite.
- Toddlers should consume 16 to 24 oz of milk per day, and may switch from drinking whole milk to drinking low-fat milk after 2 years of age. Breastfeeding can continue for up to 2 years of age or longer if desired.
- Juice consumption should be limited to 4 to 6 oz per day.
- Trans fatty acids and saturated fats should be avoided.
- Diet should include 1 cup of fruit daily.
- Food serving size should be 1 tbsp for each year of age, or ¼ to 1/3 of an adult portion.
- Toddlers generally prefer finger foods because of increasing autonomy.
- Regular mealtimes and nutritious snacks best meet nutrient needs.
- Snacks or desserts that are high in sugar, fat, or sodium should be avoided.
- Foods that are potential choking hazards (nuts, grapes, hot dogs, peanut butter, raw carrots, dried beans, tough meats, popcorn) should be avoided.
- Adult supervision should always be provided during snack and mealtimes.
- Foods should be cut into small, bite-size pieces to make them easier to swallow and to prevent choking.
- Toddlers should not be allowed to engage in drinking or eating during play activities or while lying down.
- Parents should follow the American Academy of Pediatrics guidelines for nutrition.

SLEEP AND REST

- Toddlers typically average 11 to 12 hr of sleep per day, including one nap.
- Naps often are eliminated in older toddlerhood.
- Resistance to bedtime and expression of fears are common in this age group.
- Maintaining a regular bedtime and bedtime routines are helpful to promote sleep.

DENTAL HEALTH

- Children should have an established dental provider by the age of 1 year.
- Flossing and brushing should be performed by the adult caregiver and are the best methods of removing plaque.
- Brushing should occur after meals and at bedtime. Nothing to eat or drink, except water, is given to the child after the bedtime cleaning.
- Fluoride is supplemented for children living in areas without adequate levels in drinking water.
- Early childhood caries is a form a tooth decay that develops in toddlers and is more common in children who are put to bed with a bottle of juice or milk.
- Consumption of cariogenic foods should be eliminated if possible. If not, the frequency of consumption should be limited.

INJURY PREVENTION Qs

Aspiration of foreign objects
- Small objects (grapes, coins, colored beads, candy) that can become lodged in the throat should be avoided.
- Toys that have small parts should be kept out of reach.
- Age-appropriate toys should be provided.
- Clothing should be checked for safety hazards (loose buttons).
- Balloons should be kept away from toddlers.
- Parents should know emergency procedures for choking.

Bodily harm
- Sharp objects should be kept out of reach.
- Firearms should be kept in locked boxes or cabinets.
- Toddlers should not be left unattended with any animals present.
- Toddlers should be taught stranger safety.

Burns
- The temperature of bath water should be checked.
- Thermostats on hot water heaters should be turned down to less than 49° C (120° F).
- Working smoke detectors should be kept in the home.
- Pot handles should be turned toward the back of the stove.
- Electrical outlets should be covered.
- Toddlers should wear sunscreen when outside.

Drowning
- Toddlers should not be left unattended in bathtubs.
- Toilet lids should be kept closed.
- Toddlers should be closely supervised when near pools or any other body of water.
- Toddlers should be taught to swim.

Falls
- Doors and windows should be kept locked.
- Crib mattresses should be kept in the lowest position with the rails all the way up.
- Safety gates should be used across the top and bottom of stairs.

Motor-vehicle injuries
- Infants and toddlers remain in a rear-facing car seat until the age of 2 years or the height and weight recommended by the manufacturer.
- Toddlers over the age of 2 years, or who exceed the height recommendations for rear-facing car seats, are moved to a forward-facing car seat.
- Safest area for infants and children is the backseat of the car.
- Do not place rear-facing car seats in the front seat of vehicles with deployable passenger airbags.

Poisoning
- Exposure to lead paint should be avoided. Safety locks should be placed on cabinets that contain cleaners and other chemicals.
- The phone number for a poison control center should be kept near the phone.
- Medications should be kept in childproof containers, away from the reach of toddlers.
- A working carbon monoxide detector should be placed in the home.

Suffocation
- Plastic bags should be avoided.
- Crib mattresses should fit tightly.
- Crib slats should be no farther apart than 6 cm (2.375 in).
- Pillows should be kept out of cribs.

Application Exercises

1. A nurse is assessing a 2½-year-old toddler at a well-child visit. Which of the following findings should the nurse report to the provider?

   A. Height increased by 7.5 cm (3 in) in the past year.

   B. Head circumference exceeds chest circumference.

   C. Anterior and posterior fontanels are closed.

   D. Current weight equals four times the birth weight.

2. A nurse is providing education about developmental milestones of a toddler with a newly licensed nurse. Sort the following developmental milestones according to the child's age: 12 months or 24 months.

   A. Ability to run

   B. Kicks a ball

   C. Attempts to build a tower of 2 blocks

   D. Walks up a couple of stairs

   E. Eats with a spoon

   F. Drinks from a lidless cup

   G. Place a block in a container

3. A nurse is performing a developmental screening on an 18-month-old. Which of the following skills should the nurse expect the toddler to be able to perform? (Select all that apply.)

   A. Removes few articles of their clothing

   B. Attempts using a spoon

   C. Walks independently without holding onto furniture

   D. Jumps off ground using both feet

   E. Turns pages in book one at time

4. A nurse is providing teaching about growth and development characteristics with the guardian of a toddler who is 2 years of age. Which of the following statements by the guardian should the nurse identify indicates an understanding of the teaching?

   A. "My child should be able to kick a ball."

   B. "My child should be able to turn the pages in a book one at a time."

   C. "My child should be able turn the doorknob."

   D. "My child should be able to speak about 100 words."

5. A nurse is providing anticipatory guidance to the caregivers of a toddler. Which of the following should the nurse include? (Select all that apply.)

   A. Develop food habits that will prevent dental caries.

   B. A decrease in appetite is common in toddlers

   C. Expression of bedtime fears is common.

   D. Expect behaviors associated with negativism and ritualism.

   E. Annual screenings for phenylketonuria are important.

6. A community health nurse is preparing an injury prevention program for the caregivers of toddlers who live in the community. Which of the following should the nurse include in the program?

   A. Hot water heater thermostats should be set below 49° C (120° F).

   B. Swimming lessons should begin at the age of 5.

   C. Crib mattresses should be kept in the middle position.

   D. Firearms do not need to be locked away as long as the child cannot reach them.

Application Exercises Key

1. A. Toddler height should increase by 7.5 cm (3 in) each year. Therefore, do not report this finding to the provider.
   B. **CORRECT:** The head and chest circumference should be equal by 1 to 2 years of age, with the chest circumference continuing to increase in size until it exceeds the head circumference. Therefore, report this finding to the provider.
   C. The posterior fontanel closes by the age of 6 to 8 weeks, and the anterior fontanel closes by 12 to 18 months. Therefore, do not report this finding to the provider.
   D. The current weight should be four times the birth weight at the age of 2½ years. Therefore, do not report this finding to the provider.

   Ⓝ *NCLEX® Connection: Management of Care, Collaboration with Multidisciplinary Team*

2. **12 MONTHS:** C, F, G; **24 MONTHS:** A, B, D, E

   Expected developmental milestones can vary according to the child's age. According to the CDC, a child who is 1 year of age can attempt to build a tower of two blocks, drink from a lidless cup, and place a block in a container. Also, according to the CDC, a child who is 2 years of age can run, kick a ball, walk up a couple of stairs, and eat with a spoon.

   Ⓝ *NCLEX® Connection: Health Promotion and Maintenance, Health Promotion/Disease Prevention*

3. B, C. **CORRECT:** A nurse should expect a toddler who is 18 months of age can attempt to use a spoon and walk independently.
   A, D, E. The nurse should expect a toddler who is 30 months age to remove few articles of their clothing, turn pages in a book one at a time, and jump of the ground by using both feet.

   Ⓝ *NCLEX® Connection: Health Promotion and Maintenance, Developmental Stages and Transitions*

4. A. **CORRECT:** When evaluating outcomes after providing teaching about growth and development characteristics with the guardian of a 2-year-old toddler, the nurse should identify that the statement, "My child should be able to kick a ball" indicates understanding of the expected growth and development information provided by the nurse.
   B, C. Turning the pages in a book one at a time and turning a doorknob are activities that a child who is 30 months of age is expected to perform.
   D. A child who speaks one hundred or more words is appropriate for a child who is greater than 30 months of age.

   Ⓝ *NCLEX® Connection: Health Promotion and Maintenance, Aging Process*

5. A, B, C, D. **CORRECT:** When taking action and providing anticipatory guidance to the caregivers of a toddler, the nurse should include the development of food habits that will prevent dental caries and that the child may express bedtime fears and show behaviors that are associated with negativism and ritualism. The nurse should also inform that caregivers that toddlers often experience a physiologic anorexia causing food intake to decrease.
   E. Annual screening for phenylketonuria should not be included as this is a screening that is performed on the newborn, not the toddler.

   Ⓝ *NCLEX® Connection: Management of Care, Collaboration with Multidisciplinary Team*

6. A. **CORRECT:** The community health nurse should include in the injury prevention program that the thermostats of hot water heaters should be kept below 49° C (120° F) to prevent burns.
   B. The nurse should include in the injury prevention program that while not a guaranteed protection against drowning, the American Academy of Pediatrics recommends swimming lesson for children as young as one year of age as an added layer of protection.
   C. The nurse should include in the injury prevention program that crib mattresses should be lowered as the child ages to prevent climbing out of the crib and falling.
   D. The nurse should include in the injury prevention program that toddlers are naturally curious and love to climb and explore areas that may be unsafe. It is not uncommon for a toddler to climb on top of objects that caregivers may have considered out of reach of the toddler. Therefore, firearms should always be kept unloaded, in a locked safe or cabinet to prevent accidental firearm injury.

   Ⓝ *NCLEX® Connection: Management of Care, Collaboration with Multidisciplinary Team*

Active Learning Scenario

A nurse is conducting a well-child visit with a 2-year-old toddler. Use the ATI Active Learning Template: Growth and Development to complete this item.

DEVELOPMENTAL STAGE: Identify the toddler's developmental stage according to Piaget and Erikson.

NUTRITION: List three concepts to include in teaching with the family.

INJURY PREVENTION: Identify two injury prevention methods to include in teaching with the family for each of the following categories.

- Bodily harm
- Drowning
- Burns
- Falls

Active Learning Scenario Key

Using the ATI Active Learning Template: Growth and Development

DEVELOPMENTAL STAGE
- Piaget: Preoperational stage
- Erikson: Autonomy vs. shame and doubt

NUTRITION
- May switch from whole milk to low fat milk after the age of 2 years.
- Trans fatty acids and saturated fats should be avoided.
- Diet should include 1 cup of fruit daily.
- Limit fruit juice to 4 to 6 oz per day.
- Cut food into small, bite-size pieces to prevent choking.
- Do not allow drinking or eating during play activities or while lying down.

INJURY PREVENTION
- Bodily harm
  - Keep sharp objects out of reach.
  - Lock firearms in a cabinet or box.
  - Teach toddler stranger safety.
  - Do not leave toddler unattended with animals.
- Drowning
  - Do not leave toddler unattended in bathtub.
  - Keep toilet lids closed.
  - Begin teaching toddler water safety and to swim.
  - Keep bathroom doors closed.
- Burns
  - Check bath water temperature prior to toddler contact with water.
  - Set hot water heaters to less than 49° C (120° F) .
  - Keep pot handles pointed to back of stove when cooking.
  - Cover electrical outlets.
  - Keep working smoke detectors in the home.
  - Apply sunscreen when toddler will be outside.
- Falls
  - Keep doors and windows locked.
  - Place crib mattresses in lowest position with rails all the way up.
  - Use safety gates at the top and bottom of stairs.

Ⓝ *NCLEX® Connection: Health Promotion and Maintenance, Aging Process*

CHAPTER 5

Health Promotion of Preschoolers (3 to 6 Years)

EXPECTED GROWTH AND DEVELOPMENT

PHYSICAL DEVELOPMENT

WEIGHT: Preschoolers should gain about 2 to 3 kg (4.5 to 6.5 lb) per year.

HEIGHT: Preschoolers should grow about 6.4 to 9 cm (2.5 to 3.5 in) per year.

5.1 Average Height And Weight By Age

	3-YEAR-OLD	4-YEAR-OLD	5-YEAR-OLD
WEIGHT	14.5 kg (32 lb)	16.5 kg (36.5 lb)	18.5 kg (41 lb)
HEIGHT	95 cm (37.5 in)	103 cm (40.5 in)	110 cm (43.5 in)

Preschoolers' bodies evolve away from the characteristically unsteady wide stances and protruding abdomen of the toddler, into a more graceful, erect posture, and physical stance.

DEVELOPMENTAL SKILLS

Preschoolers should show improvement in fine motor skills, which will be displayed by activities like copying figures on paper and dressing independently.

COGNITIVE DEVELOPMENT Q EBP

Piaget: preoperational phase
The preconceptual thought transitions to the phase of intuitive thought around the age of 4 years. The phase of intuitive thought lasts until the age of 7 years.

- The preschooler moves from totally egocentric thoughts to social awareness and the ability to consider the viewpoints of others.
- Preschoolers make judgments based on visual appearances. Variations in thinking during this age include:
  ○ **Magical thinking:** Thoughts are all powerful and can cause events to occur.
  ○ **Animism:** Ascribing lifelike qualities to inanimate objects.
  ○ **Centration:** Focus on one aspect instead of considering all possible alternatives.
  ○ **Time:** Preschoolers begin to understand the sequence of daily events. Time is best explained to them in relation to an event. By the end of the preschool years, children have a better comprehension of time-oriented words.

Language development

- The vocabulary of preschoolers increases to more than 2,100 words by the end of the fifth year.
- Preschoolers speak in sentences of three to four words at the ages of 3 and 4 years, and four to five words at the age of 4 to 5 years.
- This age group enjoys talking, and language becomes their primary method of communication.
- Names familiar objects, body parts, animals and family members. Imitates new words proficiently.

PSYCHOSOCIAL DEVELOPMENT Q EBP

Erikson: initiative vs. guilt
- Preschoolers become energetic learners, despite not having all the physical abilities necessary to be successful at everything.
- Guilt can occur when preschoolers believe they have misbehaved or when they are unable to accomplish a task.
- Guiding preschoolers to attempt activities within their capabilities while setting limits is important.

Kohlberg: moral development
- Preschoolers at 2 to 4 years old have a basic understanding of moral judgment, and actions are taken based on whether it will result in a reward or punishment.
- Preschoolers at 4 to 6 years old primarily take actions based on satisfying personal needs yet understand the concepts of justice and fairness.

Body-image changes

- Preschoolers begin to recognize differences in appearances and identify what is considered acceptable and unacceptable.
- By the age of 5 years, preschoolers begin comparing themselves with peers.
- Poor understanding of anatomy makes intrusive experiences (injections or cuts) frightening to preschoolers. Therefore, preschoolers believe it is important to use bandages after an injury.

Social development

- Preschoolers generally do not exhibit stranger anxiety and have less separation anxiety.
- Changes in daily routine are tolerated, but they can develop more imaginary fears.
- Prolonged separation (during hospitalization) can provoke anxiety. Favorite toys and appropriate play should be used to help ease preschoolers' fears.
- Pretend play is healthy and allows preschoolers to determine the difference between reality and fantasy.

5.2 Gross Motor Skills By Age

	MOTOR (FINE AND GROSS)	COGNITIVE	LANGUAGE	SOCIAL	CLIENT EDUCATION
3 YEARS	Strings beads or other items together Puts on some clothes independently Uses a fork Rides a tricycle Stands on one foot for a few seconds Jumps off a bottom step Builds a tower with 9-10 blocks	Returns demonstration of the drawing of a circle Avoids touching hot objects after receiving a warning	Combines 3-4 words to create simple sentence Talks in conversation with others using back-and-forth exchanges Says first name after being asked	Calms down within 10 minutes after being left in the care of others Notices other children and joins them in play	Encourage child to play with others Give child healthy and simple food choices Teach child opposites, counting numbers Play matching games with child Encourage child to say their name and age Limit screen time to less than 1 hour per day under supervision, if desired
4 YEARS	Catches a large ball Serves themselves food or pours their drinking liquids, with supervision Unbuttons some buttons Holds crayon or pencil between fingers and thumb	Names a few colors Tells what comes next in a well-known story Draws a person with three or more body parts	Says simple sentences with four or more words Says some words from a song, story, or nursery rhyme Talks about at least one thing that happened during their day, like "I played soccer." Answers simple questions like "What is a coat for?" or "What is a crayon for?"	Pretends to be something else during play Inquires about playing with other children Comforts others who are hurt or sad Likes to assist others Changes behavior based on their location (library, grocery store)	Reinforce positive behaviors in a positive manner Allow child to play with others Provide calm, quiet environment during bedtime Provide response when child ask questions Allow child to help with simple chores Encourage the counting items
5 YEARS	Buttons some buttons Hops/skips on one foot Throws a ball overhead Laces shoes	Counts to 10 Identifies some numbers between 1 and 5 and letters when pointed to Uses words about time Pays attention for 5 to 10 minutes during activities. Writes some letters of their name	Tells a story with at least two events Uses or identifies simple rhymes Answers simple questions about a book or story Keeps a conversation going with more than three back-and-forth exchanges	Follows rules or takes turns when playing with other children Sings, dances, or acts in front of others Performs simple chores at home	Teach child about safe touching Allow child to perform tasks independently Use words to assist child with understanding of time Allow time for active play daily Allow for creative play time

Information adopted from the Centers for Disease Control and Prevention, CDC's Developmental Milestones 2022 Update

AGE-APPROPRIATE ACTIVITIES Q EBP

Parallel play shifts to associative play during the preschool years. Play is not highly organized, but cooperation does exist between children. Appropriate activities include:

- Playing ball
- Putting puzzles together
- Riding tricycles
- Playing pretend and dress–up activities
- Role playing
- Hand puppets
- Painting
- Simple sewing
- Reading books
- Wading pools
- Sand boxes
- Skating
- Computer programs
- Musical toys
- Electronic games

HEALTH PROMOTION

IMMUNIZATIONS

The Centers for Disease Control and Prevention (CDC) immunization recommendations for healthy preschoolers 3 to 6 years of age include: Q EBP

- **4 TO 6 YEARS:** Diphtheria and tetanus toxoids and pertussis (DTaP); measles, mumps, and rubella (MMR); varicella; and inactivated poliovirus (IPV)
- **3 TO 6 YEARS:** Yearly seasonal influenza vaccine; inactivated influenza vaccine; or live, attenuated influenza vaccine by nasal spray

Follow the current CDC recommendations for administration of the COVID–19 vaccine to children 3 to 6 years of age.

NUTRITION

- Preschoolers who are mildly active require an estimated caloric intake range from 1200 to 1400 kcal/day.
- Finicky eating can remain a behavior in preschoolers, but often by 5 years of age they become more willing to sample different foods.
- Preschoolers need 13 to 19 g/day of protein (2- to 4-oz equivalents), in addition to 700 to 1000 mg/day of calcium and19 to 25 g/fay of fiber.
- Total fat should be 30% of total caloric intake over several days.
- With obesity rates in young children increasing, the American Academy of Pediatrics recommends a 5-2-1-0 framework, which includes that preschoolers have 5 servings of fruits and vegetables per day, 2 hr or less of screen time, 0 servings of sugar-sweetened beverages, and 1 hr of physical activity per day. **Q**SDoH
- Parents should follow the American Academy of Pediatrics' healthy diet recommendations.

SLEEP AND REST

- On average, preschoolers need about 12 hr of sleep per day, and infrequently take daytime naps.
- Sleep disturbances frequently occur during early childhood, and problems range from difficulty going to bed to night terrors. Recommended interventions vary but can include the following.
  - Keep a consistent bedtime routine.
  - Use a night light in the room.
  - Provide the child with a favorite toy.
  - Leave a drink of water by the bed.
  - Reassure preschoolers who are frightened but discourage sleeping with parents.
  - Ignore attention-seeking behaviors.

DENTAL HEALTH

- Eruption of deciduous (primary) teeth is finalized by the beginning of the preschool years.
- To prevent dental caries, parents should assist and supervise brushing and flossing to ensure it is performed correctly.
- Trauma to teeth is common in preschoolers and should be immediately evaluated by a dentist.

INJURY PREVENTION Qs

Bodily harm
- Firearms should be kept in locked cabinets or containers.
- Preschoolers should be taught stranger safety.
- Preschoolers should be taught to wear protective equipment (helmet, pads).
- Preschoolers are less prone to falls due to improved fine and gross motor skills, coordination, and balance.

Burns
- Hot water thermostats should be set at or below 49° C (120° F).
- Working smoke detectors should be kept in the home.
- Preschoolers should have sunscreen applied when outside.

Drowning
- Preschoolers should not be left unattended in bathtubs.
- Preschoolers should be closely supervised when near the pool or any other body of water.
- Preschoolers should be taught to swim.

Motor-vehicle injuries
- Preschoolers should use a federally approved car restraint according to the manufacturer recommendations.
- When the forward-facing car seat is outgrown, the preschooler transitions to a booster seat.
- It is recommended that children use an approved car restraint system until they achieve a height of 145 cm (4 feet, 9 in) or 8 to 12 years old.
- Safest area for children is the backseat of the car.
- Supervise preschool-age children when playing outside, and do not allow them to play near a curb or parked cars.
- Teach pedestrian safety rules to preschool-age children.
  - Stand back from curb while waiting to cross the street.
  - Before crossing the street, look left, then right, then left again.
  - Travel on the left, facing traffic, when there are no sidewalks.
  - At night, wear light-colored clothing with fluorescent materials attached.

Active Learning Scenario

A nurse is providing anticipatory guidance to the parents of a preschool-age child. Use the ATI Active Learning Template: Growth and Development to complete this item.

PHYSICAL DEVELOPMENT: Identify general expectations for height and weight during the preschool years.

COGNITIVE DEVELOPMENT: List two concepts related to language development in preschool-age children.

AGE-APPROPRIATE ACTIVITIES: List five activities appropriate for preschool-age children.

INJURY PREVENTION: Identify two pedestrian safety rules parents should teach children.

Active Learning Scenario Key

Using the ATI Active Learning Template:
Growth and Development

PHYSICAL DEVELOPMENT
- Weight: Preschoolers should gain about 2 to 3 kg (4.5 to 6.5 lb) per year.
- Height: Preschoolers should grow about 6.2 to 9 cm (2.4 to 3.5 in) per year.

COGNITIVE DEVELOPMENT
- Vocabulary increases to more than 2,100 words by the end of the fifth year.
- Speak in sentences of three to four words at the ages of 3 and 4 years.
- Speak in sentences of four to five words at the age of 4 to 5 years.
- Enjoy talking, and language becomes primary method of communication.

AGE-APPROPRIATE ACTIVITIES
- Putting puzzles together
- Playing ball
- Playing pretend and dress-up activities
- Painting
- Role playing
- Riding tricycles
- Simple sewing
- Reading books
- Sandboxes
- Wading pools
- Skating
- Computer programs
- Musical toys
- Electronic games

INJURY PREVENTION
- Stand back from curb while waiting to cross the street.
- Before crossing the street, look left, then right, then left again.
- Walk on the left, facing traffic, when there are no sidewalks.
- At night, wear light-colored clothing with fluorescent materials attached.

Ⓝ *NCLEX® Connection: Health Promotion and Maintenance, Developmental Stages and Transitions*

Application Exercises

1. A nurse is performing a developmental screening on a preschooler. Sort the following findings by the nurse into the correct motor skills categories: Gross Motor Skills or Fine Motor Skills

   A. Jumps off bottom step

   B. Catches ball reliably

   C. Uses scissors to cut out a picture

   D. Copies a circle

   E. Walks backwards with heel to toe

   F. Rides a tricycle

   G. Laces shoes

   H. Prints first name

2. A nurse is performing a developmental screening on a 3-year-old child. Which of the following skills should the nurse expect the child to perform?

   A. Ride a tricycle

   B. Hop on one foot

   C. Jump rope

   D. Throw a ball overhead

3. A nurse is conducting a well-child visit with a 5-year-old child. Which of the following immunizations should the nurse plan to administer to the child? (Select all that apply.)

   A. Diphtheria, tetanus, pertussis (DTaP)

   B. Inactivated poliovirus (IPV)

   C. Measles, mumps, rubella (MMR)

   D. Pneumococcal (PCV)

   E. Haemophilus influenzae type B (Hib)

4. A nurse is preparing an education program for a group of caregivers of preschool-age children about promoting optimum nutrition. Which of the following information should the nurse include in the teaching?

   A. Total fat intake should equal 20% of total daily caloric intake.

   B. Average calorie intake should be 1,400 calories per day.

   C. Daily intake of fruits and vegetables should total 2 servings.

   D. Healthy diets include a total of 8 g protein each day.

5. A nurse is providing teaching to the caregiver of a preschool-age child about methods to promote sleep. Which of the following statements by the caregiver indicates an understanding of the teaching?

   A. "I will sleep in the bed with my child if they wake up during the night."

   B. "I will let my child stay up an additional 2 hours on weekend nights."

   C. "I will let my child watch television for 30 minutes just before bedtime each night."

   D. "I will keep a dim lamp on in my child's room during the night."

1. **GROSS MOTOR SKILLS:** A, B, E, F;
   FINE MOTOR SKILLS: C, D, G, H

   Gross motor skills are those that the preschooler demonstrates and shows improvement in as their muscle strength increases and their sense of balance continues to advance. Therefore, the nurse should identify that jumping off of a bottom step, reliably catching a ball, walking backwards with heel to toe, and riding a tricycle are all examples of gross motor skills. Fine motor skills are those that involve the use of the hands and fingers when trying to pinch, grasp, or manually manipulate an object. Preschoolers show advancement in their ability to use their fine motor skills through their advancing ability to manipulate objects using their hands and fingers. Therefore, the nurse should identify that using scissors to cut out a picture, copying a circle, lacing their shoes, and printing their name are all examples of fine motor skills.

   Ⓝ *NCLEX® Connection: Health Promotion and Maintenance, Developmental Stages and Transitions*

2. A. **CORRECT:** The nurse should expect a 3-year-old child to be able to ride a tricycle.
   B. The nurse should expect a 4-year-old child, not a 3-year-old child, to hop on one foot.
   C. The nurse should expect a 5-year-old child, not a 3-year-old child, to be able to jump rope
   D. The nurse should expect a 4-year-old child, not a 3-year-old child, to be able to throw a ball overhead.

   Ⓝ *NCLEX® Connection: Health Promotion and Maintenance, Developmental Stages and Transitions*

3. A. **CORRECT:** DTaP is a recommended immunization for 4- to 6-year-olds, and should be administered by the nurse.
   B. **CORRECT:** IPV is a recommended immunization for 4- to 6-year-olds, and should be administered by the nurse.
   C. **CORRECT:** MMR is a recommended immunization for 4- to 6-year-olds, and should be administered by the nurse.
   D. PCV is given as a series of immunizations in the first 15 months of life, and is not recommended for 4- to 6-year-olds.
   E. Hib is given as a series of immunizations in the first 15 months of life, and is not recommended for 4- to 6-year-olds.

   Ⓝ *NCLEX® Connection: Health Promotion and Maintenance, Health Promotion/Disease Prevention*

4. A. Total fat should be 30% of total caloric intake over several days, not 20% of total daily caloric intake; therefore, the nurse should not include this information in the teaching.
   B. **CORRECT:** When generating solutions for an educational program for caregivers of preschool-aged children, the nurse should recognize that preschoolers should consume an average of 1,200 to 1,400 calories/day; therefore, the nurse should include this information in the teaching.
   C. Preschool-age children should consume a total of 5, not 2, servings of fruits and vegetables per day; therefore, the nurse should not include this information in the teaching..
   D. Healthy diets include 13 to 19 g protein each day, not 8 g of total protein each day; therefore, the nurse should not include this information in the teaching.

   Ⓝ *NCLEX® Connection: Basic Care and Comfort, Nutrition and Oral Hydration*

5. A. The statement "I will sleep in the bed with my child if they wake up during the night" does not indicate an understanding of the teaching. The child should not be allowed to sleep in the same bed as the caregiver.
   B. The statement "I will let my child stay up an additional 2 hours on weekend nights" does not indicate an understanding of the teaching. The caregiver should maintain a consistent bedtime routine and avoid allowing the child to stay up past a reasonable hour.
   C. The statement "I will let my child watch television for 30 minutes just before bedtime each night" does not indicate an understanding of the teaching. Watching television prior to bed can cause the child to resist and delay sleep.
   D. **CORRECT:** When evaluating outcomes after providing teaching to the caregiver of a preschool-aged child about methods to promote sleep, the nurse should recognize that the statement "I will keep a dim lamp on in my child's room during the night" indicates an understanding of the teaching. Leaving a light on in the child's room is an appropriate method to promote sleep for a preschool-age child.

   Ⓝ *NCLEX® Connection: Basic Care and Comfort, Rest and Sleep*

CHAPTER 6

Health Promotion of School-Age Children (6 to 12 Years)

EXPECTED GROWTH AND DEVELOPMENT

PHYSICAL DEVELOPMENT

Weight: School-age children will gain about 2 to 3 kg (4.4 to 6.6 lb) per year.

Height: School-age children will grow about 5 cm (2 inches) per year.

Prepubescence
- Preadolescence is typically when prepubescence occurs.
- Onset of physiologic changes begins around the age of 9 years, particularly in girls.
- Rapid growth in height and weight occurs.
- Differences in the rate of growth and maturation between boys and girls becomes apparent.
- Visible sexual maturation is minimal in boys during preadolescence.
- Permanent teeth erupt.
- Bladder capacity differs but remains greater in girls than boys.
- Immune system improves.
- Bones continue to ossify.

COGNITIVE DEVELOPMENT

Piaget: concrete operations Ⓠ EBP
- Transitions from perceptual to conceptual thinking
- Masters the concept of conservation:
  - Conservation of mass is understood first, followed by weight, and then volume
- Learns to tell time
- Classifies more complex information
- Able to see the perspective of others
- Able to solve problems

PSYCHOSOCIAL DEVELOPMENT

Erikson: industry vs. inferiority
- A sense of industry is achieved through the development of skills and knowledge that allows the child to provide meaningful contributions to society.
- A sense of accomplishment is gained through the ability to cooperate and compete with others.
- Children should be challenged with tasks that need to be accomplished, and be allowed to work through individual differences in order to complete the tasks.
- Creating systems that reward successful mastery of skills and tasks can create a sense of inferiority in children unable to complete the tasks or acquire the skills
- Children should be taught that not everyone will master every skill.

Moral development

EARLY SCHOOL-AGE YEARS
- Do not understand the reasoning behind rules and expectations for behavior.
- Believe what they think is wrong, and what others tell them is right.
- Judgment is guided by rewards and punishment.
- Sometimes interpret accidents as punishment.

LATER SCHOOL-AGE YEARS
- Able to judge the intentions of an act rather than just its consequences.
- Understand different points of view instead of just whether or not an act is right or wrong.
- Conceptualizes treating others as they like to be treated.

Self-concept development

- School-age children develop an awareness of themselves in relation to others, as well as an understanding of personal values, abilities, and physical characteristics.
- Confidence is gained through establishing a positive self-concept, which leads to feelings of worthiness and the ability to provide significant contributions.
- Parents continue to influence the school-age child's self-ideals, but by middle childhood the opinions of peers and teachers become more valuable.

Body-image changes

- Solidification of body image occurs.
- Curiosity about sexuality should be addressed with education regarding sexual development and the reproductive process.
- School-age children are more modest than preschoolers and place more emphasis on privacy issues.

Social development

- Peer groups play an important part in social development. Peer pressure begins to take effect.
- Clubs and best friends are popular.
- Bullying actions are intended to cause harm or to control someone, and are sometimes attributed to poor relationships with peers and difficulty identifying with a group.
- During early school-age years, children often prefer the company of same-sex companions, but begin developing an interest in others toward the end of the school-age years.
- Most relationships come from school associations.
- Conformity becomes evident.

AGE-APPROPRIATE ACTIVITIES Ⓠ PCC

Competitive and cooperative play is predominant.

CHILDREN FROM 6 TO 9 YEARS OF AGE
- Play simple board and number games.
- Play hopscotch.
- Jump rope.
- Collect rocks, stamps, cards, coins, or stuffed animals.
- Ride bicycles.
- Build simple models.
- Join organized sports (for skill building).

CHILDREN FROM 9 TO 12 YEARS OF AGE
- Make crafts.
- Build models.
- Collect things/engage in hobbies.
- Solve jigsaw puzzles.
- Play board and card games.
- Join organized competitive sports.

HEALTH PROMOTION

IMMUNIZATIONS

The Centers for Disease Control and Prevention (CDC) immunization recommendations for healthy school-age children 6 to 12 years of age include: Q EBP
- If not given between 4 and 5 years of age, children should receive the following vaccines by 6 years of age: diphtheria and tetanus toxoids and pertussis (DTaP); inactivated poliovirus; measles, mumps, and rubella (MMR); and varicella.
- Yearly seasonal influenza vaccine: inactivated influenza vaccine (IIV) or live, attenuated influenza vaccine (LAIV) by nasal spray.
- 11 to 12 years: tetanus and diphtheria toxoids and pertussis vaccine (Tdap); human papillomavirus (HPV) vaccine, and meningococcal vaccine.
- Follow the current CDC guidelines for administration of the COVID-19 vaccine to children 6 to 12 years of age.

HEALTH SCREENINGS

Scoliosis: School-age children should be screened for scoliosis by examining for a lateral curvature of the spine before and during growth spurts. Screening can take place at schools or at health care facilities.

NUTRITION

- By the end of the school-age years, children should eat adult portions of food. They need quality nutritious snacks.
- Obesity is an increasing concern of this age group that predisposes children to low self-esteem, diabetes, heart disease, and high blood pressure. Advise parents to: Q EBP
  - Avoid using food as a reward.
  - Emphasize physical activity.
  - Ensure that child consumes a balanced diet. (The U.S. Department of Agriculture has healthy dietary recommendations.)
  - Reinforce to children to make healthy food selections for meals and snacks.
  - Limit eating fast-food.
  - Avoid skipping meals.
  - Model healthy behaviors.

SLEEP AND REST

- Required sleep is highly variable in the school-age years, and is dependent on the following:
  - Age
  - Level of activity
  - Health status
- Approximately 9 hr of sleep is needed each night at the age of 11 years.
- Resistance to bedtime is sometimes experienced around the age of 8 and 9 years, and again around the age of 11 years, but is typically resolved by the age of 12 years.

DENTAL HEALTH

- The first permanent teeth erupt around 6 years of age.
- Children should brush after meals and snacks, and at bedtime.
- Children should floss daily.
- Children should have regular checkups.
- If necessary, children should have regular fluoride treatments.

INJURY PREVENTION Qs

Bodily harm
- Keep firearms in locked cabinets or boxes.
- Identify safe play areas. Q SDoH
- Teach stranger safety to children.
- Teach children to wear helmets and/or pads when roller skating, skateboarding, bicycling, riding scooters, skiing, and snowboarding.

Burns
- Teach fire safety and potential burn hazards.
- Keep working smoke detectors in the home.
- Children should use sunscreen when outside.
- Teach safety precautions for children to take while cooking.

Drowning
- Children should be supervised when swimming or when near a body of water.
- Children should be taught to swim.
- Check depth of water before allowing children to dive.
- Encourage breaks to prevent children from becoming over-tired.
- Children should wear proper flotation devices when swimming or boating.

Motor-vehicle injuries
- Children should use an approved car restraint system until they achieve a height of 145 cm (4 feet, 9 inches). Qs
- Teach children appropriate seat belt use when no longer using a car restraint system or booster seat.
- Safest area for children is the backseat of the car.
- Never let children ride in the bed of a pickup truck.
- Reinforce safe pedestrian behaviors.

Poisoning/substance misuse Qs
- Cleaners and chemicals should be kept in locked cabinets or out of reach of younger children.
- Children should be taught to say "no" to substance misuse.

Application Exercises

1. A nurse is discussing prepubescence and preadolescence with a group of guardians of school-age children. Which of the following information should the nurse include in the discussion?

   A. Initial physiologic changes appear during early childhood.

   B. Changes in height and weight occur slowly during this period.

   C. Growth differences between boys and girls become evident.

   D. Sexual maturation becomes highly visible in boys.

2. A nurse is assessing the psychosocial development of a group of children who are school-aged. Sort the statements made by the children into the correct developmental category: Moral, Self-Concept, or Social.

   A. "Cross the street without looking is wrong because my mom said so."

   B. "I had to start wearing make-up to hang out with the popular kids."

   C. "It is very important to me what my friends think about me."

   D. "I joined the chess club because my best friend did."

   E. "Others will be nice to you if you are nice to them."

   F. "I feel good about myself when I make a good grade on a test."

3. A nurse is providing education about age-appropriate activities for the caregivers of a 6-year-old child. Which of the following activities should the nurse include in teaching?

   A. Jumping rope

   B. Playing card games

   C. Solving jigsaw puzzles

   D. Joining competitive sports

4. A nurse is conducting a well-child visit with a child who is scheduled to receive the recommended immunizations for 11- to 12-year-olds. Which of the following immunizations should the nurse administer? (Select all that apply.)

   A. Inactivated influenza (IIV)

   B. Pneumococcal (PCV)

   C. Meningococcal (MCV4)

   D. Tetanus and diphtheria toxoids and pertussis (Tdap)

   E. Rotavirus (RV)

5. A nurse is teaching a course about safety during the school-age. Which of the following information should the nurse include in the course? (Select all that apply.)

   A. Gating stairs at the top and bottom

   B. Wearing helmets when riding bicycles or skateboarding

   C. Riding safely in bed of pickup trucks

   D. Implementing firearm safety

   E. Wearing seat belts

Active Learning Scenario

A nurse is providing anticipatory guidance to the guardians of a school-age child. Use the ATI Active Learning Template: Growth and Development to complete this item.

DEVELOPMENTAL STAGE: Identify the child's developmental stage according to Piaget and Erikson.

PHYSICAL DEVELOPMENT: Identify three facts relevant to the child's physical development.

NUTRITION: List three strategies the family can implement to reduce the risk of obesity.

Active Learning Scenario Key

Using the ATI Active Learning Template:
Growth and Development

DEVELOPMENTAL STAGE
- Piaget: concrete operations
- Erikson: industry vs. inferiority

PHYSICAL DEVELOPMENT
- Will gain about 2 to 3 kg (4.4 to 6.6 lb) per year.
- Will grow about 5 cm (2 in) per year.
- Bladder capacity is variable with each child.
- Immune system improves.
- Bones continue to ossify.

NUTRITION
- Avoid using food as a reward.
- Emphasize physical activity.
- Ensure a balanced diet is consumed.
- Teach children to select healthy foods and snacks.
- Avoid eating fast foods frequently.
- Avoid skipping meals.
- Model healthy behaviors.

Ⓝ *NCLEX® Connection: Health Promotion and Maintenance, Developmental Stages and Transitions*

1. A. Initial physiologic changes appear toward the end of middle childhood, around the age of 9 years.
   B. Changes in height and weight occur rapidly during this time period.
   C. **CORRECT:** When taking action and discussing prepubescence and preadolescent with caregivers of school-aged children, the nurse should include that growth differences between male and female children become evident during prepubescence and preadolescence.
   D. Visible sexual maturation is minimal in boys.

   Ⓝ *NCLEX® Connection: Health Promotion and Maintenance, Developmental Stages and Transitions*

2. **MORAL:** A,E; **SELF-CONCEPT:** C,F; **SOCIAL:** B,D

   During the school-aged years, children understand the way that they are supposed to behave and act, but they may not understand the reasons behind expected behaviors. If an adult tells them to do something or if there is a disagreement with an adult, in the school-aged child's mind, the adult is right, and they are wrong. School-aged children also begin to understand that how they treat others impacts the way others treat them in return; therefore, the nurse should sort the following statements by the children into the "Moral" category: "Crossing the street without looking is wrong because my mom said so" and "Others will be nice to you if you are nice to them."

   During the school-aged years, children begin to place a greater focus on what peers, rather than parents and caregivers think about them. Children also begin to gain confidence through the establishment of a positive self-concept. A positive self-concept is fostered through making good grades, positive comments made by teachers and peers, and feeling as though they have made positive contributions to their environment; therefore, the nurse should sort the following statements by the children into the "Self-concept" category: "It is very important to me what my friends think about me" and "I feel good about myself when I make a good grade on a test."

   During the school-aged years, children have a great need to gain social status and feel a sense of belonging. Because of this, school-aged children begin to conform to the influences the children around them to gain acceptance. School-aged children also begin to have a greater interest in organized clubs and having one "best friend" that they consider their go to person; therefore, the nurse should sort the following statements by the children into the "Social" category: "I had to start wearing make-up to hang out with the popular kids" and "I joined the chess club because my best friend did."

   Ⓝ *NCLEX® Connection: Health Promotion and Maintenance, Health Promotion/Disease Prevention*

3. A. **CORRECT:** Jumping rope is a recommend activity for a 6-year-old, along with playing hopscotch, riding bicycles, and joining organized sports.
   B. Playing card games is not an appropriate activity for a 6-year-old child.
   C. Solving jigsaw puzzles is not an appropriate activity for a 6-year-old child.
   D. Joining an organized competitive sport is an appropriate activity for a child who is 9 to 12 years old.

   Ⓝ *NCLEX® Connection: Basic Care and Comfort, Developmental Stages and Transitions*

4. A. **CORRECT:** The nurse should administer the IIV, MCV4, and Tdap to a child who is scheduled to receive recommended immunizations for 11- to 12-year old's.
   B. PCV is recommended as a series of immunizations in the first 15 months of life.
   C. **CORRECT:** The nurse should administer the IIV, MCV4, and Tdap to a child who is scheduled to receive recommended immunizations for 11- to 12-year old's.
   D. **CORRECT:** The nurse should administer the IIV, MCV4, and Tdap to a child who is scheduled to receive recommended immunizations for 11- to 12-year old's.
   E. RV is recommended as a series of immunizations in the first 6 months of life.

   Ⓝ *NCLEX® Connection: Safety and Infection Control, Accident/Error/Injury Prevention*

5. A. Gating stairs at the top and bottom should not be included in the teaching. This is appropriate information to include when teaching about safety during infant and toddler years.
   B. **CORRECT:** When teaching about safety in the school-age years, include information about wearing helmets when riding bicycles or skateboarding.
   C. The nurse should teach that it is never safe to ride in the bed of a pickup truck.
   D. **CORRECT:** The nurse should include information about implementing firearm safety when teaching about safety in the school-age years.
   E. **CORRECT:** The nurse should include information about wearing seat belts when teaching about safety in the school-age years.

   Ⓝ *NCLEX® Connection: Safety and Infection Control, Accident/Error/Injury Prevention*

CHAPTER 7

Health Promotion of Adolescents (12 to 20 Years)

EXPECTED GROWTH AND DEVELOPMENT

PHYSICAL DEVELOPMENT

- The final 20% to 25% of height is achieved during puberty.
- Acne can appear during adolescence.
- Females stop growing at about 2 to 2.5 years after the onset of menarche. They grow 5 to 20 cm (2 to 8 in) and gain 7 to 25 kg (15.5 to 55 lb).
- Males stop growing at around 18 to 20 years of age. They grow 10 to 30 cm (4 to 12 in) and gain 7 to 30 kg (15.5 to 66 lb).
- In females, sexual maturation occurs in the following order.
  - Breast development
  - Pubic hair growth (some females experience hair growth before breast development)
  - Axillary hair growth
  - Menstruation
- In males, sexual maturation occurs in the following order.
  - Testicular enlargement
  - Pubic hair growth
  - Penile enlargement
  - Axillary hair growth
  - Facial hair growth
  - Vocal changes

COGNITIVE DEVELOPMENT

Piaget: formal operations
- Able to think through more than two categories of variables concurrently
- Capable of evaluating the quality of their own thinking
- Able to maintain attention for longer periods of time
- Highly imaginative and idealistic
- Increasingly capable of using formal logic to make decisions
- Think beyond current circumstances
- Able to understand how the actions of an individual influence others
- Able to think in terms of abstract possibilities and hypothetical situations

PSYCHOSOCIAL DEVELOPMENT

Erikson: identity vs. role confusion
- Adolescents often try different roles and experiences to develop a sense of personal identity and come to view themselves as unique individuals.
- Group identity: Adolescents become part of a peer group that greatly influences behavior.

Psychological health

- Swings or variations in emotions are common during early adolescence, with outward expressions of emotions.
- During middle adolescence, introspection is increased.
- Stability of emotions and anger management are usually developed by the later adolescent years.

Sexual identity

- Begins with close, same-sex friendships during early adolescence, which sometimes involve sexual experimentation driven by curiosity.
- Self-exploration occurs through masturbation.
- Transition from friendships to intimate relationships during adolescence.
- In late adolescence, sexual identity typically is formed through the integration of sexual experiences, feelings, and knowledge.

Autonomy

- Emotional autonomy: independent decision-making regarding relationships
- Behavioral autonomy: ability to make independent decisions
- Suggest parental guidance and input

Health perceptions

Adolescents can view themselves as invincible to bad outcomes of risky behaviors.

Moral development

- Solve moral dilemma using internalized moral principles.
- Question relevance of existing moral values to society and individuals.

Religion and spirituality

- Adolescents' views regarding religion and spirituality become more personalized, with decreased focus on religious tradition.
- As self-identity develops, adolescents either reject or accept traditional beliefs of their families.

Self-concept development

- View themselves in relation to similarities with peers during early adolescence.
- View themselves according to their unique characteristics as the adolescent years progress.

Body-image changes

- Base their own normality on comparisons with peers.
- The image established during adolescence is retained throughout life.

Social development

- Peer relationships develop. These relationships act as a support system for adolescents.
- Best-friend relationships are more stable and longer-lasting than they were in previous years.
- Parent-child relationships change to allow a greater sense of independence.

AGE-APPROPRIATE ACTIVITIES Qᴘᴄᴄ

- Nonviolent video games
- Nonviolent music
- Sports
- Caring for a pet
- Career-training programs
- Reading
- Social interaction (going to movies, school dances, electronic messaging, and social media)

HEALTH PROMOTION

IMMUNIZATIONS

Centers for Disease Control and Prevention (CDC) recommendations for healthy adolescents 13 to 18 years old include catch-up doses of any recommended immunizations not received at 11 to 12 years old. Qᴇʙᴘ

- Yearly seasonal influenza vaccine: Inactivated influenza vaccine or live, attenuated influenza vaccine by nasal spray. Recommendation can be season-specific.
- Meningococcal vaccine: Receive 2nd dose at 16 years of age if received 1st dose received at 11-12 years of age.
- Follow the current CDC recommendations for administration of the COVID-19 vaccine to adolescents 12 to 20 years of age.

HEALTH SCREENINGS

- Scoliosis: annual screenings for adolescents (risk for idiopathic scoliosis). These screenings should include an examination for a lateral curvature of the spine before and during growth spurts. Screenings can take place at school or at a health care facility.
- Annual height and weight for BMI calculations, BP checks for hypertension screening
- Hemoglobin and hematocrit.
- Universal lipid screenings.
- Screenings for STIs if sexually active.

NUTRITION

- Rapid growth and high metabolism require increases in quality nutrients, and make adolescents unable to tolerate caloric restrictions.
  - During times of rapid growth, additional calcium, iron, protein, and zinc are needed.
  - Inadequate intake of folic acid, vitamin B_6, vitamin A, iron, calcium, and zinc is common.
- Overeating and undereating present challenges during the adolescent years.
  - Yearly assessments of height, weight, and BMI for age are needed in order to identify nutritional issues and intervene early.
- Overweight and obesity rates are of particular concern; anorexia and bulimia are common in this age group as well.
- Advise parents to:
  - Avoid using food as a reward.
  - Emphasize physical activity.
  - Ensure that a balanced diet is consumed by following the U.S. Department of Agriculture's healthy diet recommendations.
  - Encourage adolescents to make healthy food selections for meals and snacks.

SLEEP AND REST

- Adolescents should get about 9 hours of sleep each night.
- Sleep habits change with puberty due to increased metabolism and rapid growth.
- Adolescents tend to stay up late, sleep in later in the morning, and can sleep more than during the school-age years.
- During periods of active growth, the need for sleep increases. Sleep habits can change with puberty due to increased metabolism and rapid growth during the adolescent years.
- Sleep deprivation is a concern with many adolescents; discuss the importance of sleep and encourage adequate rest.

DENTAL HEALTH

- Corrective appliances are most common with this age group.
- Adolescents should brush after meals and snacks, and at bedtime.
- Adolescents should floss daily.
- Adolescents should have regular checkups.
- If necessary, adolescents should have regular fluoride treatments.

SEXUALITY

- Provide adolescents with accurate information and discuss what is heard from peers.
- Discuss abstinence and safe sexual behaviors (oral, vaginal, or anal).
- Provide information about preventing sexually transmitted infections and pregnancy. Perform STI screenings for at-risk adolescents.

- Promote an atmosphere where adolescents are comfortable asking questions.
- Assist adolescents with problem-solving and decision-making skills.
- Ask adolescents about risky sexual behaviors and discuss the need for mutual consent prior to sexual contact.
- LGBTQIA Qpcc
  - Increase incidence of high-school students identifying as LGBTQIA
  - Ask adolescent their gender pronouns
  - Risk of bullying, physical/sexual violence, substance use, suicidal behaviors, STIs
  - Refer to LGBTQIA support groups
  - Provide sensitive and non-judgmental care

INJURY PREVENTION Qs

Bodily harm
- Adolescents should have annual psychologic screenings to identify depression, anxiety, suicidal ideations, and substance use.
- Keep firearms unloaded and in a locked cabinet or box.
- Teach proper use of sporting equipment prior to use.
- Insist on helmet use and/or pads when roller skating, skateboarding, bicycling, riding scooters, skiing, and snowboarding.
- Be aware of changes in mood. Monitor for self-harm in adolescents who are at risk. Watch for the following.
  - Poor school performance
  - Lack of interest in things that were of interest to the adolescent in the past
  - Social isolation
  - Disturbances in sleep or appetite
  - Expression of suicidal thoughts
- Discuss non-violent conflict resolution strategies.
- Discuss bullying, including cyberbullying.
- Warn about the risk of sexual predators, who often communicate through electronic interactions.

Burns
- Teach fire safety.
- Adolescents should apply sunscreen when outside.
- Adolescents should avoid tanning beds.

Drowning
- Teach adolescents to swim.
- Teach adolescents not to swim alone.

Motor-vehicle injuries
- Encourage attendance at drivers' education courses. Emphasize the need for adherence to seat belt use.
- Insist on helmet use with bicycles, motorcycles, skateboards, roller skates, and snowboards.
- Discourage use of cell phones while driving and enforce laws regarding use.
- Teach the dangers of combining substance use with driving.
- Role model desired behavior.

Substance use disorder
- Monitor for indications of substance use disorder in adolescents who are at risk. Ask adolescents during health screening about alcohol, tobacco, and marijuana use, including the frequency of use.
- Discuss the risks of smoking and using smokeless tobacco or nicotine-containing products, including electronic cigarettes.
- Emphasize the short-term effects of substance use on school or work performance.

Active Learning Scenario

A nurse is preparing an educational program for a group of caregivers of adolescents. Use the ATI Active Learning Template: Growth and Development to complete this item.

DEVELOPMENTAL STAGE: Identify adolescent developmental stages according to Piaget and Erikson.

COGNITIVE DEVELOPMENT: List five cognitive developmental tasks the adolescent should accomplish.

INJURY PREVENTION: Identify three injury prevention methods in each of the following categories.

- Bodily harm
- Motor vehicle injuries

Active Learning Scenario Key

Using the ATI Active Learning Template: Growth and Development

DEVELOPMENTAL STAGE
- Piaget: formal operations
- Erikson: identity vs. role confusion

COGNITIVE DEVELOPMENT
- Able to think through more than two categories of variables concurrently
- Capable of evaluating the quality of own thinking
- Able to maintain attention for longer periods of time
- Highly imaginative and idealistic
- Increasingly capable of using formal logic to make decisions
- Think beyond current circumstances
- Understand how the actions of an individual influence others

INJURY PREVENTION
- Bodily injury
  - Keep firearms unloaded and in a locked cabinet or box.
  - Teach proper use of sporting equipment prior to use.
  - Insist on helmet use and/or pads when roller skating, skateboarding, bicycling, riding scooters, skiing, and snowboarding.
  - Be aware of changes in mood. Continuously monitor adolescents at risk for self-harm.
- Motor vehicle injuries
  - Encourage attendance at drivers' education courses.
  - Emphasize the need for adherence to seat belt use.
  - Discourage use of cell phones while driving and enforce laws regarding use.
  - Teach the dangers of combining substance use with driving.
- Role model desired behavior.

Ⓝ *NCLEX® Connection: Health Promotion and Maintenance, Developmental Stages and Transitions*

1. A nurse is providing education about the order of sexual maturation to a group of caregivers who have adolescent children. When teaching the caregivers, in which order should the nurse place sexual maturation of the male adolescent?

   A. Testicular enlargment

   B. Vocal changes

   C. Pubic hair growth

   D. Penile enlargement

   E. Growth of axillary hair

2. A nurse is providing teaching about expected changes during puberty to a group of guardians of early adolescent females. Which of the following statements by one of the guardians should the nurse identify as indicating an understanding of the teaching?

   A. "Females usually stop growing about 2 years after they have had their first menstrual period."

   B. "Females are expected to gain about 65 pounds during puberty."

   C. "Females experience menstruation prior to breast development."

   D. "Females typically grow more than 10 inches during puberty."

3. A nurse is assisting with providing anticipatory guidance to the parents of an adolescent. Which of the following screenings should the nurse recommend to the parents that the adolescent ? (Select all that apply.)

   A. Body mass index

   B. Blood lead level

   C. 24-hr dietary recall

   D. Weight

   E. Scoliosis

4. A nurse is caring for an adolescent whose guardian expresses concerns about the child sleeping such long hours. Which of the following conditions should the nurse inform the guardian as requiring additional sleep during adolescence?

   A. Sleep terrors

   B. Rapid growth

   C. Elevated zinc levels

   D. Slowed metabolism

1. A, C, D, E, B

   When providing education to the caregivers regarding sexual maturation of the adolescent male, the nurse should inform the caregivers that testicular enlargement occurs first, followed by pubic hair growth, penile enlargement, growth of axillary hair, and vocal changes.

   Ⓝ *NCLEX® Connection: Health Promotion and Maintenance, Developmental Stages and Transitions*

2. A. **CORRECT:** The nurse should identify that the statement, "Females usually stop growing about 2 years after they have had their first menstrual period" indicates understanding of the teaching. Females usually stop growing about 2 years after menarche, or having their first period.

   B. The nurse should identify that the statement, "Females are expected to gain about 65 pounds during puberty" does not indicate understanding of the teaching. Females are expected to gain 7 to 25 kg (15.5 to 55 lb) during puberty.

   C. The nurse should identify that the statement, "Girl's experience menstruation prior to breast development" does not indicate understanding of the teaching. Breast development is usually the first manifestation of sexual maturity in females, and appears before menstruation.

   D. The nurse should identify that the statement, "Females typically grow more than 10 inches during puberty "does not indicate understanding of the teaching. Females typically grow 5 to 20 cm (2 to 8 in) during puberty.

   Ⓝ *NCLEX® Connection: Health Promotion and Maintenance, Health Screening*

3. A, D, E. **CORRECT:** Annual screenings for an adolescent client include body mass index, weight, and scoliosis. The body mass index, and weights are useful to detect unexpected findings and provide the opportunity to educate about heart health. Annual scoliosis screening is recommended to detect idiopathic scoliosis and allows for prompt management of the condition.

   B. Blood lead level screenings are recommended for younger children.

   C. A 24-hr dietary recall is not an annual recommended screening for an adolescent, it is used to unexpected findings with conditions related to nutrition.

   Ⓝ *NCLEX® Connection: Basic Care and Comfort, Rest and Sleep*

4. A. Sleep terrors occur most often in preschool-age children, and do not contribute to the adolescent's need for additional sleep; therefore, the nurse should not include this as a condition that increases sleep requirements for the adolescent.

   B. **CORRECT:** The nurse should inform the caregivers that rapid growth and an increased metabolism during the adolescent years results in the need for additional sleep.

   C. Zinc levels do not typically elevate during the adolescent years, and do not contribute to the adolescent's need for additional sleep. Zinc is often identified as deficient due to inadequate dietary intake during adolescence; therefore, the nurse should not include this as a condition that increases sleep requirements for the adolescent.

   D. An increased metabolism contributes to the adolescent's need for additional sleep.

   Ⓝ *NCLEX® Connection: Health Promotion and Maintenance, Developmental Stages and Transitions*

When reviewing the following chapters, keep in mind the relevant topics and tasks of the NCLEX outline, in particular:

Psychosocial Integrity

END OF LIFE CARE: Recognize the need for and provide psychosocial support to family/caregiver.

GRIEF AND LOSS: Inform the client of expected reactions to grief and loss.

STRESS MANAGEMENT: Recognize nonverbal cues to physical and/or psychological stressors.

Basic Care and Comfort

NONPHARMACOLOGICAL COMFORT INTERVENTIONS
Recognize differences in client perception and response to pain.

Plan measures to provide comfort interventions to clients with anticipated or actual impaired comfort.

Pharmacological and Parenteral Therapies

MEDICATION ADMINISTRATION
Educate the client about medications.

Prepare and administer medications, using rights of medication administration.

PARENTERAL/INTRAVENOUS THERAPIES: Prepare the client for intravenous catheter insertion.

PHARMACOLOGICAL PAIN MANAGEMENT
Administer and document pharmacological pain management appropriate for client age and diagnoses.

Assess client need for administration of a PRN pain medication.

CHAPTER 8 # Safe Administration of Medication

Growth and organ system maturity affect the metabolism and excretion of medications in infants and children.

Administration of medications to the pediatric population can be challenging, and requires nursing patience and creativity.

Pediatric dosages are based on age, body weight, and body surface area

ASSESSMENT

- Medication and food allergies
- Appropriateness of medication dose for the child's age and weight
- Child's developmental age
- Child's physiological and psychological condition
- Tissue and skin integrity when administering intramuscular (IM), subcutaneous, and topical medications
- IV patency when administering intravenous (IV) medications

NURSING INTERVENTIONS

MEDICATION ADMINISTRATION

- Calculate the safe dosage for medication. Qs
- Notify the provider if medication dosage is determined to be outside the safe dosage range, and for any questions about medication preparation or route.
- Double-check high-risk and facility-regulated medications with another nurse.
- Use two client identifiers prior to administration: client name and date of birth. Use guardian(s) for verification of infants or nonverbal children. Two identifiers from the ID band must be confirmed: client name, date of birth, or hospital identification number. Computers may also be used to scan the child's ID band for electronic record updating.
- Determine parental involvement with administration.
- Allow the child to make appropriate choices regarding administration (choosing the left or right leg, whether the guardian or nurse will administer the medication).
- Prepare the child according to age and developmental stage.

Oral

This route of medication administration is preferred for children. Available in preparations (liquids, chewables, and meltaways).

- Determine the child's ability to swallow pills.
- Use the smallest measuring device for doses of liquid medication. Use an oral medication syringe for smaller amounts, and a medication cup for larger amounts.
- Avoid measuring liquid medication in a teaspoon or tablespoon.
- Use rigid plastic cups instead of paper cups for liquid medications.
- Avoid mixing medication with formula or putting it in a bottle of formula because the infant might not take the entire feeding, and the medication can alter the taste of the formula.
- Hold the infant in a semi-reclining position similar to a feeding position.
- Hold the small child in an upright position to prevent aspiration.
- Administer the medication in the side of the mouth in small amounts. This allows the infant or child to swallow.
- Only use the droppers that come with the medication for measurement.
- Stroke the infant under the chin to promote swallowing while holding cheeks together.
- Teach the child to swallow tablets that aren't available in liquid form and can't be crushed. Teach in short sessions using verbal instruction, demonstration, and positive reinforcement.
- Provide atraumatic care.
  - Mix the medication in a small amount of sweet nonessential food (applesauce or sherbet).
  - Offer juice, a soft drink, or snack after administration.
  - Add flavoring to medications as available.
  - Use a nipple to allow the infant to suck the medication.
  - Reward small child with a prize or sticker afterwards.
- Administer medications via a feeding tube.
  - Confirm placement.
  - Use liquid formulation.
  - Do not add medication to the formula bag.
  - If administering several medications, flush tubing with water after the administration of each medication.

Optic

- Place the child in a supine or sitting position.
- Extend the child's head and ask the child to look up.
- Pull the lower eye lid downward and apply medication in the conjunctiva pocket.
- Administer ointments from the inner to outer canthus of the eye preferably before nap or bedtime.
- Provide atraumatic care.
  - If infants clench their eyes closed, place the drops in the nasal corner. When the infant opens his eyes, the medication will enter the eye.
  - Apply light pressure to the lacrimal conjunctiva of the eye for 1 min to prevent unpleasant taste.
  - Play games with younger children.

Otic

- Place the child in a prone or supine position with the affected ear upward.
- Children younger than 3 years: pull the pinna downward and straight back.
- Children older than 3 years: pull the pinna upward and back.
- Provide atraumatic care.
  - Allow refrigerated medications to warm to room temperature prior to administration.
  - Massage the outer area for a few minutes following administration.
  - Play games with younger children.
  - Praise child after procedure.

Nasal

- Remove mucus prior to administration.
- Position the child with the head hyperextended.
- Use a football hold for infants.
- Provide atraumatic care.
  - Insert the tip into the naris vertically, then angle it prior to administration.
  - Play games with younger children.

Aerosol

- Use a mask for younger children.
- Provide atraumatic care.
  - Allow guardians to hold the child during treatment.
  - Use distraction.

Rectal

- Provide lubrication to the medication by using warm water or other lubricant, if the medication is not pre-lubricated.
- Insert beyond both rectal sphincters (small child less than 0.5 inches, older child 1 inch).
- Hold the buttocks gently together for 5 to 10 min.
- If necessary to half the dose, cut the medication lengthwise.
- Provide atraumatic care.
  - Perform the procedure quickly.
  - Use distraction.

Transdermal/topical

- Ensure the skin is dry and intact.
- Apply to the body or major muscle (try to hide from smaller children).
- Assess skin site of administration regularly.
- Rotate sites frequently.

Injection

- Change needle if it pierced a rubber stopper on a vial.
- Secure the infant or child prior to injections.
- Assess the need for assistance.
- Avoid tracking of medication.
- When selecting sites, consider the following.
  - Medication amount, viscosity, and type
  - Muscle mass, condition, access of site, and potential for contamination
  - Treatment course and number of injections
  - Age and size of child

Intradermal

- Administer on the inside surface of the forearm.
- Use a TB syringe with 26- to 30-gauge needle with an intradermal bevel.
- Insert needle at 15° angle.
- Do not aspirate.

Subcutaneous

Give anywhere there is adequate subcutaneous tissue. Common sites are the lateral aspect of the upper arm, abdomen, and anterior thigh.

- Inject volumes of less than 0.5 mL.
- Use a 1 mL syringe with a 26- to 30-gauge needle.
- Insert at a 90° angle. Use a 45° angle for children who are thin.
- Check policy for aspiration practices.

Intramuscular

Use a 22- to 25-gauge, 5/8 to 1.5-inch needle.

Vastus lateralis
- This is the recommended site in infants and small children who have minimal muscle mass.
- Position the child supine, side-lying, or sitting.
- Inject up to 0.5 mL for infants.
- Inject up to 2 mL for children.

Ventrogluteal
- Position the child supine, side-lying, or prone.
- Inject 0.5 to 1 mL, depending on muscle size of infant.
- Inject up to 2 mL in children.

Deltoid
- Explain the procedure to the child and guardians.
- Position the child sitting or standing.
- Inject up to 1 mL.
- Provide atraumatic care
  - Apply lidocaine and prilocaine topical ointment to the site for 60 min prior to injection.
  - Change needle after puncturing a rubber stopper.
  - Use the smallest gauge of needle possible. Ⓠpcc
  - Use therapeutic hugging
  - Secure the child firmly to decrease movement of the needle while injecting.
  - Use distraction.
  - Encourage guardians to hold the child after.
  - Offer praise
  - Use play therapy.
  - Offer sucrose pacifiers to infants.

Intravenous

Assess venipuncture site per facility protocol and prior to administration of medications

Peripheral venous access devices (also called intermittent infusion devices, peripheral/saline/heparin locks)
- Use a 24- to 22-gauge catheter.
- Use for continuous and intermittent IV medication administration.
- Short-term IV therapy can be completed at home with the assistance of a home health nurse.

Central venous access devices (CVADs)

- Short term: non-tunneled catheter or peripherally inserted central catheters (PICC) require an x-ray to verify placement prior to use
- Long term: tunneled catheter or implanted infusion ports
- Provide atraumatic care
  - Insert a PICC before multiple peripheral attempts.
  - Use a transilluminator to assist in vein location.
  - Avoid terminology (a "bee sting" or "stick").
  - Attach an extension tubing to decrease movement of the catheter.
  - Use play therapy.
  - Apply lidocaine and prilocaine topical ointment to the site for 60 min prior to attempt.
  - Keep equipment out of site until procedure begins.
  - Perform procedure in a treatment room. Qᴘᴄᴄ
  - Use nonpharmacologic therapies.
  - Allow guardians to stay if they prefer.
  - Use therapeutic holding.
  - Avoid using the dominant or sucking hand.
  - Cover site with a protective cover that allows visibility of the IV site.
  - Swaddle infants.
  - Offer nonnutritive sucking to infants before, during, and after the procedure.
  - Teach guardians how to properly care for device.

Active Learning Scenario

A nurse is planning to initiate IV access for a toddler. What actions should the nurse plan to take? Use the ATI Active Learning Template: Basic Concept to complete this item.

NURSING INTERVENTIONS: Describe 10 atraumatic care interventions.

Active Learning Scenario Key

Using the ATI Active Learning Template: Basic Concept

NURSING INTERVENTIONS

- Decide to insert a peripherally inserted catheter before multiple peripheral attempts.
- Use a transilluminator to assist in vein location.
- Avoid terminology such as a "bee sting" or "stick."
- Attach extension tubing to decrease movement of the catheter.
- Use play therapy.
- Apply lidocaine and prilocaine topical ointment to the site for 60 min prior to attempts.
- Keep equipment out of sight until procedure begins.
- Perform the procedure in a treatment room.
- Use nonpharmacologic therapies.
- Allow caregivers to stay if they prefer.
- Use therapeutic holding.
- Avoid using the dominant or sucking hand.
- Cover site with a colorful wrap.
- Swaddle infants.
- Offer nonnutritive sucking to infants before, during, and after the procedure.

Ⓝ *NCLEX® Connection: Pharmacological and Parenteral Therapies, Parenteral/Intravenous Therapies*

Intraosseous

- A temporary route of administration for use in an emergent situation in which venous access cannot be obtained.
- Use an intraosseous or large bore needle that is inserted into the tibia.
- Monitor site for infection, leakage of fluid.
- Monitor distal pulses, temperature of leg, and color frequently.
- Risk for compartment syndrome

Application Exercises

1. A nurse is teaching a guardian of an infant about administration of oral medications. Which of the following should the nurse include in the teaching? (Select all that apply.)

   A. Use a universal dropper for medication administration.

   B. Ask the pharmacy to add flavoring to the medication.

   C. Add the medication to a formula bottle before feeding.

   D. Use the nipple of a bottle to administer the medication.

   E. Hold the infant in an semi-reclining position.

2. A nurse is preparing to administer medication to a preschool-aged child. Which of the following actions should the nurse plan to take? (Select all that apply.)

   A. Ask the caregiver to state the child's name.

   B. Allow the caregiver to administer the medication.

   C. Calculate the safe dosage of the medication.

   D. Let the child pick a toy to hold during administration of the medication.

   E. Offer juice after the medication is administered.

3. A nurse is caring for an infant who needs otic medication. Which of the following is an appropriate action for the nurse to take?

   A. Hold the infant in an upright position.

   B. Pull the pinna downward and straight back.

   C. Hyperextend the infant's neck.

   D. Ensure that the medication is cool.

4. A nurse is preparing to administer a hepatitis B immunization to an infant who is 9-months-old. Which site should the nurse use to administer the immunization?

   A. Deltoid

   B. Vastus lateralis

   C. Dorsogluteal

   D. Ventrogluteal

5. A nurse is planning to administer the influenza vaccine to a toddler. Which of the following actions should the nurse take?

   A. Administer subcutaneously in the abdomen.

   B. Use a 20-gauge needle.

   C. Divide the medication into two injections.

   D. Place the child in the supine position.

Application Exercises Key

1. **B, D, E. CORRECT:** When taking action, or implementing interventions, the nurse should provide education to clients and caregivers that will promote positive client care outcomes. In this situation, the nurse should instruct the guardian to ask the pharmacy to add flavoring to the medication, use a nipple of a bottle to administer the medication, and hold the infant in a semi-reclining position when administering the medication. These actions provide atraumatic care to the infant and promote safe, successful medication administration.
   A. The nurse should not include use of a universal dropper for medication administration. Liquid and suspension medications have different viscosities, and droppers do not have a standard opening; therefore, a universal dropper is not an accurate way to measure medications.
   C. The nurse should not include adding medication to a bottle of formula to the teaching. The infant may not finish the entire bottle of formula which will result in administration of incorrect medication doses.

   Ⓝ *NCLEX® Connection: Pharmacological and Parenteral Therapies, Medication Administration*

2. **C, D, E. CORRECT:** When generating solutions for client care, the nurse should identify evidence-based nursing actions that will effectively address the clinical situation. In this situation, the nurse should plan to calculate the safe dosage of the medication prior to administration, allow the child to pick a toy to hold on to during administration of the medication, and offer the child juice to drink after the medication is administered.
   A. The nurse should ask the child, not the caregiver for the child's name.
   B. Before allowing the caregiver to administer the medication, the nurse would need to assess the caregiver's willingness and ability to administer the medication.

   Ⓝ *NCLEX® Connection: Pharmacological and Parenteral Therapies, Expected Actions/Outcomes*

3. A. The nurse should position the infant supine or prone, not upright, when administering otic medications.
   B. CORRECT: When taking action, the nurse should promptly and accurately perform nursing actions that promote positive client care outcomes. In this client care situation, the nurse should pull the pinna of the ear downward and straight back to straighten the ear canal and allow the medication to flow into the ear.
   C. The nurse should not hyperextend the infant's neck. This action could occlude the airway and should not be performed during otic medication administration.
   D. The nurse should allow the otic medication to warm up to room temperature to prevent stimulating vertigo and provide atraumatic care.

   Ⓝ *NCLEX® Connection: Pharmacological and Parenteral Therapies, Medication Administration*

4. A. The deltoid site is not recommended for use in children who are less that 18-months-of age due to the small muscle mass and the potential for damage to the radial and axillary nerve; therefore, the nurse should not select this site.
   B. CORRECT: The CDC, World Health Organization, and the American Academy of Pediatrics recommend that the vastus lateralis muscle be used to administer IM injections to infants. Additionally, the vastus lateralis site is the desired administration site for biological medications such as immunizations.
   C. The dorsogluteal is contraindicated as an IM injection site due to its proximity to the sciatic nerve. Additionally, the dorsogluteal site is unsafe for infants due to the decreased mass of the muscle; therefore, the nurse should not select this site.
   D. The ventrogluteal site may be used in infants; however, this is not the preferred site to use when administering an immunization; therefore, the nurse should not select this site.

   Ⓝ *NCLEX® Connection: Pharmacological and Parenteral Therapies, Medication Administration*

5. A. The influenza vaccination is administered intramuscularly, not subcutaneously, using a 22- to 25-gauge needle. The total volume of the influenza vaccination is 0.5 mL, which can be administered safely in one dose into the vastus lateralis muscle.
   B. The influenza vaccination is administered intramuscularly, not subcutaneously, using a 22- to 25-gauge needle. The total volume of the influenza vaccination is 0.5 mL, which can be administered safely in one dose into the vastus lateralis muscle.
   C. The influenza vaccination is administered intramuscularly, not subcutaneously, using a 22- to 25-gauge needle. The total volume of the influenza vaccination is 0.5 mL, which can be administered safely in one dose into the vastus lateralis muscle.
   D. CORRECT: When generating solutions for client care, the nurse should identify evidence-based nursing actions that will effectively address the clinical situation. In this situation, the nurse should plan to place the child in the supine position to access the injection site and maintain safety for the toddler.

   Ⓝ *NCLEX® Connection: Pharmacological and Parenteral Therapies, Expected Actions/Outcomes*

CHAPTER 9

Pain Management

Assessment of pain depends on the child's cognitive, emotional, and physical development.

Atraumatic care is the use of interventions that minimize or eliminate physical and psychological distress.

Pain is managed by atraumatic, nonpharmacological, and pharmacological interventions.

INFLUENTIAL FACTORS

Influential factors that can have a positive or negative effect on the client's personal pain perception
- Age
- Development stage
- Chronic or acute disease
- Prior experiences with pain
- Personality
- Dynamics (living arrangement and personal stressors)
- Culture
- Socioeconomic status ⓆSDoH

ASSESSMENT

EXPECTED FINDINGS

Developmental characteristics

Young infant
- Loud cry
- Rigid body or thrashing
- Local reflex withdrawal from pain stimulus
- Expressions of pain (eyes tightly closed, mouth open in a squarish shape, eyebrows lowered and drawn together)
- Lack of association between stimulus and pain

Older infant
- Loud cry
- Deliberate withdrawal from pain
- Facial expression of pain

Toddler
- Loud cry or screaming
- Verbal expressions of pain
- Thrashing of extremities
- Attempt to push away or avoid stimulus
- Noncooperation
- Clinging to a significant person
- Behaviors occur in anticipation of painful stimulus
- Requests physical comfort

9.1 Case Study

Scenario Introduction

Tanisha is a registered nurse in a neonatal ICU. Tanisha just received a change of shift report on Makenna Jackson, a 2-week-old newborn who was diagnosed with Hirschsprung disease. Makenna underwent surgery 24 hours ago to remove the part of the bowel affected by Hirschsprung disease.

Scene 1

Tanisha: Good morning, Mr. and Mrs. Jackson. My name is Tanisha, and I will be caring for Makenna today. I need to perform an assessment on her, but first I would like to know if you have any major concerns that we need to discuss?

Mrs. Jackson: Well, I am just scared that Makenna is in pain and that we cannot tell because she is so tiny and can't tell us.

Tanisha: I understand. Let me complete my assessment, and when I finish we can talk about the things that we monitor to help us identify whether or not a baby like Makenna is in pain.

Mrs. Jackson: Ok. That would be great!

Scene 2

Tanisha: I have completed my assessment and everything with Makenna is just as we would expect. Her vital signs are within the expected range and her incision site does not show any manifestations of infection like redness, warmth, swelling, or drainage.

Mr. Jackson: What about the things that you were looking for to help you tell if Makenna is in pain?

Tanisha: When we are looking for manifestations of pain in newborns who have had surgery, we look for 5 things: crying, the need for oxygen, an increase in the heart rate or blood pressure, the expression on the baby's face, and how well the baby has slept over the last hour. Each of those five things get a score of either a 0, 1, or 2 based on what we see. A score of 4 or above indicates treatment for pain is needed.

Mr. Jackson: What was Makenna's score?

Tanisha: Why don't we look at her together and see?

Scene 3

Tanisha: Now that we have looked at Makenna together, let's talk about whether or not she's showing manifestations of pain. We saw that Makenna cries a little but is consoled easily, she does not require oxygen, her vital signs are not elevated, she grimaces every now and then, and she has woken up several times over the last hour.

Scenario Conclusion

Tanisha has completed Makenna's physical assessment and has taught her parents what to look for as indicators that Makenna may be in pain. Tanisha is now getting ready to calculate Makenna's pain score using the CRIES Neonatal Postoperative Pain Measurement Scale. Using the CRIES Neonatal Postoperative Pain Measurement Scale found below, Tanisha calculates that Makenna has a pain level of 3. Makenna's pain level does not indicate treatment for pain is needed at this time.

9.2 CRIES Neonatal Postoperative Pain Measurement Scale

	0	1	2
CRYING	No	High pitched but consolable	Inconsolable
REQUIRES OXYGEN FOR SATURATION > 95%	No	FiO2 < 30%	FiO2 > 20%
INCREASED VITAL SIGNS	No	HR or BP < 20%	HR or BP > 20%
EXPRESSION	No	Grimace	Grimace and grunt
SLEEPLESS	No	Wakes often	Contantly awake

School–age child
- Stalling behavior
- Muscular rigidity
- Any behaviors of the toddler, but less intense in the anticipatory phase and more intense with painful stimulus

Adolescent
- More verbal expressions of pain with less protest
- Muscle tension with body control

Pain intensity

- Assessment includes behavioral measures, multidimensional, and self-report.
- Self-report is used for children 4 years or older. Children under 4 are unable to accurately report their pain.
- Multiple tools have been developed and researched as reliable.

- Choose an appropriate pain tool that will adequately evaluate the infant or child's pain.
- Include the caregiver in rating the child's pain.
- Assess the location, quality, and severity of pain.

PATIENT-CENTERED CARE

NURSING CARE

- Reassess the child's pain level frequently.
- Use nonpharmacological, pharmacological, or both approaches to manage pain.
- Ask parent or caregiver to monitor their child's pain level.
- Ask the parent or caregiver their satisfaction of the pain management.

9.3 Pain assessment tool for evaluation by age

FLACC: 2 months to 7 years
Pain rated on a scale of 0 to 10.
Assess behaviors of the child.

FACE (F)
0: Smile or no expression
1: Occasional frown or grimace, withdrawn
2: Frequent or constant frown, clenched jaw, quivering chin

LEGS (L)
0: Relaxed or normal position
1: Uneasy, restless, tense
2: Kicking or legs drawn up

ACTIVITY (A)
0: Lying quietly, moves easily, normal position
1: Squirming, shifting, tense
2: Arched, ridged, or jerking

CRY (C)
0: No cry
1: Moans or whimpers, occasional complaints
2: Crying, screaming, sobbing, frequent complaints

CONSOLABILITY (C)
0: Content or relaxed
1: Reassured by occasional touching or hugging. Able to distract
2: Difficult to console or comfort

Numeric scale: 5 years and older
Pain rated on a scale of 0 to 10.
Explain to the child that 0 means "no pain" and 10 means "worst pain."
Have the child verbally report a number or point to their level of pain on a visual scale.

FACES: 3 years and older
Pain rated on a scale of 0 to 5 using a diagram of six faces.
Substitute 0, 2, 4, 6, 8, 10 for 0 to 5 to convert to the 0 to 10 scale.
Explain each face to the child; ask the child to choose a face that best describes how they are feeling.

0: No hurt	2: Hurts a little more	4: Hurts a whole lot
1: Hurts a bit	3: Hurts even more	5: Hurts worst

Oucher: 3 to 13 years
Pain rated on a scale of 0 to 5 using six photographs.
Substitute 0, 2, 4, 6, 8, 10 for 0 to 5 to convert to the 0 to 10 scale.
Have the child organize the photographs in order of no pain to the worst pain; ask the child to choose a picture that best describes how they are feeling.

0: No hurt	2: Hurts a little more	4: Hurts a whole lot
1: Hurts a bit	3: Hurts even more	5: Hurts worst

Non-communicating children's pain checklist: 3 years and older
Behaviors are observed for 10 min.
Six subcategories are each scored on a scale 0 to 3.
0: Not at all   1: Just a little   2: Fairly often   3: Very often

SUBCATEGORIES

Vocal	Facial	Body and limbs
Social	Activity	Physiological

CUTOFF SCORES
11 or higher indicates moderate to severe pain.
6 to 10 indicates mild pain.

AGE: 0   3   5   7   10   13   15   18

FLACC
FACES
OUCHER
NUMERIC SCALE
NON-COMMUNICATING CHILDREN'S PAIN CHECKLIST

- Assess the child for adverse reactions to pain medications.
- Review laboratory reports.
- Assess the child's physical functioning following pain management intervention.
- Assess for negative effects or distress the child might experience related to pain (anxiety, withdrawal, sleep disruption, fear, depression, or unhappiness).

ATRAUMATIC MEASURES

- Use a treatment room for painful procedures.
- Avoid procedures in "safe places" (the play room or the child's bed).
- Use developmentally appropriate terminology when explaining procedures.
- Offer choices to the child.
- Allow parents to stay with the child during painful procedures.
- Use play therapy to explain procedures, allowing the child to perform the procedure on a doll or toy.

PHARMACOLOGICAL MEASURES

- The World Health Organization (2012) recommends a two-step approach for pharmacological management of pain in children.
  - For children above 3 months of age with mild pain, the first step is to administer a non-opioid. Nonsteroidal anti-inflammatory drugs (NSAIDs) are frequently used for mild pain.
  - The second step for children who have moderate or severe pain is to administer a strong opioid. Morphine is the drug of choice.
- Optimal dosage of medications control pain without causing severe adverse effects.
- Select the least traumatic route for medication administration.
- Give medications routinely, vs. PRN (as needed), to manage pain that is expected to last for an extended period of time.
- Combine adjuvant medications (steroids, antidepressants, sedatives, antianxiety medications, muscle relaxants, anticonvulsants) with other analgesics.
- Use non-opioid and opioid medications.
  - Acetaminophen and NSAIDs are acceptable for mild to moderate pain.
  - Opioids are acceptable for moderate to severe pain. Medications used include morphine sulfate, hydromorphone, and fentanyl.
  - Combining a non-opioid and an opioid medication treats pain peripherally and centrally. This offers greater analgesia with fewer adverse effects (respiratory depression, constipation, nausea).

APPROPRIATE ROUTES Qs

- IM injections are not recommended for pain control in children.
- Intranasal medications are not recommended for children younger than 18 years.
- Intradermal medications are used for skin anesthesia prior to procedures.

Oral

NURSING ACTIONS
- Route is preferred due to convenience, cost, and ability to maintain steady blood levels.
- Take 1 to 2 hr to reach peak analgesic effects. Oral medications are not suited for children experiencing pain that requires rapid relief or pain that is fluctuating in nature.

Topical/transdermal

NURSING ACTIONS
Lidocaine and prilocaine is available in a cream or gel.
- Used for any procedure in which the skin will be punctured (IV insertion, biopsy) 60 min prior to a superficial puncture.
- Place an occlusive dressing over the cream after application.
- Prior to procedure, remove the dressing and clean the skin. Indication of an adequate response is reddened or blanched skin.
- Demonstrate to the child that the skin is not sensitive by tapping or scratching lightly.
- Instruct to parents to apply medication at home prior to the procedure.

Fentanyl patch

- Use for children older than 12 years of age.
- Use to provide continuous pain control. Onset of 12 to 24 hr and a duration of 72 hr.
- Use an immediate-release opioid for breakthrough pain.
- Treat respiratory depression with naloxone.

Intravenous

NURSING ACTIONS
Bolus
- Rapid pain control in approximately 5 min
- Use for medications (morphine, hydromorphone)
- Continuous: provides steady blood levels

Patient-controlled analgesia (PCA)
- Self-administration of pain medication
- Can be basal, bolus, or combination
- Has lockouts to prevent overdosing

Family-controlled analgesia
- Same concept as PCA
- Parent or caregiver manages the child's pain

Opioid adverse effects

NURSING ACTIONS
- Administer stool softeners for constipation.
- Monitor child for respiratory depression and sedation.

NONPHARMACOLOGICAL MEASURES Qpcc

Distraction
- Use play, radio, a computer game, or a movie.
- Tell jokes or a story to the child.

Relaxation
- Hold or rock the infant or young child.
- Assist older children into a comfortable position.
- Assist with breathing techniques.

Guided imagery
- Assist the child in an imaginary experience.
- Have the child describe the details.

Positive self-talk
- Have the child say positive things during a procedure or painful episode.

Behavioral contracting
- Use stickers or tokens as rewards.
- Give time limits for the child to cooperate.
- Reinforce cooperation with a reward.

Containment
- Swaddle the infant.
- Place rolled blankets around the child.
- Maintain proper positioning.

Nonnutritive sucking
- Offer pacifier with sucrose before, during, and after painful procedures.
- Offer nonnutritive sucking during episodes of pain.

Kangaroo care
- Skin-to-skin contact between infants and parents

Complementary and alternative medicine
- Offer foods, vitamins, or supplements.
- Offer massage or chiropractic options.
- Review energy-based treatments (magnets).
- Discuss mind-body techniques (hypnosis, homeopathy, or naturopathy).

COMPLICATIONS

Chronic pain syndromes: Poorly controlled pain predisposes children to chronic pain conditions.

NURSING ACTIONS
- Assess pain thoroughly and adequately.
- Administer medications in a timely manner.
- Evaluate and monitor the child's response to treatments.
- Titrate analgesic medications to achieve optimal dosing.
- Make recommendations for alternate medications if needed.

Application Exercises

1. A nurse is assessing an infant who has otitis media for pain. Which of the following are findings of pain in an infant? (Select all that apply.)
   A. Pursed lips
   B. Loud cry
   C. Lowered eyebrows
   D. Rigid body
   E. Pushes away stimulus

2. A nurse is preparing a toddler for an intravenous catheter insertion using atraumatic care. Which of the following actions should the nurse take? (Select all that apply.)
   A. Explain the procedure using the child's favorite toy.
   B. Ask the parents to leave during the procedure.
   C. Perform the procedure with the child in his bed.
   D. Allow the child to make one choice regarding the procedure.
   E. Apply lidocaine and prilocaine cream to three potential insertion sites.

3. A nurse is completing a pain assessment on a 4-month-old infant. Which of the following pain scales should the nurse use?
   A. FACES
   B. FLACC
   C. Oucher
   D. Non-communicating children's pain checklist

4. A nurse is planning care for a 12-year-old child following a surgical procedure. Which of the following actions should the nurse include in the plan of care?
   A. Administer NSAIDs for pain greater than 7 on a scale of 0 to 10.
   B. Administer intranasal analgesics PRN.
   C. Administer IM analgesics for pain.
   D. Administer IV analgesics on a schedule.

5. A nurse is planning care for an infant who is experiencing pain. Which of the following interventions should the nurse include the plan of care? (Select all that apply.)
   A. Offer a pacifier.
   B. Use guided imagery.
   C. Use swaddling.
   D. Initiate a behavioral contract.
   E. Encourage kangaroo care.

Active Learning Scenario

A nurse is reviewing pain assessment tools with a group of newly licensed nurses. What should the nurse include in the teaching? Use the ATI Active Learning Template: Nursing Skill to complete this item.

DESCRIPTION OF SKILL: Describe four pain tools used with pediatric clients.

1. B, C, D. **CORRECT:** When analyzing cues while assessing an infant for pain, the nurse should recognize that a loud cry, lowered eyebrows, and a rigid body are manifestations of pain in an infant.

   A. The nurse should not identify pursed lips as a manifestation pain in an infant. Infants who experience pain have their mouth open in a squarish shape.

   E. The nurse should not identify pushing away a painful stimulus as a manifestation of pain in an infant. Infants who experience pain exhibit a local reflex to withdraw from the stimulus.

   Ⓝ *NCLEX® Connection: Pharmacological and Parenteral Therapies, Pharmacological Pain Management*

2. A. **CORRECT:** When providing atraumatic care, the nurse should use the child's favorite toy to explain the procedure. Using the child's favorite toy helps to assist the child in managing fears about the procedure.

   B. When providing atraumatic care, the nurse should not ask the parents to leave the child during procedures. Parents should be allowed to remain with children during procedures to offer comfort.

   C. When providing atraumatic care, the nurse should not perform procedures in safe places such as the child's room or bed. The nurse should take the child to a neutral area such as a treatment room to perform painful procedures.

   D. **CORRECT:** When providing atraumatic care, the nurse should allow the child to make choices. Allowing the child to make choices offers a sense of control over the situation.

   E. **CORRECT:** When providing atraumatic care, the nurse should use a topical analgesic such as lidocaine or prilocaine cream. Using a topical analgesic decreases pain.

   Ⓝ *NCLEX® Connection: Pharmacological and Parenteral Therapies, Parenteral/Intravenous Therapies*

3. A. The FACES pain assessment scale is recommended for children 3 years or older; therefore, this is not the pain scale that the nurse should use when assessing the pain level of a 4-month-old infant.

   B. **CORRECT:** The FLACC pain assessment scale is recommended for infants and children between 2 months and 7 years of age; therefore, this is the pain scale that the nurse should use when assessing the pain level of a 4-month-old infant.

   C. The Oucher pain assessment scale is recommended for children between the ages of 3 and 13 years; therefore, this is not the pain scale that the nurse should use when assessing the pain level of a 4-month-old infant.

   D. The non-communicating children's pain checklist is recommended for non-communicating children between the ages of 3 and 18 years; therefore, this is not the pain scale that the nurse should use when assessing the pain level of a 4-month-old infant.

   Ⓝ *NCLEX® Connection: Pharmacological and Parenteral Therapies, Pharmacological Pain Management*

4. A. The nurse should not include administering NSAIDs for a pain level of 7 on a 0-10 scale. A pain scale of 7 on a scale of 0-10 indicates severe pain. The nurse should plan to administer opioids, not NSAIDs for this pain level. NSAIDs are used for mild to moderate pain.

   B. The nurse should not include administering intranasal analgesics. Intranasal analgesics are used for clients older than 18 years of age.

   C. The nurse should not include administering IM analgesics. IM analgesics are not recommended for pain management in children.

   D. **CORRECT:** When generating solutions for the care of a 12-year-old following a surgical procedure, the nurse should plan to administer IV analgesics on a schedule to achieve optimal pain management.

   Ⓝ *NCLEX® Connection: Pharmacological and Parenteral Therapies, Pharmacological Pain Management*

5. A, C, E. **CORRECT:** When generating solutions during the care of an infant who is experiencing pain, the nurse should include nonnutritive sucking, swaddling, and skin-to-skin contact as therapeutic nonpharmacological pain management strategies.

   B. Guided imagery is a nonpharmacological strategy used with children, not infants.

   D. Behavioral contracts are a nonpharmacological strategy used with children, not infants.

   Ⓝ *NCLEX® Connection: Basic Care and Comfort, Non–Pharmacological Comfort Interventions*

Active Learning Scenario Key

Using the ATI Active Learning Template: Nursing Skill

DESCRIPTION OF SKILL

FLACC (2 months to 7 years)
- Pain rated on a scale of 0 to 10.
- Assess behaviors of the child.
- Face (F)
  - 0: Smile or no expression
  - 1: Occasional frown or grimace, withdrawn
  - 2: Frequent or constant frown, clenched jaw, quivering chin
- Legs (L)
  - 0: Relaxed or normal position
  - 1: Uneasy, restless, tense
  - 2: Kicking or legs drawn up
- Activity (A)
  - 0: Lying quietly, moves easily, normal position
  - 1: Squirming, shifting, tense
  - 2: Arched, ridged, or jerking
- Cry (C)
  - 0: No cry
  - 1: Moans or whimpers, occasional complaints
  - 2: Crying, screaming, sobbing, frequent complaints
- Consolability (C)
  - 0: Content or relaxed
  - 1: Reassured by occasional touching or hugging. Able to distract
  - 2: Difficult to console or comfort

FACES (3 years and older)
- Pain rated on a scale of 0 to 5 using a diagram of six faces.
- Substitute 0, 2, 4, 6, 8, 10 for 0 to 5 to convert to the 0 to 10 scale.
- Explain each face to the child.
  - 0: No hurt
  - 1: Hurts a bit
  - 2: Hurts a little more
  - 3: Hurts even more
  - 4: Hurts a whole lot
  - 5: Hurts worst
- Ask the child to choose a face that best describes how they are feeling

Oucher (3 to 13 years)
- Pain rated on a scale of 0 to 5 using six photographs.
- Substitute 0, 2, 4, 6, 8, 10 for 0 to 5 to convert to the 0 to 10 scale.
- Have the child organize the photographs in order of no pain to the worst pain.
  - 0: No hurt
  - 1: Hurts a bit
  - 2: Hurts a little more
  - 3: Hurts even more
  - 4: Hurts a whole lot
  - 5: Hurts worst
- Ask the child to choose a picture that best describes how they are feeling.

Numeric scale (5 years and older)
- Pain rated on a scale of 0 to 10.
- Explain to the child that 0 means "no pain" and 10 means "worst pain."
- Have the child verbally report a number or point on a visual scale their pain level.

Non-communicating children's pain checklist (3 to 18 years)
- Behaviors are observed for 10 min.
- Six subcategories are scored on a scale 0 to 3.
- Subcategories are vocal, social, facial, activity, body and limbs, and physiological, each with observable behaviors to be scored.
  - 0: Not at all
  - 1: Just a little
  - 2: Fairly often
  - 3: Very often
- Cutoff scores:
  - 11 or more indicates moderate to severe pain.
  - 6 to 10 indicates mild pain.

Ⓝ *NCLEX® Connection: Pharmacological and Parenteral Therapies, Pharmacological Pain Management*

CHAPTER 10

Hospitalization, Illness, and Play

A nurse is likely to encounter children who are ill or hospitalized. When caring for these children, it is important for the nurse to understand how these events can affect the child and incorporate interventions to help the child cope.

Hospitalization and illness

- Families and children can experience major stress related to hospitalization. The nurse should monitor for evidence of stress and intervene as appropriate.
- Families should be considered clients when children are ill.
- Separation anxiety during hospitalization manifests in three behavioral responses.
  - **Protest:** screaming, clinging to parents, verbal and physical aggression toward strangers
  - **Despair:** withdrawal from others, depression, decreased communication, developmental regression
  - **Detachment:** interacting with strangers, forming new relationships, happy appearance
- Each child's understanding of illnesses and hospitalization is dependent on the child's stage of development and cognitive ability.

IMPACT BASED ON DEVELOPMENT

Infant

LEVEL OF UNDERSTANDING
- Inability to describe illness and follow directions
- Lack of understanding of the need of therapeutic procedures

IMPACT OF HOSPITALIZATION
- Experiences stranger anxiety between 6 to 8 months of age
- Displays physical behaviors as expressions of discomfort due to inability to verbalize
- Can experience sleep deprivation due to strange noises, monitoring devices, and procedures
- Can experience anxiety due to the unfamiliar environment and fear of the unknown

Toddler

LEVEL OF UNDERSTANDING
- Limited ability to describe illness
- Poorly developed sense of body image and boundaries
- Limited understanding of the need for therapeutic procedures
- Limited ability to follow directions

IMPACT OF HOSPITALIZATION
- Experiences separation anxiety
- Can exhibit an intense reaction to any type of procedure due to the intrusion of boundaries
- Behavior can regress

Preschooler

LEVEL OF UNDERSTANDING
- Limited understanding of the cause of illness but knows what illness feels like
- Limited ability to describe manifestations
- Fears related to magical thinking
- Ability to understand cause and effect inhibited by concrete thinking

IMPACT OF HOSPITALIZATION
- Can experience separation anxiety
- Can harbor fears of bodily harm
- Might believe illness and hospitalization are a punishment

School-age child

LEVEL OF UNDERSTANDING
- Beginning awareness of body functioning
- Ability to describe pain
- Increasing ability to understand cause and effect

IMPACT OF HOSPITALIZATION
- Fears loss of control
- Seeks information as a way to maintain a sense of control
- Can sense when not being told the truth
- Can experience stress related to separation from peers and regular routine

Adolescent

LEVEL OF UNDERSTANDING
- Increasing ability to understand cause and effect
- Perceptions of illness severity are based on the degree of body image changes

IMPACT OF HOSPITALIZATION
- Develops body image disturbance
- Attempts to maintain composure but is embarrassed about losing control
- Experiences feelings of isolation from peers
- Worries about outcome and impact on school/activities
- Might not adhere to treatments/medication regimen due to peer influence

Family responses

- Fear and guilt regarding not bringing the child in for care earlier
- Frustration due to the perceived inability to care for the child
- Altered family roles
- Worry regarding finances if work is missed Q̇SDoH
- Worry regarding care of other children within the household
- Fear related to lack of knowledge regarding illness or treatments
- Siblings experiencing loneliness, jealousy, guilt, fear, or anger
- Caregiver role strain, related to the impact of hospitalization on family processes

ASSESSMENT

- Child's and family's understanding of the illness or the reason for hospitalization
- Stressors unique to the child and family (needs of other children in the family, socioeconomic situation, health of other extended family members)
- Past experiences with hospitalization and illness
- Developmental level and needs of child/family
- Parenting role and the family's perception of role changes
- Support available to the child/family
- Coping strategies for periods of crisis

NURSING INTERVENTIONS

- Teach the child and family what to expect during hospitalization. Q̇PCC
- Encourage family members to stay with the child during the hospital experience to reduce the stress.
- Maintain routine as much as possible.
- Encourage independence and choices.
- Explain treatments, procedures, and cares to the child.
- Provide developmentally appropriate activities.

Infants

- Place infants whose parents are not in attendance close to nurses' stations so that their needs can be quickly met.
- Provide consistency in assigning caregivers.

Toddlers

- Encourage parents to provide routine care for the child (changing diapers and feeding).
- Encourage the child's autonomy by offering appropriate choices.
- Provide consistency in assigning caregivers.

Preschoolers

- Explain procedures using simple, clear language. Avoid medical jargon and terms that can be misinterpreted.
- Encourage independence by letting the child provide self-care.
- Encourage the child to express feelings.
- Validate the child's fears and concerns.
- Provide toys that allow for emotional expression (a pounding board to release feelings of protest).
- Provide consistency in assigning caregivers.
- Give choices when possible ("Do you want your medicine in a cup or a spoon?").
- Allow younger children to handle equipment if it is safe.

School-age children

- Provide factual information.
- Encourage the child to express feelings.
- Try to maintain a normal routine for long hospitalizations, including time for school work.
- Encourage contact with peer group.

Adolescents

- Provide factual information.
- Include the adolescent in the planning of care to relieve feelings of powerlessness and lack of control.
- Encourage contact with peer group.

Play

- Allows children to express feelings and fears.
- Facilitates mastery of developmental stages and assists in the development of problem solving abilities.
- Allows children to learn socially acceptable behaviors.
- Activities should be specific to each child's stage of development.
- Can be used to teach children.
- A means of protection from everyday stressors.

CONTENT OF PLAY

Unoccupied behavior: focusing attention on something of interest

Dramatic: pretending and fantasizing Q̇EBP

Games: imitative, formal, or competitive

SOCIAL CHARACTER OF PLAY

Onlooker: the child observing others

Solitary: the child playing alone

Parallel: children playing independently but among other children, which is characteristic of toddlers

Associative: children playing together without organization, which is characteristic of preschoolers

Team play: organized playing in groups, which is characteristic of school-age children

FUNCTIONS OF PLAY

Play helps in the development of various types of skills.
- Intellectual
- Sensorimotor
- Social
- Self-awareness
- Creativity
- Therapeutic and moral values

PLAY ACTIVITIES RELATED TO AGE

Infants

- Birth to 3 months: colorful moving mobiles, music/sound boxes
- 3 to 6 months: noise-making objects, soft toys
- 6 to 9 months: teething toys, social interaction
- 9 to 12 months: large blocks, toys that pop apart, push-and-pull toys

Toddlers

- Cloth books, puzzles with large pieces
- Large crayons and paper
- Push-and-pull toys, balls
- Tricycles
- Educational and child-appropriate shows and videos

Preschoolers

- Imitative and imaginative play
- Drawing, painting, riding a tricycle, jumping, running
- Educational and child-appropriate shows and videos

School-age children

- Games that can be played alone or with another person
- Team sports
- Musical instruments
- Arts and crafts
- Collections

Adolescents

- Team sports
- School activities
- Reading, listening to music
- Peer interactions

THERAPEUTIC PLAY

- Makes use of dolls and/or stuffed animals
- Encourages the acting out of feelings of fear, anger, hostility, and sadness
- Enables the child to learn coping strategies in a safe environment
- Assists in gaining cooperation for medical treatment

ASSESSMENT

- Developmental level of the child
- Motor skills
- Level of activity tolerance
- Child's preferences

NURSING INTERVENTIONS

- Select toys that are safe for the child.
- Consider isolation precautions and the child's illness in relation to toy selection.
- Select activities that enhance development.
- Observe the child's play for clues to the child's fears or anxieties.
- Encourage parents to bring one favorite toy from home.
- Use dolls or stuffed animals to demonstrate a procedure before it is performed.
- Provide play opportunities that meet the child's level of activity tolerance.
- Allow the child to go to the play room if able.
- Encourage the adolescent's peers to visit.
- Involve a child life specialist in planning activities.

Application Exercises

1. A nurse is teaching a group of caregivers about separation anxiety. Which of the following information should the nurse include in the teaching?

   A. It is often observed in the school-age child.

   B. Detachment is the stage exhibited in the hospital.

   C. It results in prolonged issues of adaptability.

   D. Kicking a stranger is an example.

2. A nurse is caring for a preschooler who is in an acute care facility. Which of the following should the nurse identify as an expected behavior of a preschool-age child?

   A. Describing manifestations of illness

   B. Relating fears to magical thinking

   C. Understanding cause of illness

   D. Awareness of body functioning

3. A nurse is caring for a toddler who is on a pediatric unit. Which of the following behaviors should the nurse identify as an effect of hospitalization? (Select all that apply.)

   A. Believes the experience is a punishment

   B. Experiences separation anxiety

   C. Displays intense emotions

   D. Exhibits regressive behaviors

   E. Manifests disturbance in body image

4. A nurse is teaching a parent of a toddler about parallel play in children. Which of the following statements should the nurse include in the teaching?

   A. "Children sit and observe others playing."

   B. "Children exhibit organized play when in a group."

   C. "The child plays alone."

   D. "The child plays independently when in a group."

Active Learning Scenario

A nurse working in a pediatric unit is planning play activities for a group of children of different ages. What activities should the nurse include in the plan of care? Use the ATI Active Learning Template: Basic Concept to complete this item.

RELATED CONTENT: Identify appropriate toys and activities for children in three age groups.

Active Learning Scenario Key

Using the ATI Active Learning Template: Basic Concept

RELATED CONTENT

Infants
- Birth to 3 months: colorful moving mobiles, music/sound boxes
- 3 to 6 months: noise-making objects, soft toys
- 6 to 9 months: teething toys, social interaction
- 9 to 12 months: large blocks, toys that pop apart, push-and-pull toys

Toddlers
- Cloth books
- Large crayons and paper
- Push-and-pull toys
- Tricycles
- Balls
- Puzzles with large pieces
- Educational and child-appropriate shows and videos

Preschoolers
- Imitative and imaginative play
- Drawing, painting, riding a tricycle, swimming, jumping, running
- Educational and child-appropriate shows and videos

School-age children
- Games that can be played alone or with another person
- Team sports
- Musical instruments
- Arts and crafts
- Collections

Adolescents
- Team sports
- School activities
- Reading, listening to music
- Peer interactions

Ⓝ *NCLEX® Connection: Health Promotion and Maintenance, Developmental Stages and Transitions*

Application Exercises Key

1. A. Separation anxiety is commonly observed in the toddler, not the school-aged child; therefore, the nurse should not include this in the teaching.
   B. Protest and despair are commonly observed in the hospital setting, not the detachment stage; therefore, the nurse should not include this in the teaching.
   C. Children are adaptable and permanent issues are rare; therefore, the nurse should not include this in the teaching.
   D. **CORRECT:** When taking action and teaching a group of caregivers about separation anxiety, the nurse should include in the teaching that physical aggression toward strangers is a behavior seen in the protest stage of separation anxiety; therefore, the nurse should include in the teaching that kicking a stranger is an example of separation anxiety.

   Ⓝ *NCLEX® Connection: Health Promotion and Maintenance, Developmental Stages and Transitions*

2. A. Preschool-age children have limited ability to describe manifestations of illness; therefore, the nurse should not identify this as an expected behavior of a preschool-aged child.
   B. **CORRECT:** When analyzing cues during the care of a preschool-age child in an acute care facility, the nurse should recognize that preschool-aged children are egocentric and relate fears to magical thinking.
   C. Preschool-age children have limited understanding of cause-and-effect relationship, but understand what illness feels like; therefore, the nurse should not identify this as an expected behavior of a preschool-aged child.
   D. Awareness of body functioning is a behavior of an adolescent; therefore, the nurse should not identify this as an expected behavior of a preschool-aged child.

   Ⓝ *NCLEX® Connection: Health Promotion and Maintenance, Developmental Stages and Transitions*

3. B, C, D. **CORRECT:** When analyzing cues during the care of a toddler on a pediatric unit, the nurse should identify that effects of hospitalization on a toddler include separation anxiety, displays of intense emotions, and exhibiting regressive behaviors.
   A. Preschool children believe hospitalization is a punishment.
   E. Body image disturbances can be seen in adolescents who are hospitalized, not toddlers.

   Ⓝ *NCLEX® Connection: Health Promotion and Maintenance, Developmental Stages and Transitions*

4. A. Onlooker play, not parallel play, is when a child sits and observes others playing; therefore, the nurse should not include this statement in the teaching.
   B. Team play, not parallel play, is when a child exhibits organized play in a group; therefore, the nurse should not include this statement in the teaching.
   C. Solitary play, not parallel play, is when a child plays alone; therefore, the nurse should not include this statement in the teaching.
   D. **CORRECT:** When taking action and teaching the parent of a toddler about parallel play, the nurse should include in the teaching that parallel play is when a toddler plays independently but is among other children in a group.

   Ⓝ *NCLEX® Connection: Health Promotion and Maintenance, Aging Process*

UNIT 1 FOUNDATIONS OF PEDIATRIC NURSING
SECTION: SPECIFIC CONSIDERATIONS OF PEDIATRIC NURSING

CHAPTER 11 *Death and Dying*

A nurse must meet the physical, psychological, spiritual, and emotional needs of a client and the family during illness and at the time of death. Q$_{PCC}$

Palliative care is a interprofessional approach that focuses on the improving quality of life rather than prolonging life when cures are not possible. Focus is on control of managing the client's manifestations and offering supportive care.

Hospice care specializes in the care of a client who is dying. Family members are often the primary caregivers. Nursing focus is on pain control, comfort, and allowing the client to die with dignity. Family and client needs are equal. Provide support for the family's grieving process, which can continue after the client's death.

End-of-life decisions require honest information regarding prognosis, disease progression, treatment options, and effects of treatments. These decisions are made during a highly stressful time. It is important that all health care personnel be aware of the child's and family's decisions.

Nurses can experience personal grief when caring for children with whom they have developed rapport and intimacy.

FACTORS INFLUENCING LOSS, GRIEF, AND COPING ABILITY

- Interpersonal relationships and social support networks
- Type and significance of loss
- Culture and ethnicity
- Spiritual and religious beliefs and practices
- Prior experience with loss
- Socioeconomic status Q$_{SDoH}$

GRIEF AND MOURNING

Anticipatory grief: when death is expected or a possible outcome

Complicated grief: extensive or prolonged grief
- Intense thoughts
- Distressing yearning
- Feelings of loneliness
- Distressing emotions and feelings
- Disturbances in personal activities (sleep)
- Can require referral to an expert in grief counseling

Parental grief
- Intense, long-lasting, and complex
- Secondary losses related to the death of the child (absence of hope and dreams, disruption of the family) unit, loss of identity as a parent
- Guardian can experience and express grief differently based on their role in the family.

Sibling grief
- Differs from adult/parental grief
- Reactions depend on age and developmental stage

CURRENT STAGE OF DEVELOPMENT

INFANTS/TODDLERS (BIRTH TO 3 YEARS)
- Have little to no concept of death.
- Egocentric thinking prevents their understanding death (toddlers).
- Mirror parental emotions (sadness, anger, depression, anxiety).
- React in response to the changes brought about by being in the hospital (change of routine, painful procedures, immobilization, less independence, separation from family).
- Can regress to an earlier stage of behavior.

PRESCHOOL CHILDREN (3 TO 6 YEARS)
- Egocentric thinking.
- Magical thinking allows for the belief that thoughts can cause an event (death [as a result, child can feel guilt and shame]).
- Interpret separation from parents as punishment for bad behavior.
- View dying as temporary because of the lack of a concept of time and because the dead person can still have attributes of the living (sleeping, eating, breathing).

SCHOOL-AGE CHILDREN (6 TO 12 YEARS)
- Start to respond to logical or factual explanations.
- Begin to have an adult concept of death (inevitable, irreversible, universal), which generally applies to older school-age children (9 to 12 years).
- Experience fear of the disease process, death process, the unknown, and loss of control.
- Fear often displayed through uncooperative behavior.
- Can be curious about funeral services and what happens to the body after death.

ADOLESCENTS (12 TO 20 YEARS)

- Can have an adult-like concept of death.
- Can have difficulty accepting death because they are discovering who they are, establishing an identity, and dealing with issues of puberty.
- Rely more on peers than the influence of parents, which can result in the reality of a serious illness causing adolescents to feel isolated.
- Can be unable to relate to peers and communicate with parents.
- Can become increasingly stressed by changes in physical appearance due to medications or illness than the prospect of death.
- Can experience guilt and shame.

Factors that can increase the family's potential for dysfunctional grieving following the death of a child

- Lack of a support system
- Presence of inadequate coping skills
- Association of violence or suicide with the death of a child
- Sudden and unexpected death of a child
- Lack of hope or presence of pre-existing mental health issues

ASSESSMENT

- Knowledge regarding diagnosis, prognosis, and care
- Perceptions and desires regarding diagnosis, prognosis, and care
- Nutritional status, as well as growth and development patterns
- Activity and energy level of the child
- Guardians' wishes regarding the child's end-of-life care
- Presence of advance directives
- Family coping and available support
- Stage of grief the child and family are experiencing

PHYSICAL MANIFESTATIONS OF DEATH

- Sensation of heat when the body feels cool
- Decreased sensation and movement in lower extremities
- Loss of senses (hearing is the last to be lost)
- Confusion or loss of consciousness
- Decreased appetite and thirst
- Swallowing difficulties
- Loss of bowel and bladder control
- Bradycardia, hypotension
- Cheyne-Stokes respirations
- Pooling pulmonary and pharyngeal secretions can cause the "death rattle"

NURSING INTERVENTIONS

- Allow an opportunity for anticipatory grieving, which impacts the way a family will cope with the death of a child. Qpcc
- Provide consistency among nursing personnel who are caring for the client/family.
- Encourage guardians to remain with the child.
- Attempt to maintain a normal environment.
- Communicate with the child honestly and respectfully.
- Encourage independence.

- Stay with the child as much as possible.
- Administer analgesics to control pain.
- Provide privacy.
- Soften lights.
- Offer soft music if desired.
- Assist with arranging religious or cultural rituals desired by the child and family.
- Assist the child with unfinished tasks.
- Provide support for the family and child.

PALLIATIVE CARE

- Plan care for the entire family and it's individuals, in addition to the child
- Provide an environment that is as close to being like home as possible.
- Consult with the child and family for desired measures.
- Respect the family's cultural and religious preferences and rituals. Qpcc
- Provide and clarify information and explanations.
- Encourage physical contact; address feelings; and show concern, empathy, and support.
- Provide comfort measures (warmth, quiet, noise control, dry linens).
- Provide frequent mouth care and oral hygiene.
- Provide adequate nutrition and hydration.
- Control pain.
  - Give medications on a regular schedule.
  - Treat breakthrough pain.
  - Increase doses as necessary to control pain.
  - Encourage use of relaxation, imagery, and distraction to help manage pain.

CARE FOR GRIEVING FAMILIES DURING THE DYING PROCESS

- Provide information to the child and family about the disease, medications, procedures, and expected events.
- Encourage and support loved ones to participate in caring for the child.
- Encourage family to remain near the child as much as possible or desired.
- Encourage the child's independence and control as developmentally and physically appropriate.
- Allow for visitation of family and friends as desired.
- Emphasize open, honest communication among the child, family, and health care team.
- Provide support to the child and family with decision-making.
- Provide opportunities for the child and family to ask questions.
- Assist caregivers to cope with their feelings and help them to understand the child's behaviors.
- Use books, movies, art, music, and play therapy to stimulate discussions and provide an outlet for emotions.
- Provide and encourage professional support and guidance from a trusted member of the health care team.
- Remain neutral and accepting.

- Give reassurance that the child is not in pain and that all efforts are being made to maintain comfort and support of the child's life.
- Recognize and support the individual differences of grieving. Advise families that each member can react differently on any given day.
- Give families privacy, unlimited time, and opportunities for any cultural or religious rituals. Respect the family's decisions regarding care of the child.
- Encourage discussion of special memories and people, reading of favorite books, providing favorite toys/objects, physical contact, sibling visits, and continued verbal communication, even if the client seems unconscious.

AFTER DEATH

- Allow family to stay with the body as long as they desire.
- Allow family to rock the infant/toddler, if desired.
- Remove tubes and equipment.
- Offer to allow family to assist with preparation of the body.
- Assist with preparations involving the death ritual.

- Encourage family to prepare siblings for the funeral and related death rituals.
- Remain with the family and offer support.
- Allow family to share stories about the child's life.
- Refer to the child by name.
- Allow all family members to communicate feelings.

SELF-CARE FOR NURSES

- Express personal feelings of loss to someone who can offer support.
- Maintain good general health.
- Develop the ability for empathy.
- Take time off from work as needed.
- Develop well-rounded interests.
- Develop professional and social support systems.
- Focus on the positive aspects of caring for children who are dying.
- Attend funeral services if desired.
- Maintain contact with the family.
- Other useful techniques include:
  - Mindfulness meditation
  - Focus on positive and rewarding aspects of nursing

Application Exercises

1. A nurse is providing teaching to a guardian about complicated grief. Which of the following statements should the nurse make?
   - A. "Complicated grief occurs when little time is spent thinking about the loss."
   - B. "Personal activities are rarely affected when experiencing complicated grief."
   - C. "Guardians will experience complicated grief together."
   - D. "Counseling can be helpful in resolving complicated grief."

2. A nurse is teaching the caregiver of a preschool child about factors that affect the child's perception of death. Which of the following factors should the nurse include in the teaching?
   - A. Preschool children have no concept of death.
   - B. Preschool children perceive death as temporary.
   - C. Preschool children often regress to an earlier stage of behavior.
   - D. Preschool children experience fear related to the disease process.

3. A nurse is caring for a child who is dying. Which of the following should the nurse identify as manifestations of impending death? (Select all that apply.)
   - A. Heightened sense of hearing
   - B. Tachycardia
   - C. Difficulty swallowing
   - D. Sensation of being cold
   - E. Cheyne-Stokes respirations

4. A nurse is reviewing palliative care with an assistive personnel (AP) who is assisting with the care of a child who has a terminal illness. Which of the following statements by the AP indicates an understanding of palliative care?
   - A. "I'm sure the family is hopeful that the new medication will stop the illness."
   - B. "I'll miss working with this client now that only nurses will be caring for the child."
   - C. "I will get all the client's personal objects out of the room."
   - D. "I will listen and respond as the family talks about their child's life."

5. A charge nurse in a hospice care office is planning an in-service to provide coping strategies to nurses who care for dying children. Which of the following are strategies should the nurse include in the in-service? (Select all that apply.)
   - A. Remain in contact with the family after their loss.
   - B. Develop a professional support system.
   - C. Take time off from work.
   - D. Suggest that a hospital representative attend the funeral.
   - E. Demonstrate feelings of sympathy toward the family.

Application Exercises Key

1. A. A guardian who experiences complicated grief has frequent, intrusive thoughts that persist for more than a year after the loss; therefore, the nurse should not include this statement when providing teaching to the guardian.
   B. A guardian who is experiencing complicated grief experiences intense emotions that affect personal activities; therefore, the nurse should not include this statement when providing teaching to the guardian.
   C. Guardians grieve differently, and not all will experience complicated grief; therefore, the nurse should not include this statement when providing teaching to the guardian.
   D. **CORRECT:** Guardians who experience complicated grief often benefit from professional counseling; therefore, the nurse should include this statement when providing teaching to the guardian . The nurse should also collaborate with the provider to refer the guardian to an expert in grief counseling if complicated grief is identified.

   Ⓝ *NCLEX® Connection: Psychosocial Integrity, Grief and Loss*

2. A. Toddlers, not preschoolers have no concept of death; therefore, the nurse should not include this information in the teaching.
   B. **CORRECT:** Preschool children perceive death as temporary because they have no concept of time; therefore, the nurse should include this information in the teaching.
   C. Toddlers, not preschoolers, often regress to an earlier stage of behavior; therefore, the nurse should not include this information in the teaching.
   D. School-age children, not preschoolers, experience fear related to the disease process; therefore, the nurse should not include this information in the teaching.

   Ⓝ *NCLEX® Connection: Psychosocial Integrity, Grief and Los*

3. C, E. **CORRECT:** When analyzing cues while caring for a child who is dying, the nurse should identify that difficulty swallowing and Cheyne-Stokes respirations as manifestations of impending death.
   A. A decrease in the senses of smell, sight, and hearing are physical manifestations of approaching death, not a heightened sense of hearing.
   B. Bradycardia, not tachycardia, is a physical manifestation of approaching death..
   D. Client's experience a sensation of heat even though the body feels cool to touch as a physical manifestation of approaching death.

   Ⓝ *NCLEX® Connection: Basic Care and Comfort, System-Specific Assessments*

4. A. Palliative care is provided when there is no longer hope for a disease cure; therefore, this statement by the AP does not indicate an understanding of palliative care.
   B. Palliative care focuses on providing consistency among the interprofessional team and is not limited to care provided only by nurses; therefore, this statement by the AP does not indicate an understanding of palliative care.
   C. Palliative care focuses on offering support and a comfortable environment as the dying process occurs; therefore, this statement by the AP does not indicate an understanding of palliative care.
   D. **CORRECT:** Palliative care focuses on the process of dying and grieving, which includes using therapeutic communication; therefore, this statement by the AP indicates an understanding of palliative care.

   Ⓝ *NCLEX® Connection: Basic Care and Comfort, Non-Pharmacological Comfort Interventions*

5. A, B, C. **CORRECT:** Maintaining contact with the family after their loss, developing professional support systems, and taking time off of work are strategies that the nurse can use to cope with the stresses associated with care of the dying child.
   D. Attending funeral services of children that they have cared for has been identified as a strategy that nurses can use to cope with the stresses associated with care of the dying child, not suggesting that a hospital representative attend funeral services.
   E. Demonstrating feelings of empathy, not sympathy, toward the family has been identified as a strategy that nurses can use to cope with the stresses associated with care of the dying child.

   Ⓝ *NCLEX® Connection: Psychosocial Integrity, End of Life Care*

Active Learning Scenario

A nurse is planning care for a client who is nearing the end of life. What interventions should the nurse include in the plan of care? Use the ATI Active Learning Template: Basic Concept to complete this item.

NURSING INTERVENTIONS: Describe at least eight nursing interventions to be used.

Active Learning Scenario Key

Using the ATI Active Learning Template: Basic Concept
NURSING INTERVENTIONS
- Allow an opportunity for anticipatory grieving, which affects the way a family will cope with the death of a child.
- Provide consistency among nursing staff caring for the client and family.
- Encourage loved ones to remain with the client.
- Attempt to maintain a normal environment.
- Communicate with the client honestly and respectfully.
- Encourage independence.
- Stay with the client as much as possible.
- Administer analgesics to control pain.
- Provide privacy.
- Soften lights.
- Offer soft music if desired.
- Assist with arranging religious or cultural rituals desired by the client and family.
- Assist the client with unfinished tasks.
- Provide support for the family and client.

Ⓝ *NCLEX® Connection: Psychosocial Integrity, Grief and Loss*

When reviewing the following chapters, keep in mind the relevant topics and tasks of the NCLEX outline, in particular:

Pharmacological and Parenteral Therapies

EXPECTED ACTIONS/OUTCOMES: Evaluate client response to medication.

Reduction of Risk Potential

DIAGNOSTIC TESTS: Monitor the results of diagnostic testing and intervene as needed.

POTENTIAL FOR ALTERATIONS IN BODY SYSTEMS
Compare current client data to baseline client data.

Identify client potential for aspiration.

POTENTIAL FOR COMPLICATIONS OF DIAGNOSTIC TESTS/ TREATMENTS/PROCEDURES: Use precautions to prevent injury and/or complications associated with a procedure or diagnosis.

THERAPEUTIC PROCEDURES: Educate client about treatments and procedures.

Physiological Adaptation

ALTERATIONS IN BODY SYSTEMS: Provide care to the client who has experienced a seizure.

ILLNESS MANAGEMENT: Educate client regarding an acute or chronic condition.

UNEXPECTED RESPONSE TO THERAPIES
Assess the client for unexpected adverse response to therapy.

Recognize signs and symptoms of client complications and intervene.

CHAPTER 12 # Acute Neurologic Disorders

Meningitis is an inflammation of the meninges, which are the connective tissues that cover the brain and spinal cord. Meningitis is caused by bacteria, a virus, or fungus in the cerebrospinal fluid (CSF).

Meningitis

Viral (aseptic) meningitis usually requires supportive care for recovery.

Bacterial (septic) meningitis is a contagious infection. Prognosis depends on how quickly care is initiated.

ASSESSMENT

RISK FACTORS

VIRAL MENINGITIS
Many viral illnesses (cytomegalovirus, herpes simplex virus, enterovirus, HIV, and arbovirus)

BACTERIAL MENINGITIS
- Infections caused by bacterial agents: *Neisseria meningitidis* (meningococcal), *Streptococcus pneumoniae* (pneumococcal), *Haemophilus influenzae* type B (Hib), *Escherichia coli*
  - Incidence of bacterial meningitis has decreased in all age groups except infants under the age of 2 months since the introduction of the Hib and pneumococcal conjugate vaccines (PCV). Ⓠ EBP
- Injuries that provide direct access to CSF (skull fracture, penetrating head wound)
- Crowded living conditions

EXPECTED FINDINGS
- Photophobia
- Vomiting
- Irritability
- Headache

PHYSICAL ASSESSMENT FINDINGS
Manifestations of viral and bacterial meningitis are similar.

Newborns
- No illness is present at birth, but it progresses within a few days.
- Manifestations are vague and difficult to diagnose.
  - Poor muscle tone, weak cry, poor suck, refuses feeding, and vomiting or diarrhea
  - Possible fever or hypothermia
- Neck is supple.
- Bulging fontanels and nuchal rigidity are late findings.

3 months to 2 years
- Seizures with a high-pitched cry
- Fever and irritability
- Bulging fontanels
- Possible nuchal rigidity
- Poor feeding
- Vomiting
- Brudzinski's and Kernig's signs not reliable for diagnosis

2 years through adolescence
- Seizures (often initial finding)
- Nuchal rigidity
- Positive Brudzinski's sign (flexion of extremities occurring with deliberate flexion of the child's neck)
- Positive Kernig's sign (resistance to extension of the child's leg from a flexed position)
- Fever and chills
- Headache
- Vomiting
- Irritability and restlessness that can progress to drowsiness, delirium, stupor, and coma
- Petechiae or purpuric-type rash (with meningococcal infection)
- Involvement of joints (with meningococcal and *Hib*)
- Chronic draining ear (with pneumococcal infection)

LABORATORY TESTS
- Blood cultures are sometimes positive when the CSF culture is negative.
- Collect complete blood counts.
- CSF analysis indicative of meningitis.
  - BACTERIAL
    - Cloudy color
    - Elevated WBC count
    - Elevated protein content
    - Decreased glucose content
    - Positive Gram stain
  - VIRAL
    - Clear color
    - Slightly elevated WBC count
    - Normal or slightly elevated protein content
    - Normal glucose content
    - Negative Gram stain

DIAGNOSTIC PROCEDURES

Lumbar puncture

This is the definitive diagnostic test for meningitis.
- The provider inserts a spinal needle into the subarachnoid space between L3 and L4, or L4 and L5 vertebral spaces.
- Measures spinal fluid pressure and collects CSF for analysis.

NURSING ACTIONS
- Have the client void prior to the procedure.
- Assist the provider with the procedure.
- A topical anesthetic cream (lidocaine and prilocaine) can be applied over the biopsy area 45 min to 1 hr prior to the procedure. Qᴘᴄᴄ
- Place the client in the side-lying position with the head flexed and knees drawn up toward the chest, and assist in maintaining the position. Use distraction methods as necessary.
- The client can be sedated with fentanyl and midazolam.
- The provider cleans the skin and injects a local anesthetic.
- The provider takes pressure readings and collects three to five test tubes of CSF.
- Pressure and an elastic bandage are applied to the puncture site after the needle is removed.
- Position child according to facility policy after procedure.
- Label specimens appropriately, and deliver them to the laboratory.
- Monitor the site for bleeding, hematoma, or infection.

CT scan or MRI

Performed to identify increased intracranial pressure (ICP) or an abscess.

NURSING ACTIONS
- Assist with positioning.
- Administer sedatives as prescribed.

PATIENT-CENTERED CARE

NURSING CARE
- The presence of petechiae or a purpuric-type rash requires immediate medical attention. Qᴇʙᴘ
- Isolate the client as soon as meningitis is suspected, and maintain droplet precautions per facility protocol.
  - Droplet precautions require a private room or a room with clients who have an infection from the same microorganism, ensuring that each client has his or her own designated equipment.
  - Providers and visitors should wear a mask.
  - Maintain respiratory isolation for a minimum of 24 hr after initiation of antibiotic therapy.
- Monitor vital signs, urine output, fluid status, pain level, and neurologic status.
- Monitor and treat fever.
- For newborns and infants, monitor head circumference and fontanels for presence of or changes in bulging.
- Correct fluid volume deficits and then restrict fluids until no evidence of increased ICP and blood sodium levels are within the expected range.
- Maintain NPO status if the client has a decreased level of consciousness. As the client's condition improves, advance to clear liquids and then a diet the client can tolerate.
- Decrease environmental stimuli.
  - Provide a quiet environment.
  - Minimize exposure to bright light (natural and electric).
- Provide comfort measures.
  - Keep the room cool.
  - Position the client without a pillow, and slightly elevate the head of the bed. The client can also be positioned side-lying to reduce neck discomfort.
- Maintain safety (keep the bed in a low position, implement seizure precautions). Qs
- Keep the family informed of the client's condition.

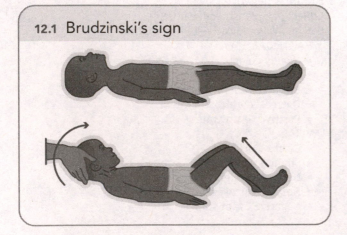

12.1 Brudzinski's sign

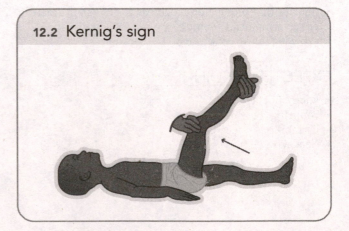

12.2 Kernig's sign

MEDICATIONS

Antibiotics

Administer IV antibiotics for bacterial infections. Length of therapy is determined by the client's condition and CSF results (normal blood glucose levels, negative culture). Therapy can last up to 21 days depending on the which infectious organism is present.

NURSING ACTIONS
- Assess for allergies.
- Provide support for the client and family.
- Educate the family about the need to complete the entire course of medication.

Corticosteroids: dexamethasone

- Not indicated for viral meningitis.
- Assists with initial management of increased ICP, but might not be effective for long-term complications.
- Most effective for reducing neurologic complications in children who have infections caused by Hib.

NURSING ACTIONS
- Assess for effectiveness of medication.
- Provide support for the client and family.
- Educate on administration and possible adverse effects of the medication.

CLIENT EDUCATION
- Early and complete treatment is necessary for upper respiratory infections.
- Maintain appropriate immunizations for the client. Children should receive the Hib and PCV vaccines at 2, 4, and 6 months of age, then again between 12 and 15 months of age.

COMPLICATIONS

Increased intracranial pressure

Could lead to neurologic dysfunction

NURSING ACTIONS
- Monitor for manifestations of increased ICP. Qs
  - **Newborns and infants:** bulging or tense fontanels, increased head circumference, high-pitched cry, distended scalp veins, irritability, bradycardia, and respiratory changes
  - **Children:** increased irritability, headache, nausea, vomiting, diplopia, seizures, bradycardia, and respiratory changes
- Provide interventions to reduce ICP (positioning; avoidance of coughing, straining, and bright lights; minimizing environmental stimuli).

Hearing Loss

NURSING ACTIONS
- Coordinate referrals for auditory evaluation after discharge.

Active Learning Scenario

A nurse is admitting a client who has bacterial meningitis. Use the ATI Active Learning Template: System Disorder to complete this item.

ALTERATION IN HEALTH (DIAGNOSIS)

RISK FACTORS: List 3 risk factors for both bacterial and viral meningitis.

EXPECTED FINDINGS: Identify four.

LABORATORY TESTS: List two results indicative of bacterial meningitis.

NURSING CARE: List 5 nursing interventions.

Active Learning Scenario Key

Using the ATI Active Learning Template: System Disorder

ALTERATION IN HEALTH (DIAGNOSIS): Bacterial meningitis is an inflammation of the meninges, which are the connective tissues that cover the brain and spinal cord risk factors

VIRAL MENINGITIS: Many viral illnesses (cytomegalovirus, herpes simplex virus, enterovirus, HIV, and arbovirus)

BACTERIAL MENINGITIS
- Infections caused by bacterial agents: Neisseria meningitidis (meningococcal), Streptococcus pneumoniae (pneumococcal), Haemophilus influenzae type B (Hib), Escherichia coli
- Injuries that provide direct access to CSF (skull fracture, penetrating head wound)
- Crowded living conditions

EXPECTED FINDINGS
- Photophobia
- Vomiting
- Irritability
- Headache

LABORATORY TESTS
- CSF analysis indicative of bacterial meningitis.
  - Cloudy color
  - Elevated WBC count
  - Elevated protein content
  - Decreased glucose content
  - Positive Gram stain

Ⓝ *NCLEX® Connection: Physiological Adaptation, Pathophysiology*

Application Exercises

1. A nurse is assisting with the development of an in-service about viral and bacterial meningitis. The nurse should include that the introduction of which of the following immunizations decreased the incidence of bacterial meningitis in children? (Select all that apply.)

   A. Inactivated polio vaccine (IPV)

   B. Pneumococcal conjugate vaccine (PCV)

   C. Diphtheria and tetanus toxoids and acellular pertussis vaccine (DTaP)

   D. *Haemophilus influenzae* type B (Hib) vaccine

   E. Trivalent inactivated influenza vaccine (TIV)

2. A nurse is assessing a 4-month-old infant who has meningitis. Which of the following manifestations should the nurse expect?

   A. Depressed anterior fontanel

   B. Constipation

   C. Presence of the rooting reflex

   D. High-pitched cry

3. A nurse is reviewing the cerebral spinal fluid analysis for a group of clients who have suspected meningitis. Sort the following analysis findings by the nurse into the correct meningitis category: Viral Meningitis or Bacterial Meningitis.

   A. Cloudly color

   B. Elevated protein content

   C. Negative gram stain

   D. Clear color

   E. Decreased glucose content

   F. Normal glucose content

   G. Positive gram stain

4. A nurse is caring for a client who has suspected meningitis and a decreased level of consciousness. Which of the following actions should the nurse take?

   A. Place the client on NPO status.

   B. Prepare the client for a liver biopsy.

   C. Position the client dorsal recumbent.

   D. Put the client in a protective environment.

Application Exercises Key

1. **B, D. CORRECT:** When developing an educational program about viral and bacterial meningitis, the nurse should include that the PCV and Hib vaccines provided immunity against the bacteria's that caused the illness decreasing the incidence of bacterial meningitis in children.
   A. The nurse should not include the IPV vaccine because it does not decrease the incidence of bacterial meningitis.
   C. The nurse should not include the DTaP vaccine because it does not decrease the incidence of bacterial meningitis.
   E. The nurse should not include the TIV because it does not decrease the incidence of bacterial meningitis.

   Ⓝ NCLEX® Connection: Health Promotion and Maintenance, Health Promotion/Disease Prevention

2. A. The nurse should expect a 4-month-old infant who has meningitis to have a bulging anterior fontanel, not a depressed anterior fontanel.
   B. The nurse should expect vomiting, not constipation, as an expected finding in a 4-month-old infant who has meningitis.
   C. The nurse should identify that the rooting reflex is an expected finding in infants until the age of 3 to 4 months and is not a manifestation of meningitis.
   D. **CORRECT:** When recognizing cues during the assessment of a 4-month-old infant who has meningitis, the nurse should expect a high-pitched cry as a manifestation of meningitis.

   Ⓝ NCLEX® Connection: Reduction of Risk Potential, Diagnostic Tests

3. **VIRAL MENINGITIS:** C, D, F;
   BACTERIAL MENINGITIS: G, E, A, B

   When reviewing cerebral fluid analysis, the nurse should identify that the cerebral spinal fluid of a client who has bacterial meningitis will be cloudy, have an elevated protein content, decreased glucose content, and a positive gram stain. The cerebral spinal fluid of a client who has bacterial meningitis will also have elevated WBC. When reviewing cerebral fluid analysis, the nurse should identify that the cerebral spinal fluid of a client who has viral meningitis will be clear, have a negative gram stain, and have normal glucose content. The cerebral spinal fluid of a client who has viral meningitis will also have slightly elevated WBC and normal to slightly elevated protein content.

   Ⓝ NCLEX® Connection: Physiological Adaptation, Alterations in Body Systems

4. A. **CORRECT:** When taking action for the client who has suspected bacterial meningitis and a decreased level of consciousness, the nurse should place the client on NPO status to decrease the client's risk of aspiration.
   B. The nurse should expect a client who has Reye syndrome to require a liver biopsy, not a client who has suspected meningitis.
   C. The nurse should position the client without a pillow and slightly elevate the head of the bed to prevent increasing intracranial pressure. The nurse should not place the client in dorsal recumbent position.
   D. The nurse should place a client who has suspected meningitis on droplet precautions for at least 24 hr after the initiation of antibiotic therapy. Clients who are immunocompromised require a protective environment.

   Ⓝ NCLEX® Connection: Physiological Adaptation, Alterations in Body Systems

CHAPTER 13 Seizures

Seizures are abnormal, involuntary, excessive electrical discharges of neurons within the brain.

Seizures are classified according to their type and etiology. Focal seizures involve one area of the brain. Generalized seizures involve the entire brain.

A diagnosis of epilepsy is made if a client has two unprovoked seizures at least 24 hr apart, or if a single unprovoked seizure occurs during a time period of 10 years following two unprovoked seizures.

ASSESSMENT

RISK FACTORS FOR SEIZURES

- Some seizures have no known etiology
- Febrile episode
- Cerebral edema
- Intracranial infection or hemorrhage
- Brain tumors or cysts
- Anoxia
- Toxins or drugs
- Lead poisoning QSDoH
- Tetanus, *Shigella*, or *Salmonella*
- Metabolic conditions

RISK FACTORS FOR EPILEPSY

- Trauma
- Hemorrhage
- Congenital defects
- Anoxia
- Infection
- Toxins
- Hypoglycemic injury
- Uremia
- Migraine
- Cardiovascular dysfunction

EXPECTED FINDINGS

Generalized

Tonic–clonic seizure (previously referred to as grand mal)
- Onset without warning QEBP
- Most prevalent of all seizure types
- Tonic phase (10 to 20 seconds)
  - Eyes roll upward
  - Loss of consciousness
  - Tonic contraction of entire body, with arms flexed and legs, head and neck extended
  - Mouth snaps shut and tongue can be bitten
  - Thoracic and abdominal muscles contract
  - Possible piercing cry
  - Flushing
  - Loss of swallowing reflex and increased salivation
  - Apnea leading to cyanosis
- Clonic phase (typically 30 to 50 seconds; can last 30 min or longer)
  - Violent jerking movements of the body
  - Trunk and extremities experience rhythmic contraction and relaxation
  - Can having foaming in the mouth
  - Can be incontinent of urine and feces
  - Gradual slowing of movements until cessation
- Postictal state (30 min to several hours)
  - Remains semiconscious but arouses with difficulty
  - Confused for several hours
  - Impairment of fine motor movements
  - Lack of coordination
  - Possible vomiting, headache, visual or speech difficulties
  - Sleeps for several hours
  - Feels tired and can complain of sore muscles
  - No recollection of the seizure

13.1 Tonic-clonic seizure

tonic phase

piercing cry
cyanosis
generalized stiffening
of body and limbs,
back arched

clonic phase

salivary frothing
incontinence
clonic jerks of limbs,
body, and head

**postictal
confusional fatigue**

limbs and body limp

Absence seizure (previously referred to as petit mal)
- Onset between ages of 4 to 12 years and ceases by the teenage years
- Loss of consciousness lasting 5 to 10 seconds
- Motionless, blank stare
- Affects schoolwork, which is often first indication of a problem
- Minimal or no change in behavior
- Resembles daydreaming or inattentiveness
- Can drop items being held, but the child seldom falls
- Automatisms: Lip smacking, twitching of eyelids or face, or slight hand movements
- Unable to recall episodes, but can be momentarily confused
- Can immediately resume previous activities

Myoclonic seizure
- Variety of seizure episodes
- Symmetric or asymmetric involvement
- Brief contractions of muscle or groups of muscle
- Can involve only the face and trunk or one or more extremities
- No postictal state
- Might not lose consciousness

Atonic or akinetic seizure
- Also known as "drop attacks"
- Onset between 2 and 5 years of age
- Muscle tone is lost for a few seconds, which often causes a fall
- A period of confusion follows
- If seizures are frequent, child should wear a helmet to prevent injury

FOCAL

Focal seizures with motor manifestations
- Aversive seizure (most common): Eyes and head turn away from the side of focus, with or without loss of consciousness
- Rolandic (Sylvan) seizure: Tonic–clonic movements involving the face, salivation, arrested sleep, and most common during sleep

Focal seizure with sensory manifestations
- Tingling, numbness or pain in one area of the body then spreading to other parts, with visual sensations
Motor development (hypertonia or posturing)

Focal seizures with impaired awareness
- Altered behavior
- Inability to respond to the environment
- Impaired consciousness but regains in less than 5 min
- Confusion and inability to recall event
- Aura: warning of onset of seizure activity that can be a strange feeling in the throat, an odor, or taste. It can also produce auditory or visual hallucinations, feelings of fear, distorted sense of time and self

Unclassified

West syndrome (infantile spasms)
Rare disorder of unknown origin with a peak onset between 4 and 8 months of age. Rarely occurs after 2 years of age.
- Sudden, brief, symmetric muscle contractions
- Flexed head, extended arms with legs drawn up
- Possible eye deviation or nystagmus
- Possible cry or irritability during or after seizure spasms
- Can occur as a single event or in a cluster of up to 150 seizures
- Treated with adrenocorticotropic hormone (ACTH)

Lennox–Gastaut syndrome
- Mixture of different seizures in child with cognitive deficits
- Aggressive and hyperactive behavior
- Difficult to treat
- Poor prognosis

Febrile seizures
- Associated with as sudden spike in temperature as high as 38.9° to 40° C. (102° to 104° F)
- Duration of 15 to 20 seconds

TREATMENT
- After seizure subsides, take actions to reduce fever
- Administer acetaminophen or ibuprofen when the child has a fever
- If child is unable to swallow, administer acetaminophen suppository
- Dress the child in light clothing

LABORATORY TESTS

Depend on age, history, and physical condition.
- Lead level
- WBC
- Blood glucose
- Metabolic panel
- Chromosomal analysis
- Toxicology screen

DIAGNOSTIC PROCEDURES

Electroencephalogram (EEG)
Records electrical activity and can identify the origin of seizure activity.
- Can be monitored during sleep, when awake, and with stimulation and hyperventilation.
- Test can last 1 hr to multiple periods and days of monitoring.
- Can be performed with video monitoring.
- A normal EEG does not rule out seizures.

CLIENT EDUCATION
- Remain still during the procedure.
- If prescribed, withhold sleep from child prior to the test.
- Strobe lights or hyperventilation may be used to induce a seizure.
- The test will not be painful.
- Abstain from caffeine for several hours prior to the procedure.
- Wash hair (no oils or sprays) before and after the procedure to remove electrode gel.

Magnetic resonance imaging (MRI)

More detailed and used to detect malformations, cortical dysplasia, or tumors.

Lumbar puncture

Measures spinal fluid pressure and detects infection (meningitis).

Computed tomography (CT) scan

Detects hemorrhage, infarction or malformations.

PATIENT-CENTERED CARE

NURSING CARE

Initiate seizure precautions for any child at risk.
- Pad side rails of bed, crib, and wheelchair.
- Keep bed free of objects that could cause injury.
- Have suction and oxygen equipment available.

During a seizure

- Protect from injury. If child is on the floor, place blanket under head.
- Maintain a position to provide a patent airway.
- Be prepared to suction oral secretions.
- Turn child to a side–lying position (decreases risk of aspiration).
- Loosen restrictive clothing.
- Do not attempt to restrain the child.
- Do not attempt to open the jaw or insert an airway during seizure activity. (This can damage teeth, lips, or tongue). Do not put anything in the child's mouth.
- Remove the child's glasses.
- Prepare to administer oxygen.
- Remain with the child.
- Note onset, time, and characteristics of seizure.
- Remain calm and reassure caregivers.

Postseizure

- Maintain the child in a side–lying position to prevent aspiration and to facilitate drainage of oral secretions.
- Check breathing, vital signs, and position of head and tongue.
- Assess the head and body for injuries, including the mouth (tongue, teeth).
- Perform neurologic checks.
- Allow for rest if necessary.
- Reorient and calm the client (due to agitation or confusion).
- Maintain seizure precautions, including placing the bed in the lowest position and padding the side rails to prevent future injury.
- Note the time of the postictal period.
- Remain with the client.
- Do not offer food or liquids until completely awake and swallowing reflex has returned.
- Encourage client to describe the period before, during, and after the seizure activity.

- Determine if the client experienced an aura, which can indicate the origin of seizure in the brain.
- Try to determine the possible trigger (fatigue or stress).
- Document the onset and duration of seizure and client findings/observations prior to, during, and following the seizure (level of consciousness, apnea, cyanosis, motor activity, incontinence).

MEDICATIONS

Antiepileptic drugs (AEDs)

EXPECTED EFFECT: Decrease incidence and severity of seizures.

Diazepam, phenytoin, carbamazepine, valproic acid, and fosphenytoin sodium, topiramate, lamotrigine, clonazepam
- Medication selection is based on the client's age, type of seizure, and other medical factors.
- A single medication is initiated at low dosage and gradually increased until seizures are controlled.
- A second medication can be added to achieve seizure control.

NURSING ACTIONS
- Monitor for seizure control.
- Assess allergies.
- Monitor for adverse effects.
- Monitor therapeutic blood medication levels for required medications.

CLIENT EDUCATION
- Take medications at the same time every day to enhance effectiveness.
- Be aware of medication and food interactions that are specific to each medication.
- Observe for adverse effects of the medications.
- Dosage can need to be increased as the child grows.
- Blood cell counts, urinalysis, and liver function tests will need to be obtained at frequent intervals to determine effect on organ function.

INTERPROFESSIONAL CARE

- The school nurse should be involved in providing for the child's safety in the school setting. This can include implementation of an individualized education plan or another specialized program.
- Referral to nutrition services if a ketogenic diet is prescribed.

THERAPEUTIC PROCEDURES

Brain surgery

- Removal of a tumor, lesion, or hematoma
- **Focal resection** of an area of the brain to remove epileptogenic zone
- **Hemispherectomy:** removal of one hemisphere of the brain; procedure is reserved for catastrophic, intractable epilepsy
- **Corpus callosotomy:** separation of the connection between the two hemispheres in the brain

Vagal nerve stimulator

- Under general anesthesia, the stimulator is implanted into the left chest wall and connected to an electrode that is placed at the left vagus nerve. The device is then programmed to administer intermittent vagal nerve stimulation at a rate specific to the client's needs.
- Adjunctive therapy to reduce seizure frequency for partial onset seizures which are unmanageable with antiepileptic medications.
- In addition to routine stimulation, the client can initiate vagal nerve stimulation by holding a magnet over the implantable device at the onset of seizure activity. This will either abort the seizure or lessen its severity.
- Short-term adverse effects include throat discomfort, cough, and dysphonia.

CLIENT EDUCATION

- It is important to undergo periodic laboratory testing to monitor AED levels.
- Do not stop medications without provider authorization.
- Adhere to the medication regimen.
- Possible medication interactions include decreased effectiveness of oral contraceptives.
- Ensure the child wears a medical alert bracelet or necklace at all times.
- Refer to the state's Department of Motor Vehicles to determine laws regarding driving for adolescents who have seizure disorders.
- Children should wear safety devices (helmets) while participating in sport (biking, skiing, horseback riding).
- Do not leave the child unattended in water or permit climbing on objects taller than the child.
- Older children should be encouraged to use a shower, rather than a bathtub, and leave the bathroom door unlocked while showering.

Active Learning Scenario

A nurse is planning care for a child who has tonic-clonic seizures. What actions should the nurse include in the plan of care? Use the ATI Active Learning Template: System Disorder to complete this item.

NURSING CARE: Describe nursing actions during and after a seizure.

- Avoid triggering factors (emotional stress, sleep deprivation, bright lights, fatigue, physical abuse).
- Not all disorders that cause epilepsy will affect the child's intelligence. The child can attend regular school.
- A ketogenic diet (high-fat, low-carbohydrate, and adequate protein) can be prescribed to promote body use of fat instead of glucose for energy. This can reduce seizure frequency, especially if the child has a metabolic disorder.
  - Monitor for adverse effects of diet therapy (lethargy, kidney or bladder stones, weight loss).
- Apply the same child-rearing techniques for the child as you would for other children (establishing rules, boundaries, consequences, and rewards).

> **!** Call Emergency Medical Service if any of the following occur.
>
> - Apnea
> - Seizure lasts more than 5 min
> - Status epilepticus
> - Pupils are not equal following seizure
> - Vomiting continuously for 30 min after the seizure
> - Unresponsive to pain or difficult to arouse
> - Seizure occurs in water
> - First seizure episode

COMPLICATIONS

Status epilepticus

Status epilepticus is prolonged seizure activity lasting 30 minutes or longer or continuous seizure activity in which the client does not enter a postictal phase. This acute condition requires immediate emergent treatment to prevent loss of brain function, which can become permanent.

NURSING ACTIONS

- Maintain airway, administer oxygen, establish IV access, perform ECG monitoring, and monitor pulse oximetry and ABG results.
- Administer a loading dose of diazepam or lorazepam. Buccal, rectal or nasal medications can be given until intravenous access is established. If seizures continue after the loading dose is given, fosphenytoin followed by phenobarbital should be administered.
- Provide support for the client and family.

Developmental delays

NURSING ACTIONS

- Promote optimal development.
- Make appropriate referrals.
- Provide support for the family.

Application Exercises

1. A nurse is teaching a group of caregivers about the risk factors for seizures. Which of the following factors should the nurse include in the teaching? (Select all that apply.)

   A. Febrile episodes

   B. Hypoglycemia

   C. Sodium imbalances

   D. Low blood lead levels

   E. Presence of diphtheria

2. A nurse is caring for a child who has absence seizures. Which of the following findings should the nurse expect? (Select all that apply.)

   A. Loss of consciousness

   B. Appearance of daydreaming

   C. Dropping held objects

   D. Falling to the floor

   E. Having a piercing cry

3. A nurse is providing teaching to the guardians of a child who is to have an electroencephalogram (EEG). Which of the following statements, by a guardian indicates teaching was effective?

   A. "My child should remain quiet and still during this procedure."

   B. "I cannot wash my child's hair prior to the procedure."

   C. "I should not give my child anything to eat prior to the procedure."

   D. "This procedure will be very painful for my child."

4. A nurse is caring for a child who just experienced a generalized seizure. Which of the following is the priority action for the nurse to take?

   A. Position the child in a side-lying position.

   B. Try to determine the seizure trigger.

   C. Reorient the child to the environment.

   D. Note the time of the postictal period.

5. A nurse is reviewing treatment options with the caregiver of a child who has epilepsy and is beginning to have more frequent seizure activity. Which of the following treatment options should the nurse include in the discussion? (Select all that apply.)

   A. Vagal nerve stimulator

   B. Additional antiepileptic medications

   C. Corpus callosotomy

   D. Focal resection

   E. Radiation therapy

Active Learning Scenario Key

Using the ATI Active Learning Template: System Disorder

NURSING CARE

- During a seizure
  - Protect the child from injury. (Move furniture away, hold the child's head in lap if on the floor.)
  - Position the child to maintain a patent airway.
  - Be prepared to suction oral secretions.
  - Turn the child to the side (decreases risk of aspiration).
  - Loosen restrictive clothing.
  - Do not attempt to restrain the child.
  - Do not attempt to open the jaw or insert an airway during seizure activity. (This can damage teeth, lips, or tongue.) Do not use padded tongue blades.
  - Remove glasses.
  - Administer oxygen if needed.
  - Remain with the child.
  - Note the onset, time, and characteristics of the seizure.
- Postseizure
  - Maintain the child in a side-lying position to prevent aspiration and to facilitate drainage of oral secretions.
  - Check for breathing, check vital signs, and check position of head and tongue.
  - Assess for injuries, including the mouth.
  - Perform neurologic checks.
  - Allow the child to rest if necessary.
  - Reorient and calm the child (they can be agitated or confused).
  - Maintain seizure precautions, including placing the bed in the lowest position and padding the side rails to prevent future injury.
  - Check inside the mouth to see if the lips and tongue have been bitten.
  - Note the time of the postictal period.
  - Remain with the child.
  - Do not offer food or liquids until completely awake and has a swallowing reflex has returned.
  - Encourage the child to describe the period before, during, and after the seizure activity.
  - Determine if the child experienced an aura, which can indicate the origin of seizure in the brain.
  - Try to determine the possible trigger (fatigue or stress).
  - Document the onset and duration of seizure and client findings/observations prior to, during, and following the seizure (level of consciousness, apnea, cyanosis, motor activity, incontinence).

Ⓝ *NCLEX® Connection: Physiological Adaptation, Alterations in Body Systems*

1. A, B, C. **CORRECT:** When taking action and providing teaching to a group of caregivers about risk factors for seizures, the nurse should include that febrile episodes, hypoglycemia, hyponatremia, and hypernatremia are all risk factors for inducing seizure activity.
   D. High blood lead levels, not low blood lead levels, are a risk factor for seizure activity.
   E. Diphtheria is a respiratory illness causing difficulty breathing and is not a risk factor for seizures.

   Ⓝ *NCLEX® Connection: Physiological Adaptation, Alterations in Body Systems*

2. A, B, C. **CORRECT:** When recognizing cues during the care of a child who has absence seizures, the nurse should expect the child to have a brief loss of consciousness lasting 5 to 10 seconds, exhibit behavior that resembles daydreaming, and drop objects that are being held.
   D. The nurse should expect a child who is having a tonic-clonic seizure to fall to the floor and have a piercing cry.
   E. The nurse should expect a child who is having a tonic-clonic seizure to fall to the floor and have a piercing cry.

   Ⓝ *NCLEX® Connection: Physiological Adaptation, Alterations in Body Systems*

3. A. **CORRECT:** When evaluating the outcomes of teaching to the caregivers of a child who is to have an EEG, the nurse should identify that the following statement by the caregiver indicates understanding of the teaching: "My child should remain still during this procedure." Excessive movements during the procedure can cause false-positive results.
   B. The child's hair should be washed to remove oils that permit adherence of the EEG electrodes.
   C. Foods are not withheld prior to an EEG. Withholding food may cause hypoglycemia which could impact the results of the EEG.
   D. The procedure is not painful; however, it can cause anxiety for the child.

   Ⓝ *NCLEX® Connection: Reduction of Risk Potential, Diagnostic Tests*

4. A. **CORRECT:** When taking action for the child who has just experienced a generalized seizure, the nurse should recognize that when using the airway, breathing, and circulation priority-setting framework, the first action to take is to place the child in a side-lying position to maintain a patent airway and prevent aspiration of secretions.
   B. Determining the seizure trigger can help prevent future seizure episodes. However, it is not the priority action.
   C. Reorienting the child to the environment following a generalized seizure is an appropriate action. However, it is not the priority action.
   D. Noting the timing of the postictal period can assist with planning seizure management. However, it is not the priority action.

5. A, B, C, D. **CORRECT:** When taking action and reviewing treatment options with the caregiver of a child who has epilepsy and worsening seizure activity, the nurse should include in the discussion that implantable vagal nerve stimulators, additional antiepileptic medications, a corpus callosotomy, and a focal resection are all treatments that can improve seizure control.
   E. Radiation therapy is used in cancer treatment and is not used to control seizures.

   Ⓝ *NCLEX® Connection: Reduction of Risk Potential, Therapeutic Procedures*

UNIT 2 SYSTEM DISORDERS
SECTION: NEUROSENSORY DISORDERS

CHAPTER 14 *Head Injury*

A head injury can be from mechanical force that involves cranium, scalp, meninges, or brain. Injuries that are unintentional are the leading cause of death in children who are greater than 1 year of age.

- **Concussion** is a mild traumatic injury to the brain that alters the way the brain functions.
- **Contusion** is bruising of the cerebral tissue.
- **Laceration** is tearing of the cerebral tissue.
- **Skull fractures** are caused by direct trauma to the skull. Fractures of the skull can be linear, depressed, comminuted, basilar, open or growing.

TYPES OF SKULL FRACTURES

- **Linear fractures** are the most common and involve a single fracture beginning from the point of impact; they do not cross the suture line.
- **Depressed fractures** occur when broken bone fragments are pushed inward.
- **Comminuted fractures** are made up of more than one linear fracture, and occur following intense impact or repeated trauma to the head (abuse).
- **Basilar fractures** involve those at the anterior or posterior base of the skull.
- **Open fractures** involve a break in the scalp or mucosa of the respiratory tract and can lead to osteomyelitis.
- **Growing fractures** occur when a fracture worsens due to pressure from brain herniation, dilated ventricles or a cyst.

HEALTH PROMOTION AND DISEASE PREVENTION

- Wear helmets when skateboarding, riding a bicycle, all-terrain vehicle, or motorcycle, skiing, playing contact sports, and participating in any other sport that might lead to head injury. Qs
- Wear seat belts when driving or riding in a car.
- Avoid dangerous activities (riding a bicycle at night without a light, driving faster than the speed limit or while under the influence of alcohol or controlled substances).
- Never shake a baby because it can cause head trauma.
- Install and use car seats for children in compliance with manufacturer recommendations and laws.

ASSESSMENT

RISK FACTORS

- Lack of supervision
- Inappropriate/absent safety practices
- Improper use of safety devices (helmets, seat belts)

EXPECTED FINDINGS

- History of events leading up to the injury, including any reports of dizziness, headache, diplopia, and/or vomiting
- Amnesia (loss of memory) before or after injury
- Alcohol or ingestion of controlled substances

PHYSICAL ASSESSMENT FINDINGS
- **Loss of consciousness:** The length of time the client is unconscious is significant.
- **Minor injury**
  - Possible loss of consciousness
  - Temporary period of confusion
  - Vomiting
  - Pallor
  - Irritability
  - Lethargy
  - Drowsiness
- **Progression of injury**
  - Marked changes in vital signs
  - Altered mental status
  - Focal neurologic deficits
  - Increase in agitation

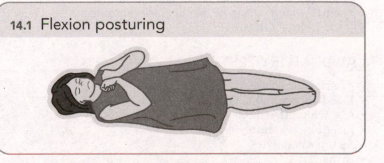

14.1 Flexion posturing

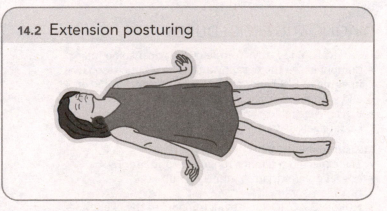

14.2 Extension posturing

- **Severe injury:** Increased intracranial pressure (ICP)
  - INFANTS: bulging fontanel, separation of cranial sutures, irritability, restlessness, increased sleeping, high-pitched cry, poor feeding, setting-sun sign, distended scalp veins
  - CHILDREN: nausea, headache, forceful vomiting, blurred vision, increased sleeping, inability to follow simple commands, decline in school performance, seizures
  - LATE FINDINGS: Alterations in pupillary response, posturing (flexion and extension), bradycardia, decreased motor response, decreased response to painful stimuli, Cheyne-Stokes respirations, optic disc swelling, decreased consciousness, coma
    - **Flexion posturing** (severe dysfunction of the cerebral cortex): Demonstrates the arms, wrists, elbows, and fingers flexed and bent inward onto the chest and the legs extended and rotated internally.
    - **Extension posturing** (severe dysfunction at the level of the midbrain): Demonstrates a backward arching of the legs and arms, flexed wrists and fingers, extended neck, clenched jaw, and possibly an arched back.
- **Skull Fractures**
  - Depressed: Skull appears misshapen
  - Basilar: Blood behind the tympanic membrane, over the mastoid process, or around the eye orbits; leakage of cerebral spinal fluid from the nose (CSF rhinorrhea), or ear (CSF otorrhea)
  - **Open:** tissue laceration over the fracture; possible CSF otorrhea or rhinorrhea
  - **Growing:** skull defect, scalp edema; neurologic changes can occur months to years after the initial injury (headache, hemiparesis, seizures, intellectual difficulty)

LABORATORY TESTS

- Arterial blood gases
- Blood alcohol and toxicology screening
- CBC with differential
- Liver function tests
- Serum electrolytes
- Urinalysis

DIAGNOSTIC PROCEDURES

- Cervical spine x-rays to rule out cervical spine injury
- Computerized tomography and/or magnetic resonance imaging of head and/or neck might be performed with and without contrast if indicated.
- Electroencephalogram (EEG) to assess for seizure activity.

Measurement of ICP

- The expected reference range is 1 to 10 mm Hg.
- A level greater than 15 mm Hg requires further assessment.
- NURSING ACTIONS: Provide support to the client and family. Qᴘᴄᴄ

PATIENT-CENTERED CARE

NURSING CARE

- Care is determined by the extent of the brain trauma.
- Ensure the spine is stabilized until a spinal cord injury is ruled out.
- Monitor vital signs, level of consciousness, pupils, ICP, motor activity, sensory perception, and verbal responses at frequent intervals. Use the Glasgow Coma Scale as indicated.
- Maintain a patent airway. Provide mechanical ventilation as indicated.
- Monitor oxygen saturation levels. Administer prescribed oxygen as indicated to maintain oxygen saturation level.
- Use padded restraints for clients who have agitation to prevent injury.
- Assess for clear fluid drainage from ears or nose (cerebral spinal fluid) and report to the provider.
- Assess for bleeding from the ear (indicates basal skull fracture) and report to the provider.
- Implement actions that will decrease ICP. Qs
  - Keep the head midline with the bed elevated to 30°, which will also promote venous drainage.
  - Avoid extreme flexion, extension, or rotation of the head and maintain in midline neutral position.
  - Keep the client's body in alignment, avoiding hip flexion/extension.
  - Minimize oral suctioning. Nasal suctioning is contraindicated.
  - Instruct the client to avoid coughing and blowing the nose, because these activities increase ICP.
- Implement measures to prevent complications of immobility (turn every 2 hr, maintain footboard and splints). Specialty beds might be used.
- Insert and maintain an indwelling urinary catheter.
- Administer stool softener to prevent straining (Valsalva maneuver).
- Provide a calm, restful environment (limit visitors, minimize noise).
- Use energy-conservation measures (alternating activities with rest periods, cluster nursing activities).
- Implement seizure precautions.
- Monitor fluid and electrolyte values and osmolarity to detect changes in sodium regulation, the onset of diabetes insipidus, or severe hypovolemia.
- Provide adequate fluids to maintain cerebral perfusion. When a large amount of IV fluids is prescribed, monitor the client for excess fluid volume, which might increase ICP.
- Maintain the client's safety (side rails up, padded side rails, call light within reach). Qs
- Provide nutritional support (parenteral nutrition, enteral nutrition). If nasogastric tube is used for nutritional support, do not overfeed due to the risk for aspiration.
- Maintain ongoing communication with the client and family.
- Instruct the family on effective ways to communicate with the child (touching, cuddling, talking, assisting with care as appropriate).

14.3 Activity Case Study

Scenario Introduction

Tina is a registered nurse who works triage in an emergency department (ED). Tina has just received Julian. Julian is a 9-year-old who was discharged from the ED 24 hours ago after being evaluated for a head injury sustained after falling from a tree.

Tina reviewed Julian's electronic medical record (EMR) and found that Julian's mother, Dia brought him to the emergency department after witnessing the fall. During the initial admission Julian's mother reported that he fell from approximately 5 feet after climbing a tree in their back yard. He reportedly lost conscious for less than a minute and was groggy but oriented upon awakening. A CT, CBC, and CMP were performed. All results were within the expected reference range. Before discharge, Julian's mother was educated regarding manifestations of increasing intracranial pressure as well as precautions to take if seizure activity developed. Julian's mother was instructed to seek immediate medical attention if seizures or manifestations of increased intracranial pressure occurred. Julian has no medical history but has had a cold for the last 2-3 days with rhinorrhea present.

Upon discharge, Julian had a closed, edematous area measuring 1.5 in x 1.5 in (3.8 cm x 3.8 cm) over the left occipital area of the skull. He reported tenderness to the area but denied headache or visual disturbances. He was oriented to person, place, and day. Demeanor was calm and cooperative. PERRLA with brisk reaction was observed. Vital signs were Temp: 37.2°C (98.9 °F), BP 104/58 mmHg, heart rate 88/min, respiratory rate 23/min, and oxygen saturation was 100% on room air.

Scene 1

Tina: Hello, Dia, I am Tina. I will be your triage nurse. I noticed that Julian was here yesterday for a head injury. What brings you back today?

Dia: Julian is just not acting right. He is irritable and said his head hurts. He also threw up right before we left the house to come back to the hospital.

Tina: You were right to bring him back to the hospital. Let me take a look at him.

Tina: Julian, can you show me where your head hurts?

Julian: It hurts everywhere.

Case Study Exercise

1. Before exiting the room in scene 2, which of the following actions should Nurse Gerad have implemented to help ensure Julian's safety? Sort each intervention into the following categories: Indicated or Contraindicated.

   A. Place the head of Julian's bed at a 30° angle

   B. Place pillows under Julian's head

   C. Keep the foot of the bed elevated

   D. Suction nasal secretions

   E. Raise the siderails of the bed

   F. Dim the lights in the room

Tina continues to assess Julian and observes that he is oriented to person, place, and day. He is irritable. The edematous area over the left occipital area is now measuring 2.5 in x 2.5 in (6.4 cm x 6.4 cm) and tender to touch. Julian rates the discomfort from the headache a 6 using the Wong Baker Faces pain rating scale. He denies visual disturbances. PERRLA with brisk reaction is observed. Vital signs are Temp: 36.8°C (98.2 °F), heart rate 92/min, respiratory rate 24/min, BP 102/53 mmHg, and oxygen saturation is 98% on room air. Julian has an occasional cough with rhinorrhea present.

Julian is admitted to a room in the ED.

Scene 2

Gerad: Hi Dia, Hi Julian, my name is Gerad. I am going to be your nurse now that you have been placed in a room. Julian, can you tell me if you are hurting anywhere right now?

Julian: My head hurts.

Dia: I am very worried about him. He just has not been acting right for the last few hours. Now he seems more sleepy than normal. What could be wrong? He was fine when we left!

Gerad: The provider wants Julian to have another CT scan to ensure that Julian has not developed any bleeding or swelling of the brain tissue. We are also going to repeat the lab work that he had yesterday. I will also need to start an IV on Julian.

Gerad: Julian, have you ever had an IV before?

Gerad explains what an IV is to Julian and initiates IV access without difficulty. Gerad explains the use of the call light to Julian and his mother and leaves the room.

Scene 3

Dia (opens the door to Julian's room and shouts): Please come quickly! Something is wrong with Julian. Gerad enters the room and finds Julian having a seizure.

Gerad presses the call light.

Gerad: I need help in here. My client is having a seizure.

Scenario Conclusion

Gerad ensures Julian's safety and monitors him until the seizure ends. After 1.5 minutes, the seizure ends and Julian enters a postictal state.

2. Which of the following client findings by Nurse Tina in scene 1 requires follow-up? (Select all that apply.)

   A. Julian's affect

   B. The edematous area on Julian's scalp

   C. Julian's blood pressure

   D. Julian's headache

   E. Julian's pupillary reaction

3. Following Julian's seizure, what is the priority action for Nurse Gerad to take?

   A. Assess vital signs

   B. Perform neurological checks

   C. Check position of the head and tongue

   D. Assess for injuries

MEDICATIONS

Mannitol: osmotic diuretic can be given IV decrease intracranial pressure and cerebral edema.

Antiepileptics: used to prevent or treat seizures that might occur.

Antibiotics: in cases of CSF leakage, lacerations, or penetrating injuries

Analgesics (acetaminophen): used for headache, pain, and fever management. Morphine and midazolam can be given as well.

THERAPEUTIC PROCEDURES

- Transfontanel percutaneous aspiration
- Subdural drains
- Placement of burr hole
- Craniotomy
  - Involves removal of part of the skull
  - The bone is replaced once the edema has resolved.
- For depressed fractures, surgery to elevate the depression

INTERPROFESSIONAL CARE

- Care for the client who has a head injury should include professionals from other disciplines as indicated. These might include physical, occupational, recreational, and/or speech therapists.
- Social services should be contacted to provide links to social service agencies and schools.
- Rehabilitation facilities are frequently used to compress the time required to recover from a head injury.

COMPLICATIONS

Epidural hematoma

Bleeding between the dura and the skull

MANIFESTATIONS: Short period of unconsciousness followed by a normal period for several hours, then lethargy or coma due to the accumulation of blood in the epidural space and compression of the brain. Vomiting can be present as well.

TREATMENT: Removal of accumulated blood or ligation of torn artery

Subdural hemorrhage

- Bleeding between the dura and the arachnoid membrane
- Might be a result of birth injury, falls, or violent shaking
- If retinal hemorrhages are observed as well, evaluate for child abuse

MANIFESTATIONS: Irritability, vomiting, increased head circumference, lethargy, anemia, seizures, coma.

TREATMENT: Subdural puncture

Cerebral edema

Can develop within 24 to 72 hr posttrauma

MANIFESTATIONS: Increased ICP, changes in cerebral flow

Brain herniation

Downward shift of brain tissue

MANIFESTATIONS: Loss of blinking, loss of gag reflex, pupils fail to react to light, Cushing's triad (systemic hypertension, bradycardia, respiratory distress), coma

---

Active Learning Scenario

A nurse is teaching a guardian of a child about complications of a head injury. What should be included in the teaching? Use the ATI Active Learning Template: System Disorder to complete this item.

COMPLICATIONS: Identify three and their corresponding manifestations.

Application Exercises

1. A nurse is caring for an adolescent who has a closed head injury. Which of the following findings should the nurse identify as manifestations of increased intracranial pressure (ICP)? (Select all that apply.)

   A. Report of headache

   B. Alteration in pupillary response

   C. Increased motor response

   D. Increased sleeping

2. A nurse is in the emergency department is assessing a child following a motor-vehicle crash. The child is unresponsive, has spontaneous respirations of 22/min, and has a laceration on the forehead that is bleeding. Which of the following actions should the nurse take first?

   A. Stabilize the child's neck.

   B. Clean the child's laceration with soap and water.

   C. Implement seizure precautions for the child.

   D. Initiate IV access for the child.

3. A nurse is caring for a child who has a head injury and is experiencing ICP. Which of the following medications should the nurse anticipate the provider prescribing?

   A. Albuterol

   B. Warfarin

   C. Mannitol

   D. Prednisone

Active Learning Scenario Key

Using the ATI Active Learning Template: System Disorder

COMPLICATIONS

Epidural hematoma
- Bleeding between the dura and the skull
- Manifestations: short period of unconsciousness followed by a normal period for several hours, then lethargy or coma due to the accumulation of blood in the epidural space and compression of the brain. Possible vomiting.

Subdural hemorrhage
- Bleeding between the dura and the arachnoid membrane
- Results from birth injury, falls, or violent shaking
- Manifestations: irritability, vomiting, increased head circumference, lethargy, coma, seizures
- Retinal hemorrhage can be an indicator of abuse.

Cerebral edema
- Develops 24 to 72 hr posttrauma
- Manifestations: increased ICP, changes in cerebral blood flow

Brain herniation
- Downward shift of brain tissue
- Manifestations: loss of blinking, loss of gag reflex, decreased pupillary response, Cushing's triad (systemic hypertension, bradycardia, respiratory distress), coma

Ⓝ *NCLEX® Connection: Physiological Adaptation, Unexpected Response to Therapies*

1. A, B, D. **CORRECT:** When analyzing cues, the nurse should identify those manifestations of increased intracranial pressure include headache, alterations in pupillary response, and increased sleeping. Other findings include a decrease in motor and sensory response.

   Ⓝ *NCLEX® Connection: Safety and Infection Control, Accident/Error/Injury Prevention*

2. A. **CORRECT:** When taking action for the child who has been in a motor-vehicle crash the nurse should identify that the child's greatest risk is for a cervical-spinal injury; therefore, the nurse should first stabilize the child's neck to prevent potential complications until a cervical-spinal injury can be ruled out. Other non-priority actions the nurse should take include cleaning the child's laceration with soap and water which can prevent infection, implementing seizure precautions which is a safety measure, and establishing IV access which allows for the administration of medications and fluids.

   Ⓝ *NCLEX® Connection: Safety and Infection Control, Accident/Error/Injury Prevention*

3. A. Albuterol is a bronchodilator that is used to manage asthma.
   B. Warfarin is an anticoagulant used to prevent thrombosis and manage atrial fib.
   C. **CORRECT:** ICP is managed by administering osmotic diuretics such as mannitol. This medication crosses the blood brain barrier and causes a reduction in ICP.
   D. Prednisone is a corticosteroid used to manage inflammation.

   Ⓝ *NCLEX® Connection: Pharmacological and Parenteral Therapies, Pathophysiology*

1. **INDICATED:** A, E, F; **CONTRAINDICATED:** B, C, D

   When taking action for a client who has sustained a head injury, the nurse should place the head of the bed at a 15-30° degree angle. This position helps to prevent a further increase in intracranial pressure by decreasing the risk for jugular compression and promoting venous drainage. The nurse should also implement seizure precautions which include raising the side rails on the bed, placing the bed in the lowest position, and padding the siderails. The lights in the room should be dimmed to help provide a calm environment and prevent further cerebral irritation. Keeping the foot of the bed elevated or placing pillows behind the knees is contraindicated because the child should be maintained in a neutral position. Nasal suctioning is contraindicated because this can cause further injury.

   Ⓝ *NCLEX® Connection: Physiological Adaptation, Unexpected Response to Therapies*

2. A, B, D. **CORRECT:** When analyzing cues, the Tina should identify that Julian's affect, the edematous area on his scalp, and his headache all require follow up. A new onset of headache and irritability are manifestations of increased intracranial pressure. Scalp edema, or hematomas, are indicators of intracranial injury and linear skull fractures. Since Julian's area of edema is increasing, follow-up is needed. Julian's blood pressure and pupillary findings are within the expected ranges and do not require follow-up.

   Ⓝ *NCLEX® Connection: Pharmacological and Parenteral Therapies, Pathophysiology*

3. C. **CORRECT:** When taking action for a child who has just had a seizure and using the airway, breathing, and circulation priority setting framework, the nurse should ensure that the airway is patent by checking the position of the head and tongue. The nurse should also position the child on their side to prevent aspiration if the child vomits. Assessing vital signs, performing neurological checks, and assessing the child for injuries are all actions that the nurse should implement after ensuring that the child has a patent airway.

   Ⓝ *NCLEX® Connection: Pharmacological and Parenteral Therapies, Pathophysiology*

UNIT 2   SYSTEM DISORDERS
SECTION: NEUROLOGIC DISORDERS

CHAPTER 15

Cognitive and Sensory Impairments

Sensory impairments in children most commonly affect the eyes and ears. Adequate vision and hearing are necessary for normal growth and development. Therefore, it is important to identify any impairments early in life.

Down syndrome is a common chromosomal abnormality that affects the child's growth and development and results in cognitive and sensory impairments.

Visual impairments

- Visual impairments encompass both partial sight and legal blindness.
- Common visual impairments in children include myopia, hyperopia, astigmatism, anisometropia, amblyopia, strabismus, cataracts, and glaucoma.

HEALTH PROMOTION AND DISEASE PREVENTION

Screen children for visual impairments yearly.

ASSESSMENT

RISK FACTORS

- Prenatal or postnatal conditions (retinopathy of prematurity, trauma, meningitis, and postnatal infections)
- Perinatal infections (herpes, rubella, syphilis, chlamydia, gonorrhea, and toxoplasmosis)
- Chronic illness (sickle cell disease, rheumatoid arthritis, retinoblastoma, albinism, and Tay-Sachs disease)

EXPECTED FINDINGS

Visual impairment manifestations

Myopia (nearsightedness)
- Sees close objects clearly, but not objects in the distance
- Headaches and vertigo
- Eye rubbing
- Difficulty reading
- Clumsiness (frequently walking into objects)
- Poor school performance

Hyperopia (farsightedness)
- Sees distant objects clearly, but not objects that are close
- Because of accommodation, not usually detected until age 7

Astigmatism
- Uneven refractive curvatures in vision in which only parts of letters on a page can be seen
- Headache and vertigo
- Appearance of normal vision because tilting the head enables all letters to be seen

Anisometropia
- Different refractive strength in each eye
- Headache and vertigo
- Excessive eye rubbing
- Poor school performance

Amblyopia (lazy eye): Reduced visual acuity in one eye

Strabismus: Esotropia (inward deviation of eye); **exotropia** (outward deviation of eye)
- Abnormal corneal light reflex or cover test
- Misaligned eyes
- Frowning or squinting
- Difficulty seeing print clearly
- One eye closed to enable better vision
- Head tilted to one side
- Headache, dizziness, diplopia, photophobia, and crossed eyes

Cataracts
- Gray opacity of the lens which prevents light from entering into the eye
- Decreased ability to see clearly
- Possible loss of peripheral vision
- Nystagmus
- Strabismus
- Absence of red reflex
- Infant: inability to reach and grab objects (a rattle toy)

Glaucoma
- Increase in ocular pressure in the eye
- Loss of peripheral vision
- Perception of halos around objects
- Red eye
- Excessive tearing (epiphora)
- Photophobia
- Spasmodic winking (blepharospasm)
- Corneal haziness
- Enlargement of the eyeball (buphthalmos)
- Possible pain
- Red reflex of the eye will appear gray to green

DIAGNOSTIC PROCEDURES

Visual screening
- This is completed using the Snellen letter, tumbling E, or picture chart (HOTV test) useful for preschoolers.
  - Place the child 10–20 feet from the chart depending on the age of the child and the type of chart used.
  - The child should be wearing glasses, if appropriate, and keep both eyes open during the screening.
  - While covering one eye, the child reads each line on the chart, starting at the bottom of the chart, until he can pass a line. The child needs to identify four of the six characters in the line correctly to pass.
  - The child is then asked to start at the top and move down until he can no longer pass a line.
  - The procedure is repeated with the other eye.
- **Partial visual impairment** is classified as visual acuity of 20/70 to 20/200.
- **Legal blindness** is classified as visual acuity of 20/200 or worse or a visual field of 20 degrees or less in the child's better eye. This is a legal definition not diagnosis.

Ocular alignment: Observed using the corneal light reflex test
- A flashlight is shone directly into the client's eye, from a distance of 16 inches.
- Reflected light should be observed in the same location on both pupils.

Cover test: Client is asked to cover each eye and observe an object at a distance of 13 inches. The cover is removed and the eye is observed for movement, which should not occur.

Peripheral vision: Evaluated by having the client fixate on an object
- A pencil is moved from beyond the field of vision into the range of peripheral vision.
- The client is asked to say stop when the object is noted in the peripheral vision. This angle is then measured.
- Each quadrant of peripheral vision is tested. The test is repeated in the other eye.
- Normal findings are 50° upward, 70° downward, 60° nasalward, and 90° temporally.

Color vision: Evaluated using the Ishihara or Hardy-Rand-Rittler test
- The client is shown a set of cards and asked to identify the number embedded in the confusion of colors.
- The client should identify all of the numbers on the cards with correct color vision.

PATIENT-CENTERED CARE

NURSING CARE

- Maintain normal to bright lighting for the child when reading, writing, or participating in any activity that requires close vision.
- Assess infants and children for visual impairments, and identify children that are high-risk.
- Observe for behaviors that suggest a decrease or loss of vision.

- Promote child's optimal development and parent-child attachment.
- Identify safety hazards, and prevent injury to the eyes (helmets, safety glasses). Qs
- Provide information regarding laser surgery for clients who have myopia, hyperopia, or astigmatism.

CLIENT EDUCATION
- Possible corrective measures include
  - Myopia: Biconcave lenses, contact lenses (adolescents), laser surgery (adolescents)
  - Hyperopia: Convex lenses, laser surgery
  - Astigmatism: Lenses that compensate for refractive errors, laser surgery
  - Anisometropia: Lenses that compensate for refractive errors, preferably corrective contacts, laser surgery
  - Amblyopia: Treat primary visual defect.
  - Strabismus: Occlusion therapy (patch stronger eye, remove patch 1 hr each day), laser surgery
  - Cataracts and glaucoma: Surgery
- Work with the child's school to make accommodations as needed.

CARING FOR A CHILD WHO HAS A VISION IMPAIRMENT
- Reassure the child and family.
- Orient the child to the surroundings and provide a safe environment.
- Promote independence and meeting developmental milestones while assisting with play and socialization. Qpcc
- Refer to educational services for visual impairment (Braille, audio tapes, special computers).
- Work with the child's school to make accommodations as needed.

Hearing impairments

Hearing impairments affect speech and the ability to clearly process linguistic sounds.

HEALTH PROMOTION AND DISEASE PREVENTION

- Screen for hearing impairments. Newborns are screened after delivery.
- Avoid hazardous noises, and wear ear protection in loud environments.

ASSESSMENT

RISK FACTORS

- Exposure to loud environmental sounds
- Pregnancy or labor and delivery factors (anatomic malformation, maternal ingestion of toxic substances during pregnancy, perinatal asphyxia, perinatal infection)
- Chronic ear infection or ototoxic medications
- Chronic conditions (Down syndrome, cerebral palsy)

TYPES OF HEARING IMPAIRMENT

- **Conductive losses** involve interference of sound transmission, which can result from otitis media, external ear infection, foreign bodies, or excessive ear wax.
- **Sensorineural losses** involve interference of the transmission along the nerve pathways, which can result from congenital defects or secondary to acquired conditions (infection, ototoxic medication, exposure to constant noise [as in a NICU]).
- **Central auditory imperception** involves all other hearing losses related to natural causes (aphasia, agnosia [inability to interpret sounds]).

EXPECTED FINDINGS

INFANTS
- Lack of startle reflex
- Failure to respond to noise
- Absence of vocalization by 7 months
- Lack of response to the spoken word
- Failure to localize sound by 6 months

OLDER CHILDREN
- Using gestures rather than talking after 15 months
- Failure to develop understood speech by 24 months
- Yelling to express emotions
- Irritability due to inability to gain attention
- Seeming shy or withdrawn
- Inattentive to surroundings
- Speaking in monotone
- Need for repeated conversation
- Speaking loudly for situation

PATIENT-CENTERED CARE

NURSING CARE

- Assess children for hearing impairment.
- Promote speech development, lip reading, and use of cued speech (hand gestures with verbal communication).
- Encourage socialization and use of aids to promote independence (flashing light when the doorbell or phone rings, telecommunication devices, closed captioning on the television).
- Refer child and family to community support groups.
- Use sign language or an interpreter if appropriate when working with a child who has hearing loss. Always talk to the child, not the interpreter.
- Assess gait/balance for instability.
- Identify safety hazards and adjust environment as needed. Qs
- Assist with the use of hearing aids.
  ○ Store batteries in a safe place.
  ○ If whistling sound present, turn down the volume or readjust the hearing aid in ear.
- Instruct families on methods to prevent further damage to hearing.

THERAPEUTIC PROCEDURES

Cochlear implants: Used for extensive hearing loss. Send impulses to the auditory nerve. Surgically implanted under skin or worn externally.

COMPLICATIONS

Delayed growth and development

Visual and hearing impairments can affect the child's speech and motor development. Identifying the impairment early can minimize this.

NURSING ACTIONS
- Encourage self-care and optimal independence.
- Make interprofessional referrals as needed (social services, speech therapy, physical therapy, occupational therapy, teachers). Qтс

CLIENT EDUCATION: Assist the family to obtain and access appropriate assistive devices.

Down syndrome

- Most common chromosomal abnormality of a generalized syndrome. Trisomy 21 is seen in 97% of cases of Down syndrome.
- Many medical conditions accompany Down syndrome (congenital heart malformation, hypotonicity, dysfunction of the immune system, thyroid dysfunction, leukemia).

ASSESSMENT

RISK FACTORS
- The cause is unclear but might be multicausal in nature.
- Maternal age greater than 35 years

EXPECTED FINDINGS
- Separated sagittal suture
- Enlarged anterior fontanel
- Small round head
- Occipital area of head flattened
- Upward, outward slant to eyes
- Small nose with depressed nasal bridge (saddle nose)
- Small ears with short pinna
- Epicanthal folds observed in ocular area
- High-arched narrow palate
- Protruding tongue
- Short, broad neck
- Shortened rib cage
- Possible congenital heart defect
- Protruding abdomen
- Incurved fifth finger (clinodactyly)
- Broad, short feet and hands with stubby toes and fingers
- Transverse palmar crease

- Large space between big and second toes with plantar crease
- Short stature
- Hyperflexibility, muscle weakness, and hypotonia
- Dry skin that cracks easily

DIAGNOSTIC PROCEDURES

PRENATAL: Testing for alpha-fetoprotein in maternal blood

INFANT: Chromosome analysis and echocardiography

CHILD: Neck x-rays prior to participation in sports

PATIENT-CENTERED CARE

NURSING CARE

- Swaddle the infant to prevent heat loss due to limp, extended body position.
- Assist family with feeding difficulties, and monitor dietary intake.
- Promote good skin care.
- Assess developmental progress at regular intervals.
- Support family at the time of diagnosis.
- Make appropriate referrals.
- Assist the parents in holding and bonding with the infant.

THERAPEUTIC PROCEDURES

Surgical interventions depend on the associated congenital anomalies. These can include cardiac defects or strabismus.

INTERPROFESSIONAL CARE

Social work, home health, school early intervention, genetic counseling, speech therapy, physical therapy, occupational therapy

NURSING ACTIONS: Listen to the concerns of the parents and discuss ethical dilemmas regarding treatment for physical defects. Provide standard postoperative care with emphasis on wound care, respiratory care, and pain management.

CLIENT EDUCATION
- Teach postoperative and home-care management.
- Reinforce the therapeutic plan of care.

CLIENT EDUCATION

- Aspirate nasal secretions.
- Change the infant's position frequently.
- Perform strategies to accommodate for the protruding tongue. A long handled spoon can be used for feeding to decrease tongue protrusion during feeding.
- Care for skin using moisturizing creams daily.
- A diet high in fiber and fluid can prevent constipation, and monitoring calorie intake can prevent obesity.

- Attend regular health care visits.
- Monitor developmental milestones.
- Monitor height and weight by plotting growth on National Center for Health Statistics or World Health Organization charts.
- Report manifestations of spinal cord compression: neck pain, loss of motor function, bladder incontinence, impaired sensations.
- Prepare for surgery for cardiac problems or strabismus if indicated.
- Evaluate eyesight and hearing frequently.
- Perform frequent thyroid functioning tests.
- Assess for atlantoaxial instability (neck pain, weakness, and torticollis).
- Perform strategies to prevent complications.

COMPLICATIONS

INTELLIGENCE: Mental capacity varies typically from mild to moderate cognitive impairment.

CONGENITAL ANOMALIES: About 40% to 45% have congenital heart disease. Other possible anomalies include hip subluxation, patella dislocation, duodenal atresia, tracheoesophageal fistula, and Hirschsprung's disease.

SENSORY PROBLEMS
- **Ocular problems** include strabismus, nystagmus, astigmatism, myopia, hyperopia, head tilt, excessive tearing, and cataracts.
- **Hearing loss** can occur due to shorter ear canals, otitis media, and impacted cerumen. Frequent otitis media, narrow canals, and impacted cerumen can contribute to the hearing problems.

OTHER PHYSICAL DISORDERS
- Frequent respiratory tract infections
- Increased incidence of leukemia
- Thyroid dysfunctions.
- Cardiac deficiencies

GROWTH: Both height and weight are reduced. Weight gain is more rapid than growth in height and can result in excessive weight by 36 months.

SEXUAL DEVELOPMENT: Male (lower fertility rates) and female genitalia can be underdeveloped and delayed.

Respiratory infections

Respiratory infections are common due to decreased muscle tone and impaired drainage of mucus associated underdeveloped nasal bone.

NURSING ACTIONS
- Rinse the child's mouth with water after feeding and at other times of the day when it is dry. Mucous membranes are dry due to constant mouth breathing, which also increases the risk for respiratory infection.
- Provide cool mist humidification to moisten secretions and clearing of the nasal passages with a bulb syringe as needed.

CLIENT EDUCATION

- Increase the oral intake of fluids.
- Rinse the client's mouth after feedings.
- Use cool mist in the room to assist in moistening secretions. Practice good hand hygiene. Dispose of contaminated tissues properly.
- Frequently reposition the child to promote respiratory function.
- Keep up to date with routine immunizations.
- Seek health care at the earliest indication of infection.
- Follow the antibiotic schedule if prescribed.

Active Learning Scenario

A nurse is planning to perform a visual screening test on a child. What nursing actions should the nurse include? Use the ATI Active Learning Template: Nursing Skill to complete this item.

DESCRIPTION OF SKILL: Explain the procedure.

OUTCOMES/EVALUATION: Describe findings that indicate visual impairment.

Active Learning Scenario Key

Using the ATI Active Learning Template: Nursing Skill

DESCRIPTION OF SKILL

- Choose appropriate chart: Snellen Letter, tumbling E, or picture chart.
- Place child 10 feet from the chart with heels on the 10-foot mark.
- Screen child wearing glasses, if appropriate.
- Child keeps both eyes open and covers one eye.
- First have the child start at the bottom and read each line, continuing up until the child can pass a line.
- Then have the child start at the top and move down until the child can no longer pass a line.
- To pass, the child needs to identify four of the six characters correctly.
- Repeat the procedure with the other eye.

OUTCOMES/EVALUATION

- Partial visual impairment is classified as visual acuity of 20/70 to 20/200.
- Legal blindness is classified as visual acuity of 20/200 or worse or a visual field of 20 degrees or less in the child's better eye.

Ⓝ *NCLEX® Connection: Health Promotion and Maintenance, Health Screening*

Application Exercises

1. A nurse is assessing a child who has myopia. Which of the following findings should the nurse expect? (Select all that apply.)
   - A. Headaches
   - B. Photophobia
   - C. Difficulty reading
   - D. Difficulty focusing on close objects
   - E. Poor school performance

2. A nurse is planning to perform a peripheral vision test on a child. Which of the following actions should the nurse take?
   - A. Place the child 10 feet away from a Snellen chart.
   - B. Show a set of cards to the child one at a time.
   - C. Cover the child's eye while performing the test on the other eye.
   - D. Have the child focus on an object while performing the test.

3. A nurse is assessing a toddler for possible hearing loss. Which of the following findings are indications of a hearing impairment? (Select all that apply.)
   - A. Uses monotone speech
   - B. Speaks loudly
   - C. Repeats sentences
   - D. Appears shy
   - E. Is overly attentive to the surroundings

4. A nurse is teaching a group of parents about possible manifestations of Down syndrome. Which of the following findings should the nurse include in the teaching? (Select all that apply.)
   - A. A large head with bulging fontanels
   - B. Larger ears that are set back
   - C. Protruding abdomen
   - D. Broad, short feet and hands
   - E. Hypotonia

5. A nurse is teaching the parent of an infant who has Down syndrome. Which of the following statements by the parent indicates an understanding of the teaching?
   - A. "I should expect him to have frequent diarrhea."
   - B. "I should place a cool mist humidifier in his room."
   - C. "I should avoid the use of lotion on his skin."
   - D. "I should expect him to grow faster in length than other infants."

1. A, C, E. **CORRECT:** When recognizing cues during the assessment of a child who has myopia, the nurse should expect the child to find reports of headaches, difficulty with reading, and poor school performance.
   B. Photophobia is a manifestation of strabismus.
   D. Difficulty focusing on close objects is a manifestation of hyperopia.

   Ⓝ *NCLEX® Connection: Health Promotion and Maintenance, Health Screening*

2. A. The nurse should plan to place the child 10 feet away from a Snellen chart when performing a visual acuity test, not a peripheral vision test.
   B. The nurse should plan to show a set of cards to the child one at a time when performing a color test, not a peripheral vision test.
   C. The nurse should plan to cover one of the child's eyes while performing testing on the other eye when completing a cover test, not a peripheral vision test.
   D. **CORRECT:** When generating solution for performing a peripheral vision test on a child, the nurse should plan to ask the child to focus on an object while bringing a pencil into the child's peripheral vision.

   Ⓝ *NCLEX® Connection: Health Promotion and Maintenance, Health Screening*

3. A, B, D. **CORRECT:** When recognizing cues, the nurse should recognize that the use of monotone speech, speaking loudly, and appearing shy and withdrawn are indicators of hearing impairment in a toddler.
   C. The nurse should recognize that repeating sentences is an expected developmental task for a toddler.
   E. The nurse should recognize that inattentiveness, not over attentiveness to surroundings, is a manifestation of a hearing impairment.

   Ⓝ *NCLEX® Connection: Basic Care and Comfort, Assistive Devices*

4. C, D, E. **CORRECT:** When taking action and teaching parents about manifestations of Down syndrome, the nurse should include protruding abdomen, broad, short feet and hands, and hypotonia as manifestations of Down syndrome.
   A. A child who has hydrocephalus, not Down syndrome, will exhibit a large head with bulging fontanels due to the increased CSF in the head.
   B. A child who has Down syndrome will exhibit small ears with a short pinna, not large set back ears.

   Ⓝ *NCLEX® Connection: Basic Care and Comfort, Illness Management*

5. A. The nurse should identify that the statement, "I should expect him to have frequent diarrhea" does not indicate understanding of the teaching. Down syndrome increases the risk for constipation, resulting in the need for additional fluid and fiber in the diet.
   B. **CORRECT:** When evaluating the outcomes of teaching to parents of an infant who have Down syndrome, the nurse should recognize the statement, "I should place a cool mist humidifier in their room" as an indicator of understanding. Down syndrome increases the risk for respiratory infections. Using a cool mist humidifier in the infant's room helps prevent respiratory infections.
   C. The nurse should identify that the statement, "I should avoid the use of lotion on their skin" does not indicate understanding of the teaching. Down syndrome causes the infant to have dry skin that cracks easily. The parent should practice good skin care, including the application of lotion.
   D. The nurse should identify that the statement, "I should expect him to grow faster in length than other infants" does not indicate understanding of the teaching. Down syndrome results in reduced growth in length for infants and height for children.

   Ⓝ *NCLEX® Connection: Basic Care and Comfort, Illness Management*

When reviewing the following chapters, keep in mind the relevant topics and tasks of the NCLEX outline, in particular:

Safety and Infection Control

STANDARD PRECAUTIONS/TRANSMISSION-BASED PRECAUTIONS/SURGICAL ASEPSIS: Understand communicable diseases and the modes of organism transmission.

Pharmacological and Parenteral Therapies

EXPECTED ACTIONS/OUTCOMES: Use clinical decision making/critical thinking when addressing expected effects/outcomes of medications.

Reduction of Risk Potential

DIAGNOSTIC TESTS: Monitor the results of diagnostic testing and intervene as needed.

LABORATORY VALUES: Identify laboratory values for ABGs, BUN, cholesterol, creatinine, glucose, glycosylated hemoglobin, hematocrit, hemoglobin, INR, platelets, potassium, PT, PTT and APTT, sodium, and WBC.

THERAPEUTIC PROCEDURES: Educate client about treatments and procedures.

Physiological Adaptation

ALTERATIONS IN BODY SYSTEMS: Provide pulmonary hygiene.

ILLNESS MANAGEMENT
Manage the care of a client who has impaired ventilation/oxygenation.

Apply knowledge of client pathophysiology to illness.

UNEXPECTED RESPONSE TO THERAPIES: Recognize signs and symptoms of client complications and intervene.

CHAPTER 16
Oxygen and Inhalation Therapy

Oxygen is used to maintain adequate cellular oxygenation. It is used in the treatment of many acute and chronic respiratory problems (hypoxemia, cystic fibrosis, asthma). Supplemental oxygen can be delivered using a variety of methods, depending on individual circumstances.

Pulse oximetry is used to monitor the effectiveness of inhalation therapies.

Common treatment methods for children who have respiratory issues (acute or chronic) are nebulized aerosol therapy, metered-dose inhaler (MDI), dry powder inhaler (DPI), chest physiotherapy (CPT), oxygen therapy, suctioning, and artificial airway.

Pulse Oximetry

Pulse oximetry is a noninvasive measurement of the oxygen saturation (SaO_2) of arterial blood.
A pulse oximeter is a device that is operated by battery or electricity and has a sensor probe that is attached securely to the child's fingertip, toe, earlobe, or around the foot with a clip or band.

INDICATIONS

Pulse oximetry is used for a variety of situations in which quick assessment of a child's respiratory status is needed.

CONSIDERATIONS

PREPROCEDURE NURSING ACTIONS

- Find an appropriate probe site. The probe site must be dry and have adequate circulation. Remove polish from nails or remove earrings if using the earlobe.
- Be sure the child is in a comfortable position and that the arm is supported if a finger is used as a probe site.

INTRAPROCEDURE NURSING ACTIONS

- Note the pulse reading and compare it with the child's radial pulse. Any discrepancy between the values warrants further assessment.
- If continuous monitoring is required, make sure the alarms are set for a low and a high limit, the alarms are functioning, and the sound is audible. Move the probe every 4 to 8 hr or per facility policy to prevent pressure necrosis in infants who have disrupted skin integrity or poor perfusion.

POSTPROCEDURE NURSING ACTIONS

Report unexpected findings to the provider.

If a child's SaO_2 is less than the expected range (usually 90% to 92%) Qs
- Confirm that the sensor probe is properly placed with the light-emitting diode (LED) placed on the top of the nail when digits are used.
- Confirm that the oxygen delivery system is functioning and that the child is receiving the prescribed oxygen flow rate. Increase oxygen rate as prescribed.
- Place the child in a semi-Fowler's or Fowler's position to maximize ventilation.
- Encourage deep breathing.
- Report significant findings to the provider.
- Remain with the child and provide emotional support to decrease anxiety.

INTERPRETATION OF FINDINGS

- The expected reference range for SaO_2 is 95% to 100%. Acceptable levels can range from 91% to 100%. Some illnesses can allow for a SaO_2 of 85% to 89%.
- Results less than 91% require nursing intervention to assist the child to regain acceptable SaO_2 levels. A SaO_2 of less than 86% is a life-threatening emergency. The lower the SaO_2 level, the less accurate the value.

Nebulized Aerosol Therapy

The process of nebulization breaks up medications into minute particles that are then dispersed throughout the respiratory tract. These droplets are much finer than those created by inhalers.

INDICATIONS

Respiratory conditions that necessitate bronchodilators, corticosteroids, mucolytics, or antibiotics.

CONSIDERATIONS

PREPARATION OF THE CLIENT

- Instruct the child and family that the treatment can take 10 to 15 min.
- Determine if the child should use a mouthpiece, mask, or blow-by.
- Perform a preprocedure assessment, including vital signs and oxygen saturation.
- Pour the medication into the small container and attach the device to an air or oxygen source.

ONGOING CARE

- Encourage the child to take slow, deep breaths by mouth.
- Monitor the child during the treatment, watching carefully for indications of local tracheal or bronchial effects (spasms, edema).
- Assess vital signs, oxygen saturation, and lung sounds at the completion of treatment.
- Assist the family with obtaining a nebulizer for home use if needed.
- Enforce recommendations for aerosolized medications.
- Monitor for adverse reactions to medications.

CLIENT EDUCATION

- Teach the family how to operate a home nebulizer.
- Teach the family about adverse effects of the prescribed medications.

Metered-Dose Inhaler or Dry Powder Inhaler

These are handheld devices that allow children to self-administer medications on an intermittent basis. (16.1)

INDICATIONS

Respiratory conditions that necessitate bronchodilators or corticosteroids

CONSIDERATIONS

Provide instructions to the child and parents for use of an MDI

- Remove the cap from the inhaler.
- Shake the inhaler five to six times.
- Attach the spacer. (Encourage a spacer for children to facilitate proper inhalation of the medication.)
- Hold the inhaler with the mouthpiece at the bottom.
- Hold the inhaler with the thumb near the mouthpiece, and the index and middle fingers at the top.

- Instruct the child on an MDI placement technique.
  - **Open-mouth method**: Hold the inhaler approximately 3 to 4 cm (1.2 to 1.6 in) away from the front of the mouth.
  - **Closed-mouth method**: Place the inhaler between the lips and instruct the child to form a seal around the MD.
- Take a deep breath and then exhale.
- Tilt the head back slightly, and press the inhaler. While pressing the inhaler, begin a slow, deep breath that lasts for 3 to 5 seconds to facilitate delivery to the air passages.
- Hold the breath for approximately 5 to 10 seconds to allow the medication to deposit in the airways.
- If an additional puff is needed, wait 1 min between puffs.
- Take the inhaler out of the mouth and slowly exhale through the nose.
- Resume normal breathing.

Provide instructions to the child and parents for the use of a DPI

- Do not shake the device.
- Take the cover off the mouthpiece.
- Follow the directions of the manufacturer for preparing the medication (turning the wheel of the inhaler).
- Exhale completely.
- Place the mouthpiece between the lips and take a deep breath through the mouth.
- Hold breath for 5 to 10 seconds.
- Take the inhaler out of the mouth and slowly exhale through pursed lips.
- Resume normal breathing.
- If more than one puff is prescribed, wait the length of time directed before administering the second puff.
- Remove the canister and rinse the inhaler, cap, and spacer once a day with warm running water. Dry the inhaler before reuse.

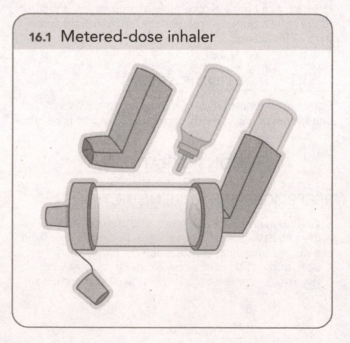

16.1 Metered-dose inhaler

COMPLICATIONS

Improper medication dosage related to improper use

- Inhalation is too rapid.
- Inability to coordinate inhalation with spray
- Not holding breath for adequate period

NURSING ACTIONS: Ensure the child uses the inhaler with proper technique.

CLIENT EDUCATION: Reinforce proper technique with client and family.

FUNGAL INFECTIONS

Fungal infections of the oral cavity can occur with corticosteroid use.

NURSING ACTIONS

- Assess mouth for manifestations of infections.
- Assist the child with rinsing his mouth after administration.

CLIENT EDUCATION: Instruct the child and guardians to clean the MDI and spacer after each use and to have the child rinse out the mouth and expectorate. Qpcc

Chest physiotherapy

Chest physiotherapy is a set of techniques that includes manual or mechanical percussion, vibration, cough, forceful expiration (or huffing), and breathing exercises, which are generally performed by respiratory therapists. Gravity and positioning loosen respiratory secretions and move them into the central airways, where they can be eliminated by coughing or suctioning to rid excessive secretions from specific areas of the lungs.

INDICATIONS

CLIENT PRESENTATION: Thick secretions with an inability to clear the airway

CONTRAINDICATION: Decreased cardiac reserves, pulmonary embolism, or increased intracranial pressure

CONSIDERATIONS

PREPROCEDURE NURSING ACTIONS

- Schedule treatments before meals or at least 1 hr after meals and at bedtime to decrease the likelihood of vomiting or aspirating.
- Administer a bronchodilator medication or nebulizer treatment prior to postural drainage if prescribed.

INTRAPROCEDURE NURSING ACTIONS

- Perform hand hygiene, provide privacy, and explain the procedure to the child and parents.
- Ensure proper positioning to promote drainage of specific areas of the lungs.
  - **Apical sections of the upper lobes**: Fowler's position
  - **Posterior sections of the upper lobes**: Sitting position with child leaning forward curled over pillows
  - **Anterior segments of both upper lobes**: Supine and rotated slightly away from side being drained
  - **Superior segments of both lower lobes**: Prone with hips elevated on pillows.
- Apply manual percussion by using cupped hand or a special device to clap rhythmically on the chest wall to break up secretions.
- Electronic percussion is applied by a vest device worn by the child.
- Individualize the position used and the duration and frequency of treatment.
- Discontinue the procedure if the child reports faintness or dizziness.

POSTPROCEDURE NURSING ACTIONS

- Perform lung auscultation and assess the amount, color, and character of the expectorated secretions.
- Document interventions and repeat the procedure as prescribed (typically three or four times per day).

Oxygen therapy

- Oxygen therapy increases the oxygen concentration of the air that is being breathed.
- Oxygen can be delivered via nasal cannula, face mask, face tent, CPAP, BiPAP, tent, hood, or mechanical ventilator. (16.2)
- Humidification of oxygen moistens the airways, which promotes loosening and mobilization of pulmonary secretions and prevents drying and injury of respiratory structures.
- While the client is receiving oxygen, continue to monitor vital signs, including SaO_2 for changes, and intervene as needed.

INDICATIONS

Hypoxemia

Hypoxemia develops when there is an inadequate level of oxygen in the blood. Hypovolemia, hypoventilation, and interruption of arterial flow can lead to hypoxemia.

EARLY MANIFESTATIONS

- Tachypnea
- Tachycardia
- Restlessness
- Pallor of the skin and mucous membranes
- Evidence of respiratory distress (use of accessory muscles, nasal flaring, tracheal tugging, adventitious lung sounds)

Late Manifestations

- Confusion and stupor
- Cyanosis of skin and mucous membranes
- Bradypnea
- Bradycardia
- Hypotension or hypertension

CONSIDERATIONS

PREPARATION OF THE CLIENT

- Warm oxygen to prevent hypothermia.
- Use a calm, nonthreatening approach.
- Explain all procedures to the child and parents.
- Place the client in semi–Fowler's or Fowler's position to facilitate breathing and to promote chest expansion.
- Ensure that equipment is working properly.

ONGOING CARE

- Provide oxygen therapy at the lowest liter flow that corrects hypoxemia.
- Assess/monitor lung sounds and respiratory rate, rhythm, and effort to determine the need for supplemental oxygen.
- Do not allow oxygen to blow directly onto infants' faces.
- Change linens and clothing frequently.
- Monitor the child's temperature closely in an oxygen tent for hypothermia.
- Assess/monitor oxygenation status with pulse oximetry and ABGs.
- Apply the oxygen delivery device prescribed.
- Provide oral hygiene as needed.
- Promote turning, coughing, deep breathing, and use of incentive spirometry and suctioning.

- Promote rest and decrease environmental stimuli.
- Provide emotional support for children who appear anxious.
- Assess nutritional status and provide supplements as prescribed.
- Assess/monitor skin integrity closely for pressure injuries. Move devices and inspect the skin several times daily. Provide moisture and pressure–relief devices as indicated.
- Assess/monitor and document response to oxygen therapy.
- Titrate oxygen to maintain the prescribed oxygen saturation.
- Discontinue oxygen gradually.

COMPLICATIONS

COMBUSTION

Oxygen is combustible. Qs

NURSING ACTIONS

- Place "No Smoking" or "Oxygen in Use" signs to alert others of the combustion hazard.
- Know where the closest fire extinguisher is located.
- Have the child wear a cotton gown, because synthetics or wools can create sparks of static electricity.
- Ensure that all electric machinery (monitors, suction machines) are grounded.
- Avoid toys that can induce a spark.
- Do not use volatile, flammable materials (alcohol, acetone) near children who are receiving oxygen.
- Educate the child and others about the fire hazards of smoking with oxygen use. QPCC

16.2 Oxygen therapy delivery systems

DELIVERY SYSTEM	NURSING ACTIONS
Oxygen hood Small plastic hood that fits over the infant's head	Use a minimum flow rate of 4 to 5 L/min to prevent carbon dioxide buildup. Ensure that neck, chin, or shoulders do not rub against the hood. Secure a pulse oximeter for continuous SaO_2 monitoring.
Nasal cannula Disposable plastic tube with two prongs for insertion into the nostrils that delivers an oxygen concentrations of 24% to 44% FiO_2 at a flow rate of 1 to 6 L/min	Nasal cannulas are safe, easy to apply, and well tolerated. The child is able to eat, talk, and ambulate while wearing a cannula. Cannulas can be used by infants and older children who are cooperative. Assess the patency of the nares. Ensure that the prongs fit in the nares properly. A nasal cannula can cause skin breakdown and dry mucous membranes. Supply the child with a water-soluble gel if the nares are dry. Provide humidification for flow rates greater than 4 L/min. Prongs can become dislodged easily. Monitor the child frequently.
Pediatric face mask Pediatric-size mask that covers the nose and mouth	Used for short-term therapy Used at a flow rate of 5 to 10 L/min to minimize carbon dioxide rebreathing. Face masks require a snug fit and might not be tolerated. Used for supplying high oxygen flow rate or for children who are mouth breathers.

Oxygen toxicity

- Oxygen toxicity can result from high concentrations of oxygen, long duration of oxygen therapy, and the child's degree of lung disease.
- Hypoventilation and increased PaCO2 levels allow for rapid progression into unconscious state.

MANIFESTATIONS: Nonproductive cough, substernal pain, nasal stuffiness, nausea, vomiting, fatigue, headache, sore throat, and hypoventilation

NURSING ACTIONS

- Use the lowest level of oxygen necessary to maintain an adequate SaO_2.
- Monitor ABGs and notify the provider if PaCO2 levels rise outside of the expected reference range.
- Decrease the oxygen flow rate gradually.

Suctioning

Suctioning can be accomplished orally, nasally, endotracheally, or through a tracheostomy tube.

INDICATIONS

To remove mucus plugs and excessive secretions

CLIENT PRESENTATION: Early manifestations of hypoxemia (restlessness, tachypnea, tachycardia, decreased SaO_2 levels), adventitious breath sounds, visualization of secretions, cyanosis, absence of spontaneous cough)

CONSIDERATIONS

Nasal suctioning

- Use clean technique.
- Use a mushroom tip catheter.

Oral suctioning

- Use clean technique.
- Use a hard catheter tip.
- Insert in sides of mouth.

Endotracheal and tracheal suctioning

PREPROCEDURE NURSING ACTIONS

- Perform hand hygiene, provide privacy, and explain the procedure to the child.
- Don the required personal protective equipment. Assist the child to a high-Fowler's or Fowler's position for suctioning if possible.
- Perform through a tracheostomy or an endotracheal tube. Select a catheter with a diameter one half the diameter of the tracheostomy tube.
- Ask for assistance if necessary.
- Hyperoxygenate and hyperventilate the child using a bag-valve-mask resuscitator or specialized ventilator function with an FiO2 of 100%.
- Obtain baseline breath sounds and vital signs, including oxygen saturation (SaO_2) by pulse oximeter. Oxygen saturation should be monitored continually during the procedure.

INTRAPROCEDURE NURSING ACTIONS

- Use correct surgical aseptic technique as identified in appropriate resources.
- Maintain ongoing assessments of oxygen status while performing the procedure.
- Limit suction time to less than 5 seconds for infants and less than 10 seconds for children.
- Allow the child to rest 30 to 60 seconds after each aspiration for oxygen saturation to return to normal.

POSTPROCEDURE NURSING ACTIONS: Document the child's response.

COMPLICATIONS

Hypoxia

NURSING ACTIONS

- Stop the procedure.
- Hyperoxygenate the child.

Artificial airways

- A tracheotomy is a sterile surgical incision into the trachea through the skin and muscles for the purpose of establishing an airway.
- A tracheotomy can be performed as an emergency procedure for epiglottitis, croup, or foreign-body aspiration, or as a scheduled surgical procedure.
- A tracheostomy is the stoma/opening that results from a tracheotomy to provide and secure a patent airway. A tracheostomy can be permanent or temporary.
- Artificial airways can be placed orotracheally, nasotracheally, or through a tracheostomy to assist with respiration.
- Pediatric tracheostomy tubes made of plastic and/or with a cuff to prevent dislodgement.

INDICATIONS

CLIENT PRESENTATION: Obstruction of the upper airway requiring the use of artificial ventilation

CONSIDERATIONS

- Assess/monitor
  - Oxygenation, ventilation (respiratory rate, effort, SaO_2), and vital signs hourly
  - Thickness, quantity, odor, and color of mucous secretions
  - The stoma and skin surrounding the stoma for manifestations of inflammation or infection (redness, swelling, or drainage)
- Provide adequate humidification and hydration to thin secretions and decrease the risk of mucus plugging.
- Suctioning only as often as necessary to maintain patency of the tube. Do not suction routinely. This can cause mucosal damage, bleeding, and bronchospasm.

- Assess/monitor the need for suctioning. Suction as necessary when assessment findings indicate the need to do so (audible/noisy secretions, crackles, restlessness, tachypnea, tachycardia, and mucus in the airway).
- Maintain surgical aseptic technique when suctioning to prevent infection.
- Provide emotional support to the child and guardians.
- Provide oral hygiene every 2 hr.
- Provide tracheostomy care as indicated by the provider.
- Check ties frequently and change if soiled.
- Keep an emergency tracheostomy tube (one size smaller) at the bedside.

CLIENT EDUCATION
- Provide discharge teaching regarding the following.
  ○ Tracheostomy care
  ○ Assess skin at the tracheostomy site for drainage or breakdown. This area should be cleaned with soap and water.
  ○ Findings that the family should immediately report to the provider (manifestations of infection or copious secretions)
  ○ Ways to promote improved nutrition
- Provide written material for parents to reinforce instructions. Qpcc

COMPLICATIONS

Accidental decannulation

Accidental decannulation in the first 72 hr after surgery is an emergency because the tracheostomy tract has not matured and replacement can be difficult.

NURSING ACTIONS: Always have an additional staff member present when moving the tube or during any situation in which decannulation can occur. Keep a new tube and obturator at the bedside.

CLIENT EDUCATION: When caring for the tube at home, have a second tube available in the event of dislodgement.

Occlusion

Occlusion is a situation in which the tube is clogged with secretions and prevents adequate air exchange.

NURSING ACTIONS: Maintain a patent airway with suctioning.

CLIENT EDUCATION: Suction to prevent occlusion.

Active Learning Scenario

A nurse is teaching a newly licensed nurse about how to care for a client who has an artificial airway. What information should be included in the teaching? Use the ATI Active Learning Template: Basic Concept to complete this item.

DESCRIPTION OF SKILL: Outline the assessment and nursing interventions for a client who has an artificial airway.

Application Exercises

1. A nurse is preparing to apply a pulse oximeter to a child who is having an acute asthma attack. In which of the following areas can the nurse correctly place the pulse oximeter? (Select all that apply.)
   A. Forearm
   B. Earlobe
   C. Cheek
   D. Foot
   E. Fingertip
   F. Toe

2. A nurse caring for a child who is receiving oxygen therapy and is on a continuous oxygen saturation monitor that is reading 89%. Which of the following actions should the nurse take first?
   A. Increase the oxygen flow rate.
   B. Encourage the child to take deep breaths.
   C. Ensure proper placement of the sensor probe.
   D. Place the child in the Fowler's position.

3. A nurse is caring for a child who is receiving a bronchodilator medication by nebulized aerosol therapy. Which of the following actions should the nurse take? (Select all that apply.)
   A. Instruct the child that the treatment will last 30 min.
   B. Obtain vital signs prior to the procedure.
   C. Tell the child to take slow deep breaths.
   D. Determine if the child should use a mask.
   E. Attach the device to an air source.

4. A nurse is planning to teach a client who has new prescription for a metered-dose inhaler how to use the inhaler. Place the following instructions for using a metered-dose inhaler in the correct order.
   A. Attach the spacer.
   B. Hold the breath for approximately 5 to 10 seconds.
   C. Hold the inhaler with the mouthpiece at the bottom
   D. Instruct the child on placement technique (open or closed mouth)
   E. Remove the cap from the inhaler.
   F. Shake the inhaler five to six times.
   G. Take a deep breath and then exhale.
   H. Take the inhaler out of the mouth and exhale slowly through the nose.
   I. Tilt the head back slightly and press the inhaler. While pressing the inhaler, begin a slow, deep breath that lasts for 3 to 5 seconds to facilitate delivery to the air passages.

5. A nurse in the emergency department is assessing a newly-admitted infant. Which of the following findings is an early indication of hypoxemia?
   A. Nonproductive cough
   B. Hypoventilation
   C. Tachypnea
   D. Nasal stuffiness

Application Exercises Key

1. B, D, E, F. **CORRECT:** The nurse should identify that the pulse oximeter probe can be placed on the child's fingertip, toe, foot, or earlobe.

2. A. Increasing the oxygen flow rate for a child who has an oxygen saturation of 89% is important but there is another action that the nurse should take first.
   B. Encouraging the child to take deep breaths to increase oxygenation is important but there is another action that the nurse should take first.
   C. **CORRECT:** When prioritizing hypothesis using the nursing process for a child who is receiving oxygen therapy and has as an oxygen saturation of 89%, the nurse should first ensure that the sensor probe is properly placed.
   D. Placing the child in Fowler's position to increase oxygenation is important but there is another action that the nurse should take first.

   Ⓝ *NCLEX® Connection: Physiological Adaptation, Illness Management*

3. B, C, D, E. **CORRECT:** When taking action for a child who is receiving a bronchodilator medication by nebulized aerosol therapy, the nurse should obtain vital signs prior to the procedure, determine if the child should use a mask, attach the device to an air source, and instruct the child to take slow deep breaths.
   A. A nebulized medication takes approximately 10 to 15 min to deliver, not 30 minutes.

   Ⓝ *NCLEX® Connection: Physiological Adaptation, Therapeutic Procedures*

4. E, F, A, C, D, G, I, B, H

   When generating solutions for inhaler use, the nurse should plan to teach the child to first remove the cap from the inhaler. After removing the cap, the child should shake the inhaler five to six time. If a spacer is being used, the child should then attach the spacer. After attaching the spacer, the child should hold the inhaler with the mouthpiece down, the thumb on the mouthpiece and the index and middle fingers on top of the mouthpiece. After preparing the inhaler, the nurse should instruct the child on inhaler placement. When the inhaler is properly placed for usage, the child should be instructed to take a deep breath, exhale, tilt the head back while pressing the inhaler and begin taking a slow, deep breath over 3 to 5 seconds. The child should hold the breath for 5 to 10 seconds before removing the inhaler and slowly exhaling through the nose.

   Ⓝ *NCLEX® Connection: Pharmacological and Parenteral Therapy, Medication Administration*

5. A. A nasal stuffiness and a nonproductive cough are manifestations of a respiratory infection.
   B. Hypoventilation is a manifestation of oxygen toxicity.
   C. **CORRECT:** When recognizing cure, the nurse should identify that tachypnea is an early indication of hypoxemia.
   D. A nasal stuffiness and a nonproductive cough are manifestations of a respiratory infection.

   Ⓝ *NCLEX® Connection: Physiological Adaptation, Illness Management*

Active Learning Scenario Key

Using the ATI Active Learning Template: Nursing Skill

ASSESSMENT
- Oxygenation, ventilation (respiratory rate, effort, SaO₂), and vital signs hourly
- Thickness, quantity, odor, and color of mucous secretions
- The stoma and skin surrounding the stoma for manifestations of inflammation or infection (redness, swelling, or drainage)
- Assess/monitor the need for suctioning. Suction as necessary when assessment findings indicate the need to do so (audible/noisy secretions, crackles, restlessness, tachypnea, tachycardia, and mucus in the airway).

INTERVENTIONS
- Provide adequate humidification and hydration to thin secretions and decrease the risk of mucus plugging.
- Suctioning only as often as necessary to maintain patency of the tube. Do not suction routinely. This can cause mucosal damage, bleeding, and bronchospasm.
- Maintain surgical aseptic technique when suctioning to prevent infection.
- Provide emotional support to the child and guardians.
- Provide oral hygiene every 2 hr.
- Provide tracheostomy care as indicated by the provider.
- Check ties frequently and change if soiled.
- Keep an emergency tracheostomy tube (one size smaller) at the bedside.

Ⓝ *NCLEX® Connection: Physiological Adaptation, Illness Managemen*

CHAPTER 17 # Acute and Infectious Respiratory Illnesses

Acute and infectious respiratory illnesses prevalent in children include tonsillitis, nasopharyngitis, pharyngitis, croup syndromes, bacterial tracheitis, bronchitis, bronchiolitis, allergic rhinitis, and pneumonia.

Tonsillitis and Tonsillectomy

Tonsils are masses of lymph-type tissue found in the pharyngeal area. They filter pathogenic organisms (viral and bacterial), which helps to protect the respiratory and gastrointestinal tracts. In addition, they contribute to antibody formation.

Tonsils are highly vascular, which helps them to protect against infection because foreign materials (viral or bacterial organisms), enter the body through the mouth.

Palatine tonsils are located on both sides of the oropharynx. These are the tonsils removed during a tonsillectomy.

Pharyngeal tonsils, also known as the adenoids, are removed during an adenoidectomy.

Enlarged tonsils
- In some instances, enlarged tonsils can block the nose and throat. This can interfere with breathing, nasal and sinus drainage, sleeping, swallowing, and speaking.
- Enlarged tonsils also can disrupt the function of the Eustachian tube, which can cause otitis media or impede hearing.

Acute tonsillitis occurs when the tonsils become inflamed and reddened. Acute tonsillitis can become chronic.

ASSESSMENT

RISK FACTORS
- Exposure to a viral or bacterial agent
- Immature immune systems (younger children)

EXPECTED FINDINGS
- Report of sore throat with difficulty swallowing
- History of otitis media and hearing difficulties

PHYSICAL ASSESSMENT FINDINGS
- Mouth odor
- Mouth breathing
- Snoring

- Nasal qualities in the voice
- Fever
- Tonsil inflammation with redness and edema
- Difficulty swallowing or eating

LABORATORY TESTS

Throat culture for group A beta-hemolytic streptococci (GABHS)

PATIENT-CENTERED CARE

NURSING CARE

Tonsillitis
- Provide treatment for manifestations of viral tonsillitis (rest, warm fluids, warm salt-water gargles).
- Administer antibiotic therapy as prescribed for bacterial tonsillitis.

MEDICATIONS

Antipyretics/analgesics: acetaminophen

Hydrocodone is indicated for the child having difficulty drinking fluids.

Antipyretics

Decrease fever and manage pain.

NURSING ACTIONS: Be aware of allergies.

CLIENT EDUCATION: Teach appropriate dosing for acetaminophen and ibuprofen.

Antibiotics

For treatment of GABHS infection

NURSING ACTIONS: Be aware of allergies.

CLIENT EDUCATION: Teach guardians to administer antibiotics for the full course of treatment.

THERAPEUTIC PROCEDURES

Tonsillectomy and/or adenoidectomy

PREOPERATIVE NURSING ACTIONS: Maintain NPO status.

POSTOPERATIVE NURSING ACTIONS
- Positioning
  ○ Place in position to facilitate drainage.
  ○ Elevate head of bed when child is fully awake.
- Assessment
  ○ Assess for evidence of bleeding, which includes frequent swallowing, clearing the throat, restlessness, bright red emesis, tachycardia, and/or pallor.
  ○ Assess the airway and vital signs.
  ○ Monitor for difficulty breathing related to oral secretions, edema, and/or bleeding.

- Comfort measures
  - Administer liquid analgesics or tetracaine lollipops as prescribed.
  - Provide an ice collar.
  - Avoid administering codeine postoperatively.
  - Offer ice chips or sips of water to keep throat moist.
  - Administer pain medication on a regular schedule.
- Diet
  - Encourage clear liquids and fluids after a return of the gag reflex, avoiding red-colored liquids, citrus juice, and milk-based foods initially.
  - Advance the diet with soft, bland foods.
- Instruction
  - Discourage coughing, throat clearing, and nose blowing in order to protect the surgical site.
  - Avoid straws as they can damage the surgical site
  - Alert guardians that there can be clots or blood-tinged mucus in vomitus.

CLIENT EDUCATION

- Notify the provider if bright red bleeding occurs.
- Get plenty of rest.
- Contact the provider if the child experiences difficulty breathing, lack of oral intake, increase in pain, and/or indications of infection.
- Ensure that the child does not put objects in the mouth.
- Administer pain medications for discomfort.
- Intake plenty of fluids, advance to a soft diet, and avoid foods that are irritating or highly seasoned.
- Limit activity to decrease the potential for bleeding.
- Full recovery usually occurs in approximately 14 days.
- Observe for manifestations of hemorrhage, dehydration, and infection, and notify the provider if necessary.

COMPLICATIONS

HEMORRHAGE

NURSING ACTIONS
- Use a good light source and possibly a tongue depressor to directly observe the throat.
- Assess for findings of bleeding (tachycardia, repeated swallowing and clearing of throat, hemoptysis). Hypotension is a late manifestation of shock.
- Contact the provider immediately if there is any indication of bleeding.

CLIENT EDUCATION: Instruct family to report indications of bleeding (frequent swallowing, clearing the throat, restlessness, bright red emesis, tachycardia, pallor).

DEHYDRATION

NURSING ACTIONS
- Encourage oral fluids.
- Monitor I&O.

CLIENT EDUCATION
- Increase intake of oral fluids.
- Observe for manifestations of dehydration.

CHRONIC INFECTION

Chronically infected tonsils with GABHS can pose a potential threat to other parts of the body. Some children who frequently have tonsillitis can develop other diseases (rheumatic fever and kidney infection).

CLIENT EDUCATION: Seek medical attention when the child presents with manifestations of tonsillitis.

Common Respiratory Illness

Disorders can affect both the upper (oronasopharynx, pharynx, larynx, and upper part of the trachea) and lower (bronchi, bronchioles, and alveoli) respiratory tracts. Infections of the respiratory tract can affect more than one area.

The information in this section is applicable to a range of common respiratory illnesses.

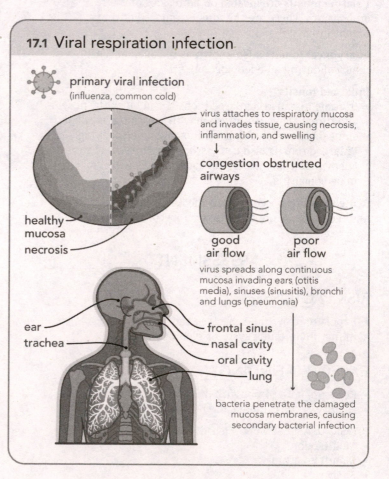

17.1 Viral respiration infection

primary viral infection
(influenza, common cold)

virus attaches to respiratory mucosa and invades tissue, causing necrosis, inflammation, and swelling

↓

congestion obstructed airways

healthy mucosa

necrosis

good air flow

poor air flow

virus spreads along continuous mucosa invading ears (otitis media), sinuses (sinusitis), bronchi and lungs (pneumonia)

ear

trachea

frontal sinus

nasal cavity

oral cavity

lung

bacteria penetrate the damaged mucosa membranes, causing secondary bacterial infection

ASSESSMENT

RISK FACTORS

Age

- Infants between 3 and 6 months of age are at increased risk due to the decrease of maternal antibodies acquired at birth and the lack of antibody protection.
- Viral infections are more common in toddlers and preschoolers. The incidence of these infections decreases by age 5.
- Certain viral agents can cause serious illness during infancy, but only cause a mild illness in older children.

Anatomy

- A short, narrow airway can become easily obstructed with mucus or edema.
- A short respiratory tract allows infections to travel quickly to the lower airways.
- Infectious agents have easy access to the middle ear through the short and open Eustachian tubes of infants and young children.

Decreased resistance

- Compromised immune system
- Anemia
- Nutritional deficiencies
- Allergies
- Chronic medical conditions (asthma, cystic fibrosis, chronic lung disease, cardiac anomalies)
- Exposure to second-hand smoke

Seasonal variables

- Children who have asthma have a greater incidence of respiratory infections during cold weather.
- Respiratory syncytial virus (RSV) and other common respiratory infections are more common during the winter and spring.
- Infections caused by Mycoplasma pneumoniae are more frequent during autumn and early winter.

EXPECTED FINDINGS

- Nursing history that includes recent infections, medications taken, immunization status, and family coping
- Reports of sore throat, decreased activity level, chest pain, fatigue, difficulty breathing, shortness of breath, cough, and decreased appetite

LABORATORY TESTS

Throat culture or rapid antigen testing to rule out GABHS infection

PATIENT-CENTERED CARE

NURSING CARE

- Closely monitor progression of illness and ensuing respiratory distress. Observe for increased heart and respiratory rate, retractions, nasal flaring, and restlessness.
- Make emergency equipment for intubation readily accessible.
- Position the child to have optimal ventilation without increasing distress that would contribute to increasing respiratory distress.
- Implement isolation precautions as indicated.

CLIENT EDUCATION

- Use a cool-air vaporizer to provide humidity.
- Rest during febrile illness.
- Maintain adequate fluid intake. Infants may be given commercially prepared oral rehydration solutions, and older children may be given sports drinks.
- Administer medications using accurate dosages and appropriate time intervals.
- Develop strategies to decrease the spread of infection. Strategies include performing good hand hygiene; covering the nose and mouth with tissues when sneezing and coughing; properly disposing of tissues; not sharing cups, eating utensils, and towels; and keeping infected children from contact with children who are well.
- Seek further medical attention for the child if manifestations worsen or respiratory distress occurs.

Nasopharyngitis

Also known as the common cold: Self-limiting virus that persists for 10 to 14 days

ASSESSMENT

EXPECTED FINDINGS

- Nasal inflammation, dryness and irritation of nasal passages and the pharynx
- Fever, decreased appetite, and restlessness

PATIENT-CENTERED CARE

NURSING CARE

- Instruct guardians about home management.
- Give antipyretic for fever.
- Encourage rest.
- Provide vaporized air (cool mist).
- Give decongestants for children older than 6 years.
- Give cough suppressants with caution (avoid over sedation).
- Antihistamines are not recommended.
- Antibiotics are not indicated.

Acute streptococcal pharyngitis

GABHS: Infection of the upper airway (strep throat)

ASSESSMENT

EXPECTED FINDINGS

- Onset is abrupt and characterized by pharyngitis, headache, fever and abdominal pain. **Qᴾᶜᶜ**
- Tonsils and pharynx can be inflamed and covered with exudate, usually appears by second day of illness.

LABORATORY TESTS

Throat culture or rapid antigen testing to determine GABHS infection

PATIENT-CENTERED CARE

NURSING CARE

- Administer antibiotics as prescribed.
  - Oral penicillin in a dose sufficient to control the acute local manifestations and is administered for at least 10 days.
  - Amoxicillin once a day for 10 days is also effective.
  - IM penicillin G benzathine is also appropriate.
  - Oral erythromycin for children allergic to penicillin.
- Administer antipyretics for fever.
- Clarithromycin, azithromycin, clindamycin, oral cephalosporins and amoxicillin with clavulanic acid are also effective to treat GABHS.
- For discomfort, apply cold or warm compresses to neck as needed.
- Encourage cool liquids or ice chips.
- Do not force eating if painful.
- Instruct parents to replace child's toothbrush after taking antibiotics for 24 hours.

Bronchitis (tracheobronchitis)

- Associated with an upper respiratory infection and inflammation of large airways
- Self-limiting

ASSESSMENT

EXPECTED FINDINGS

- Persistent dry, hacking cough as a result of inflammation
- Resolves in 5 to 10 days

LABORATORY TESTS

Test nasopharyngeal secretions

PATIENT-CENTERED CARE

NURSING CARE

- Instruct guardians about home management.
- Give antipyretics for fever.
- Give a cough suppressant.
- Provide increased humidity (cool mist vaporizer).

Bronchiolitis

- Mostly caused by respiratory syncytial virus (RSV)
- Primarily affects the bronchi and bronchioles
- Occurs at the bronchiolar level

ASESSMENT

EXPECTED FINDINGS

INITIALLY: Rhinorrhea, intermittent fever, pharyngitis, coughing, sneezing, wheezing, possible ear or eye infection

WITH ILLNESS PROGRESSION: Increased coughing and sneezing, fever, tachypnea and retractions, refusal to breastfeed or bottle feed, copious secretions

SEVERE ILLNESS: Tachypnea (greater than 70/min), listlessness, apneic spells, poor air exchange, poor breath sounds, cyanosis

LABORATORY TESTS

Test nasopharyngeal secretions using either rapid immunofluorescent antibody-direct fluorescent antibody staining or enzyme-linked immunosorbent assay techniques for RSV antigen detection.

PATIENT-CENTERED CARE

NURSING CARE

- Supplemental oxygen to maintain oxygen saturation equal to or greater than 90%.
- Encourage fluid intake if able to tolerate oral fluids. Otherwise IV fluids until acute phase has passed.
- Maintain airway.
- Medications as prescribed. Corticosteroid use is controversial. Bronchodilators are not recommended.
- Antibiotics if a coexisting bacterial infection is present
- CPT not recommended.
- Nasopharyngeal or nasal suctioning as needed.
- Encourage breastfeeding.

Allergic rhinitis

Caused by seasonal reaction to allergens most often in the autumn or spring

ASSESSMENT

EXPECTED FINDINGS

Watery rhinorrhea; nasal obstruction; itchiness of the nose, eyes, pharynx and conjunctiva; snoring; fatigue; malaise; headache; and poor performance in school

LABORATORY TESTS

Nasal smear to determine amount of eosinophils in nasal secretions, blood exam for total IgE and elevated eosinophils, skin tests and various challenge tests.

PATIENT-CENTERED CARE

NURSING CARE

Instruct guardians about home management.
- Avoid allergens.
- Give nasal corticosteroids (first-line medications used).
- Give antihistamines, beta-adrenergic decongestants, mast cell stabilizers, leukotriene modifiers, and ipratropium.

Bacterial pneumonia

- Bacterial pneumonia often caused by Streptococcus pneumoniae, Group A streptococci, Staphylococcus aureus, Mycoplasma catarrhalis, Mycoplasma pneumoniae. ⓠEBP
- Viral pneumonias are more common among children of all ages and are often accompanied by a viral upper respiratory infection

ASSESSMENT

EXPECTED FINDINGS

- High fever
- Cough that can be unproductive or productive of white sputum
- Tachypnea
- Retractions and nasal flaring
- Chest pain
- Dullness with percussion
- Adventitious breath sounds (rhonchi, fine crackles)
- Pale color that can progress to cyanosis
- Irritability, restlessness, lethargy
- Abdominal pain, diarrhea, lack of appetite, and vomiting

LABORATORY TESTS

- Radiographic examination to detect presence of infiltrates
- Gram stain and culture of sputum in older children
- Nasopharyngeal specimens
- Blood cultures
- Occasionally lung aspiration and biopsy
- Elevated antistreptolysin titer if streptococcal infection present

PATIENT-CENTERED CARE

NURSING CARE

Viral

- Administer oxygen
- Monitor continuous oximetry.
- Administer antipyretics for fever.
- Monitor I&O.
- CPT and postural drainage

Bacterial

- Encourage rest.
- Administer IV antibiotics.
- Promote increased oral intake.
- Monitor I&O.
- Administer antipyretics for fever.
- CPT and postural drainage can be helpful.
- Administer IV fluids.
- Administer oxygen.
- Monitor continuous oximetry.

CLIENT EDUCATION: The pneumococcal conjugate vaccine is encouraged for the prevention of pneumonia.

COMPLICATIONS

PNEUMOTHORAX

Accumulation of air in the pleural space

MANIFESTATIONS: Dyspnea, chest pain, back pain, labored respirations, decreased oxygen saturations, and tachycardia

NURSING INTERVENTIONS
- Prepare the client for an emergent needle aspiration to remove air in pleural space, with insertion of chest tube to closed drainage.
- Provide for chest tube management.
- Assess respiratory status.
- Administer oxygen.

PLEURAL EFFUSION

Accumulation of fluid in the pleural space

MANIFESTATIONS: Decreased breath sounds, vomiting, tachypnea, fatigue, irritability, and hypoxia

NURSING INTERVENTIONS

- Prepare the client for an emergent needle aspiration to remove fluid in the pleural space, with insertion of chest tube to closed drainage.
- Provide for chest tube management.
- Assess respiratory status.
- Administer oxygen as prescribed.

Croup syndromes: Bacterial epiglottitis (acute supraglottitis)

- Medical emergency
- Usually caused by Haemophilus influenza

ASSESSMENT

EXPECTED FINDINGS

- Drooling, agitation, absence of spontaneous cough
- Sitting upright with chin pointing out, mouth opened, and tongue protruding (tripod position)
- Dysphonia (thick, muffled voice and froglike croaking sound)
- Dysphagia (difficulty swallowing)
- Inspiratory stridor (noisy inspirations)
- Suprasternal and substernal retractions
- Sore throat, high fever, and restlessness

DIAGNOSTIC PROCEDURES

Lateral neck radiograph of the soft tissues

PATIENT-CENTERED CARE

NURSING CARE

- Protect airway.
- Avoid throat culture or using a tongue blade.
- Prepare for intubation.
- Provide humidified oxygen.
- Monitor continuous oximetry.
- Administer corticosteroids, and IV fluids as prescribed.
- Administer antibiotic therapy starting with IV, then transition to oral to complete a 10-day course, as prescribed.
- Droplet isolation precautions for first 24 hr after IV antibiotics initiated.

Croup syndromes: Acute laryngotracheobronchitis and acute spasmodic laryngitis

Acute laryngotracheobronchitis: Causative agents include RSV, influenza A and B, and Mycoplasma pneumonia, parainfluenza types 1, 2, and 3.

Acute spasmodic laryngitis
- Self-limiting illness that can result from allergens
- Characterized by paroxysmal attacks of laryngeal obstruction that occur mainly at night

ASSESSMENT

EXPECTED FINDINGS

Acute laryngotracheobronchitis
- Low-grade fever, restlessness, hoarseness, barky cough, dyspnea, inspiratory stridor, and retractions
- INFANTS AND TODDLERS: nasal flaring, intercostal retractions, tachypnea, and continuous stridor

Acute spasmodic laryngitis: Croupy barky cough, restlessness, difficulty breathing, hoarseness, and nighttime episodes of laryngeal obstruction

PATIENT-CENTERED CARE

NURSING CARE

- Provide humidity with cool mist.
- Administer oxygen if needed.
- Monitor continuous oximetry.
- Administer nebulized racemic epinephrine as prescribed.
- Administer corticosteroids: oral or IM (dexamethasone), or nebulized (budesonide).
- Encourage oral intake if tolerated.
- Administer IV fluids as prescribed.

HOME MANAGEMENT: ACUTE SPASMODIC LARYNGITIS

- Reinforce to guardians to provide cool mist for the child's room.
- Advise guardians to run hot shower and sit with their child in the steamy environment.

Influenza A and B

Mild, moderate, or severe

ASSESSMENT

EXPECTED FINDINGS

- Sudden onset of fever and chills
- Dry throat and nasal mucosa
- Dry cough
- Flushed face
- Photophobia
- Myalgia
- Fatigue

LABORATORY TESTS

- Analyze nasopharyngeal secretions for viral culture or rapid detection testing.
- Influenza A and B detected by fluorescent antibody and indirect immunofluorescent antibody staining.

PATIENT-CENTERED CARE

NURSING CARE

Instruct guardians about home management.
- Promote increased fluid intake.
- Rest.
- Acetaminophen or ibuprofen for fever.
- Give medications, as prescribed.

MEDICATIONS

Amantadine (type A)

- Shortens the length of the illness
- Administer within 24 to 48 hr of onset of manifestations.

Zanamivir (type A and B)

- Treatment of influenza for children 7 and older or for prophylaxis for children 5 and older
- Start within 48 hr of manifestations
- Inhaled two times per day for 5 days

Oseltamivir (type A and B)

- Decreases manifestations
- Give orally for 5 days
- Start within 48 hr of manifestations

Influenza vaccine (prevention)

- Inactivated influenza vaccine recommended for children 6 months and older.
- Live vaccination should not be used in children who have heart or lung disease, diabetes or kidney failure, are immunocompromised, have respiratory conditions, are pregnant, have a severe allergy to chicken eggs, or have a history of Guillain–Barré syndrome. Qs
- Clients who have experienced a severe allergic reaction to eggs should receive the influenza vaccine in a medical setting that is able to manage severe allergic reactions should they occur.

SARS-CoV-2 Infection (COVID-19)

ASSESSMENT

EXPECTED FINDINGS

- Fever
- Cough
- Shortness of breath
- Muscle aches
- Sore throat
- Headache
- Nausea and vomiting
- Diarrhea
- Loss of taste or smell

LABORATORY TESTS

- Analyze nasopharyngeal secretions for detection of SARS–CoV–2 antigen.
- Nucleic acid amplification testing for detection of RNA.

PATIENT-CENTERED CARE

NURSING CARE

- Instruct caregivers about home management.
- Provide information on isolation precautions.
- Administer ibuprofen and acetaminophen as prescribed for fever and discomfort.
- Teach caregivers the manifestations illness progression
  - Difficulty breathing
  - Reports of chest pain or pressure
  - Cyanosis in the face and lips
  - Decreased urine output
  - Confusion
  - Difficulty tolerating oral fluids
- Increase fluid intake.
- Provide popsicles or ice for sore throat.

MEDICATIONS

- Administration of antiviral and monoclonal antibody therapy are determined on a case by case basis

PATIENT EDUCATION

Instruct caregivers about prevention of SARS-CoV-2 infection.

- Frequent hand hygiene
- Maintain distance of at least 6 ft from others when indicated
- Wear facemask when indicated
- Avoid touching face, mouth, and eyes
- Obtain COVID-19 vaccination according to current CDC guidelines
- The following vaccines are currently available for children greater than or equal to 5 years old
- Refer to CDC guidelines for various age groups
- Not recommended for children less than 6 months of age
- Current recommendations are as follows: 2- dose mRNA vaccine (recommend doses given 4-8 weeks apart); 3-dose mRNA vaccine (recommend dose 1-2 to be administered 3-8 weeks apart; dose 2 to 3 to be administered at least 8 weeks to 5 months apart)
- Age 6 months to 5 years: 2-dose mRNA vaccine (at least 4-8 weeks apart); 3-dose mRNA vaccine (dose 1 to 2 at least 3-8 weeks apart; dose 2 to 3 at least 8 weeks apart
- Age 5 to 11 and 12-17 years: appropriate dose given intramuscularly in the deltoid. 2- dose mRNA vaccine (recommend doses given 4-8 weeks apart); 3-dose mRNA vaccine (recommend dose 1-2 to be administered 3-8 weeks apart; dose 2 to 3 to be administered at least to 5 months apart

Active Learning Scenario

A nurse is teaching a guardian of a child who has an infectious respiratory illness. What should the nurse include in the teaching? Use the ATI Active Learning Template: Basic Concept to complete this item.

RELATED CONTENT: Identify at least three strategies to decrease the spread of infection.

Application Exercises

1. Sort the following postoperative nursing actions for the child who has had a tonsillectomy into the indicated or contraindicated category.
   A. Administer codeine as prescribed
   B. Administer pain medications on a regular schedule
   C. Elevate the head of the bed
   D. Encourage turning, coughing, and deep breathing
   E. Monitor for frequent swallowing
   F. Provide ice chips
   G. Provide straws for liquids

2. A nurse is caring for a child who has bronchiolitis. Which of the following actions should the nurse take? (Select all that apply.)
   A. Initiate airborne precautions.
   B. Initiate chest percussion and postural drainage.
   C. Administer humidified oxygen.
   D. Suction the nasopharynx as needed.
   E. Administer oral penicillin.

3. A nurse is assessing a child who has epiglottitis. Which of the following findings should the nurse expect? (Select all that apply.)
   A. Hoarseness and difficulty speaking
   B. Difficulty swallowing
   C. Low-grade fever
   D. Drooling
   E. Dry, barking cough
   F. Stridor

4. A nurse is teaching a group of caregivers about influenza. Which of the following information should the nurse include in the teaching?
   A. "Amantadine will prevent the illness."
   B. "Children who are 3 months or older should receive the inactivated influenza vaccine."
   C. "Zanamivir can be given to children 1 year and older."
   D. "Oseltamivir should be given within 48 hours of onset of manifestations."

Application Exercises Key

1. **INDICATED:** B, C, E, F; **CONTRAINDICATED:** A, D, G

   When reviewing nursing actions for a child who has just had a tonsillectomy the following actions should be place in the indicated category: Elevate the head of the bed, provide ice chips, monitor for frequent swallowing, and administer pain medications on a regular schedule. These actions work to promote drainage, provide comfort, and monitor for manifestations of hemorrhage. Encouraging turning, coughing, and deep breathing, administering codeine as prescribed, and providing straws for liquids are contraindicated. To prevent injury to the surgical site, coughing and use of straws are discouraged. Codeine is contraindicated in children who have had a tonsillectomy due to the risk for respiratory depression caused by rapid metabolism of the medication.

   Ⓝ *NCLEX® Connection: Physiological Adaptation, Alterations in Body Systems*

2. C, D. **CORRECT:** When taking action for the child who has bronchiolitis the nurse should administer humidified oxygen and suction the nasopharynx as needed. Humidified oxygen provides moisture to the airway and suctioning the nasopharynx assists the child with clearing secretions.
   A. Airborne precautions are not indicated for a child who has bronchiolitis. However, the child who has bronchiolitis caused by the respiratory syncytial virus should be placed on contact precautions.
   B. Chest percussion and postural drainage are not indicated for a child who has bronchiolitis.
   E. Antibiotics are not indicated for a child who has bronchiolitis.

   Ⓝ *NCLEX® Connection: Physiological Adaptation, Alterations in Body Systems*

3. B, D, F. **CORRECT:** When recognizing cues, the nurse should identify difficulty swallowing, drooling, and stridor as manifestations of epiglottitis.
   A. A thick and muffled voice, not hoarseness, is a manifestation of epiglottitis.
   C. A high fever, not a low-grade fever, is a manifestation of epiglottitis.
   E. Dry, barking cough is a manifestation of croup, not epiglottitis.

   Ⓝ *NCLEX® Connection: Physiological Adaptation, Medical Emergencies*

4. A. Amantadine can shorten, but not prevent, the length of the illness.
   B. The inactivated influenza vaccine should be administered to children 6 months and older, not to children who are 3 months or older.
   C. Zanamivir is approved for children over the age of 5 years, not for children who are 1 year and older.
   D. **CORRECT:** When taking action and teaching about the influenza vaccine, the nurse should include that oseltamivir decreases flu manifestations when started within the first 48 hours that manifestations occur.

   Ⓝ *NCLEX® Connection: Physiological Adaptation, Alterations in Body Systems*

Active Learning Scenario Key

Using the ATI Active Learning Template: Basic Concept

RELATED CONTENT
- Perform appropriate hand hygiene.
- Cover the nose and mouth with tissues when sneezing and coughing.
- Dispose of tissues properly.
- Do not share cups, eating utensils, or towels.
- Keep infected children from contact with children who are well.

Ⓝ *NCLEX® Connection: Safety and Infection Control, Standard Precautions/Transmission-Based Precautions/Surgical Asepsis*

Asthma

Asthma is a chronic childhood inflammatory disorder of the airways that results in intermittent and reversible airflow obstruction of the bronchi and bronchioles. It causes school absences and is considered one of the leading causes of hospitalizations among children. The obstruction occurs because the mast cells release histamines and leukotrienes which causes inflammation or airway hyper-responsiveness. The different types of asthma include: intrinsic (no prior history of asthma), extrensic (exposure to an allergen), exercise induced, and medication induced. Asthma diagnoses are classified into one of four categories based on effects on the child: intermittent, mild persistent, moderate persistent, and severe persistent. (18.1) Q EBP

ASSESSMENT

RISK FACTORS

- Family history of asthma or allergies
- Assigned sex at birth: (boys affected more than girls until adolescence, then the incidence is greater among girls)
- Exposure to tobacco smoke
- Low birth weight
- Race: Black
- Being overweight

TRIGGERS TO ASTHMA

- Allergens
  - Indoor: mold, cockroach antigen, dust, dust mites, animal dander
  - Outdoor: grasses, pollen, trees, shrubs, molds, spores, air pollution, weeds
  - Irritants: Tobacco smoke, wood smoke, odors, sprays
- Exercise
- Cold air or changes in weather or temperature
- Environmental change (new home or school)
- Infections/viruses (colds)
- Animals: dogs, cats, horses, rodents
- Medications: Aspirin, NSAIDs, antibiotics, beta blockers
- Strong emotions: Fear, anger, laughing, crying
- Conditions: GERD, tracheoesophageal fistula
- Foods: nuts, eggs, dairy products
- Endocrine factors: Menses, pregnancy, thyroid disease

EXPECTED FINDINGS

- Chest tightness
- History regarding current and previous asthma exacerbations
  - Onset and duration
  - Precipitating factors
  - Changes in medication regimen
  - Medications that relieve manifestations
  - Other medications
  - Self–care methods used to relieve manifestations
  - Home/school environment
  - Heating/cooling source in the home

PHYSICAL ASSESSMENT FINDINGS

- Dyspnea
- Cough
- Audible wheezing
- Coarse lung sounds, wheezing throughout possible crackles
- Mucus production
- Short, panting speech
- Restlessness, irritability
- Anxiety
- Sweating
- Use of accessory muscles
- Decreased oxygen saturation (low SaO_2)
- Tripod positioning
- Retractions when sitting
- Inaudible breath sounds or crackles (severe obstruction)

18.1 Effects of asthma on the child

		Intermittent	Mild persistent	Moderate persistent	Severe persistent
FREQUENCY OF FINDINGS		0 to 2 times/week	More than twice/ week, but not daily	Daily	Continually
NIGHTTIME FINDINGS	0- to 4-year-old	None	1 to 2 times/month	3 to 4 times/month	Frequent
	5- to 11-year-old	Two times a month or less	3 to 4 times/month	More than once/ week, but not daily	
ACTIVITY LIMITATIONS		None	Minor	Some	Extreme
USE OF A SHORT-ACTING BETA AGONIST		Less than twice/week	More than 2 days/ week, but not daily	Daily	Several times/day

LABORATORY TESTS

CBC with differential (increased WBC, eosinophils, neutrophils)

DIAGNOSTIC PROCEDURES

Pulmonary function tests (PFTs) (different tests such as spirometry, peak expiratory flow rates, bronchoprovocation, fractional exhaled nitric oxide)
- The most accurate tests for diagnosing asthma and its severity Q**EBP**
- Baseline test at time of diagnosis
- Repeat testing after treatment is initiated and child is stabilized
- Test every 1 to 2 years

Spirometry
- Assists with diagnosis of asthma and determines how well asthma is managed
- Blow into a spirometer (how much air inhaled, how much air is exhaled, and how fast you can exhale)
- If results are decreased, provider may administer a bronchodilator and repeat testing

Peak expiratory flow rates (PEFR)
- Uses a flow meter to measure the amount of air that can be forcefully exhaled in 1 second
- Each child needs to establish personal best

Bronchoprovocation testing
- Exposure to methacholine, cold air, or histamine
- Exercise challenge

Fractional exhaled nitric oxide (FeNO)
- Determines airway inflammation by measuring amount of nitric oxide in your breath
- Blow into handheld device that measures the results

Skin prick testing: Identify allergens that trigger asthma.

Chest x-ray: Showing hyperexpansion and infiltrates

PATIENT-CENTERED CARE

NURSING CARE

- Avoid allergens whenever possible.
- Assess airway patency, respiratory rate, symmetry, effort, and use of accessory muscles.
- Auscultate breath sounds in all lung fields.
- Monitor for shortness of breath, dyspnea, and audible wheezing. An absence of wheezing can indicate severe constriction of the alveoli.
- Monitor vital signs and oxygen saturation.
- Check CBC and chest x-ray results, possible ABGs.
- Position the child to maximize ventilation.
- Administer oxygen therapy as prescribed. Keep endotracheal intubation equipment nearby. Q**s**
- Initiate and maintain IV access as prescribed.

- Maintain a calm and reassuring demeanor.
- Encourage appropriate vaccinations and prompt medical attention for infections.
- Administer medications. The provider can prescribe antibiotics if a bacterial infection is confirmed.
- Teach the family and the child about when to use each of the prescribed medications (rescue medications vs. maintenance medications).

THERAPEUTIC MANAGEMENT

MEDICATIONS
A stepwise approach is used for treatment based upon the severity.

Bronchodilators (inhalers)

Short-acting beta2 agonists (SABA) (albuterol, levalbuterol, terbutaline)
- Used for acute exacerbations
- Prevention of exercised-induced asthma

Long-acting beta2 agonists (LABA) (formoterol, salmeterol)
- Used to prevent exacerbations, especially at night, and reduce use of SABA.
- Must be used along with anti-inflammatory therapy.
- Cannot be used to treat acute exacerbations.

Cholinergic antagonists (anticholinergic medications; atropine, ipratropium) block the parasympathetic nervous system, providing relief of acute bronchospasms.

NURSING ACTIONS
- Instruct the child and family in the proper use of metered-dose inhaler or nebulizer.
- Monitor the child for dizziness, nasal dryness, sore throat, vision changes, cardiac and CNS stimulation when taking ipratropium.

CLIENT EDUCATION
- Older children who are taking ipratropium can suck on hard candies to help with dry mouth.
- Administer prior to exercise or activity
- Rinse mouth after using inhaler.
- Monitor for irritably, tremors, insomnia, and nervousness while taking this medication.

Anti-inflammatory agents

Decrease airway inflammation.

Corticosteroids can be given parenterally (methylprednisolone), orally (prednisone), or by inhalation (fluticasone).
- Oral systemic steroids can be given for short periods (3 or 10 days).
- Inhaled corticosteroids are administered daily as a preventive measure.
- Monitor child's growth (can suppress bone growth).

Leukotriene modifiers (zafirlukast, montelukast)
Decrease in airway resistance

Mast cell stabilizers (cromolyn) Long term control

Monoclonal antibodies (omalizumab, reslizumab) are used to treat moderate to severe persistent allergic asthma uncontrolled by inhaled corticosteroids in children 12-years-old and older.

- Monitor for hypersensitivity reaction during administration.

Combination medications contain an inhaled corticosteroid and a LABA (fluticasone/salmeterol)

NURSING ACTIONS

- Observe the oral mucosa for infection secondary to use of inhaled medication.
- Assess weight, blood pressure, electrolytes, glucose, and growth with oral corticosteroid use.

CLIENT EDUCATION

- Drink plenty of fluids to promote hydration.
- Take oral corticosteroids with food.
- Rinse the mouth after the use of a corticosteroid inhaler.
- Watch for redness, sores, or white patches in the mouth, and report them to the provider.
- Follow prescription for medication administration (dosage, tapering off medication, length of time to take).

Xanthine derivatives (theophylline/aminophylline): dilates the airways, used when the child is not responding to maximum therapy.

- Monitor theophylline blood levels frequently (narrow therapeutic window and the risk for toxicity.)

INTERPROFESSIONAL CARE

- Consult respiratory services for inhalers and breathing treatments. **Qrc**
- Contact nutritional services for weight loss or gain related to medications or diagnosis.
- Consult rehabilitation if the child has prolonged weakness and needs assistance with increasing level of activity.

CLIENT EDUCATION

- Identify personal triggering agents.
- Avoid triggering agents.
- Ensure the family and child has an asthma action plan.
- Properly self-administer medications (nebulizers, inhalers, and spacer).
- Use a peak flow meter. (Encourage to use at the same time each day.)
  - Ensure the marker is zeroed.
  - Have the child stand up straight.
  - Remove gum or food from mouth.
  - Close lips tightly around the mouthpiece (ensure the tongue is not occluding).
  - Blow out as hard and as quickly as possible.
  - Read the number on the meter.
  - Repeat these steps two more times for a total of three attempts (wait at least 30 seconds between attempts.)
  - Record highest number.
- Keep a record of PEFR results. Readings over time show the child's "best" efforts, and provide a warning of increased airway impairment.

- Learn how to interpret PEFR results and what measures to take for their zone. **(18.2)**
- Learn how to recognize an asthma exacerbation (decreased PEFR, increased use of SABA, difficulty speaking or eating). **Qs**
- Perform infection prevention techniques.
  - Promote good nutrition.
  - Reinforce importance of good hand hygiene.
  - Reduce allergens in the child's environment
- Perform prompt medical attention for infections.
- Keep immunizations, including seasonal influenza and pneumonia vaccines, up to date.
- Perform regular exercise as part of asthma therapy.
  - Promotes ventilation and perfusion
  - Maintains cardiac health
  - Enhances skeletal muscle strength
- Children can require medication before exercise to prevent induced spasms of the bronchus.

COMPLICATIONS

Status asthmaticus

A life-threatening episode of airway obstruction that is often unresponsive to common treatment. It is considered a prolonged severe asthma attack.

MANIFESTATIONS include wheezing, labored breathing, nasal flaring, lack of air movement in lungs, use of accessory muscles, inability to speak in full sentences distended neck veins, tachycardia, tachypnea, hypoxia, diaphoresis, and risk for cardiac and respiratory arrest.

NURSING ACTIONS

- Monitor oxygen saturations continuously.
- Place on continuous cardiorespiratory monitoring.
- Position the child sitting upright, standing, or leaning slightly forward.
- Administer humidified oxygen.
- Administer three nebulizer treatments of a beta$_2$ agonist, 20 to 30 min apart or continuously. Ipratropium bromide can be added to the nebulizer to increase bronchodilation.
- Obtain IV access.
- Monitor ABGs and blood electrolytes.

18.2 Analysis of peak flow rates according to colored zones

	% OF PERSONAL BEST	ANALYSIS
GREEN	80% to 100%	Good control. Follow routine plan.
YELLOW	50% to 79%	Caution. This zone warns of an acute attack. Use maintenance medications. Notify provider if the peak flow rate stays in this zone.
RED	Less than 50%	Emergent action needed. Use a short-acting bronchodilator. Notify provider if the peak flow rate does not improve.

- Administer corticosteroid.
- Prepare for emergency intubation.
- Magnesium sulfate IV decreases inflammation and improves pulmonary function and peak flow rate among children who have moderate to severe asthma when treated in the emergency department or pediatric ICU.
- Heliox (a mixture of helium and oxygen) can be administered via a non–rebreathing mask to decrease airway resistance and work of breathing
- Ketamine: Smooth muscle relaxant that decreases airway resistance

Respiratory failure

Persistent hypoxemia related to asthma can lead to respiratory failure.

NURSING ACTIONS
- Monitor oxygenation levels and acid–base balance.
- Prepare for intubation and mechanical ventilation as indicated.

18.3 Case Study

Scenario Introduction

Pauline is a school nurse at an elementary school in a small, underserved, rural community. Pauline has just received Colton Weeks to her office. Colton was brought to the nurses' office by a teacher after he reported being short of breath and needing his inhaler. Colton is 8 years old and a new student at the school who was enrolled one month ago.

Scene 1

Pauline: Colton, can you tell me what is going on?

Colton: I was playing….and it started getting hard to breathe….so I told the teacher.

Pauline: Ok, Colton, sit right here for me. I need to listen to your lungs and count how fast you are breathing.

Pauline assesses Colton. His respiratory rate is 29/min with mild sub-clavicular and intercostal retractions. His oxygen saturation is 92% and he has expiratory wheezing with a nonproductive cough. His heart rate is 115/min and regular.

Pauline retrieves Colton's albuterol inhaler and spacer and notices that the albuterol inhaler is expired. Pauline administers albuterol to Colton using an inhaler from the school's medication cabinet.

Scene 2

Pauline reassess Colton and notes that his respirations are 25/min, no retractions observed. His oxygen saturation level is 96% with an occasional expiratory wheeze noted upon auscultation. Cough is unchanged. Heart rate is 110/min and regular.

Pauline: Colton, do you have an albuterol inhaler at home?

Colton: Yes.

Pauline: How often do you use it?

Colton: My dad gives me one puff in the morning before school. He is afraid we will run out and not be able to get more.

Scene 3

After determining that it is safe to send Colton back to class, Pauline calls Mr. Weeks, Colton's dad.

Pauline: Hello Mr. Weeks, this is Pauline, Colton's school nurse. I just wanted to let you know that I had to administer albuterol to Colton today at school. He is ok and has returned to class. I noticed that his albuterol was expired. He also mentioned that he only gets one puff in the morning before school and that there is some worry about running out of his medication and not being able to get more.

Mr. Weeks: Thank you for calling me. Yes, that is true. Colton's mother passed away 6 months ago. She always took care of that kind of stuff. I just moved here with Colton and his sister a month ago. I can't find a job and I am having a really hard time trying to figure all of this out.

Scenario Conclusion

Pauline continues the conversation with Colton's dad. She learns that Colton's dad has been without a job since Colton's mother passed away and that they moved to be closer to family; however, the family has not been a source of support. Mr. Weeks and the children are currently living in low-income public housing. The children have no health insurance. Mr. Weeks is concerned about finding a job because he has no formal education though he reports a stable job history. Mr. Weeks is open to any help that Pauline can provide.

Case Study Exercises

1. As a school nurse, Pauline is concerned about the Social Determinants of Health (SDOH) that are impacting this situation. Match the SDOH identified by Pauline to the correct categories.

   A. Mr. Weeks is currently unemployed.

   B. Mr. Weeks has no formal education.

   C. The children are uninsured.

   D. Mr. Weeks and the children currently live in public housing.

   E. The family has not been a source of support for Mr. Weeks and the children.

   1. Neighborhood and Build Environment
   2. Social and Community Context
   3. Education Access and Quality
   4. Economic Stability
   5. Health Care Access and Quality

2. For each SDOH identified, provide an example of how it directly impacts Colton and his asthma.

3. Pauline is exploring available community resources that she can refer Mr. Weeks to that will assist him in providing adequate health care for Colton and his sister. Identify some community resources related to SDOH that would be beneficial for Mr. Weeks and the children.

Application Exercises

1. A nurse is discussing risk factors for asthma with a group of newly licensed nurses. Which of the following risk factors should the nurse include in the teaching? (Select all that apply.)

   A. Family history of asthma

   B. Family history of allergies

   C. Exposure to smoke

   D. Low birth weight

   E. Being underweight

2. A nurse is assessing a child who has an acute exacerbation of asthma. Which of the following findings should the nurse expect? (Select all that apply.)

   A. Oxygen saturation 96%

   B. Wheezing

   C. Retraction of sternal muscles

   D. Bronchovesicular breath sounds

   E. Cough

3. A nurse is teaching an adolescent about the correct use of their asthma medications. Which of the following medications should the nurse instruct the adolescent to use before exercise?

   A. Fluticasone/salmeterol

   B. Montelukast

   C. Prednisone

   D. Albuterol

4. A nurse is teaching a child who has asthma how to use a peak flow meter. Which of the following information should the nurse include in the teaching? (Select all that apply.)

   A. Zero the meter before each use.

   B. Record the average of the attempts.

   C. Perform three attempts.

   D. Deliver a long, slow breath into the meter.

   E. Sit in a chair with feet on the floor.

5. A nurse is planning care for a child who has an exacerbation of asthma. Which of the following interventions should the nurse include in the plan of care? (Select all that apply.)

   A. Perform chest percussion.

   B. Place the child in an upright position.

   C. Monitor oxygen saturation.

   D. Administer bronchodilators.

   E. Administer dornase alfa daily.

Active Learning Scenario

A nurse is teaching a child about asthma triggers. What information should the nurse include in the teaching? Use the ATI Active Learning Template: System Disorder to complete this item.

CLIENT EDUCATION: List at least eight possible asthma triggers.

Case Study Exercises Key

1. A, 4; B, 3; C, 5; D,1; E, 2

   When recognizing cues, the nurse should identify and match the following SDOH: Mr. Weeks being unemployed is an example of Economic Stability; Mr. Weeks having no formal education is an example of Education Access and Quality; the children being uninsured, living in a rural, underserved neighborhood, and Mr. Weeks having difficulty navigating the health care system are examples of Health Care Access and Quality; living in a new neighborhood and living in public housing are examples of Neighborhood and Built Environment; and no family support is an example of Social and Community Context.

   Ⓝ *NCLEX® Connection: Safe and Effective Care Environment, Management of Care*

2. Mr. Weeks' unemployment impacts his ability to pay for visits to the provider, purchase required medications, secure safe housing, and provide transportation to provider visits. The inability to pay for provider visits and medications, as well as potential transportation problems may result in seeking healthcare for Colton after he has become too sick for outpatient treatment causing admission to an acute care facility further straining the limited resources that Mr. Weeks has available.

   Living in low-income public housing places the family at a greater risk for living near pollution sources that impact air quality. Poor air quality can have a negative impact on Colton's asthma control.

   Mr. Weeks' educational level may impact his health literacy and his ability to navigate the health care system causing frustration. This could result in Colton not receiving all of the resources that are available to achieve optimal care for his asthma.

   The children being uninsured impacts their access to care as well as the ability to obtain prescribed medications and treatments.

   Mr. Weeks moved his children to be closer to family. The family members could serve as a resource for Mr. Weeks and the children by providing guidance about community resources. According to Mr. Weeks, this has not happened. Social support of the family for Mr. Weeks and the children could greatly impact health-promoting practices and improve the outcomes for care for Colton.

   Ⓝ *NCLEX® Connection: Safe and Effective Care Environment, Management of Care*

3. When generating solutions for Mr. Weeks and the children to help address SDOH, the nurse should plan referrals to community resources that will help provide Mr. Weeks with the resources needed to provide adequate health care for the children. These resources include the local Medicaid office, health departments and free clinics, employment and training programs, community health education programs, and parental support groups.

   Ⓝ *NCLEX® Connection: Safe and Effective Care Environment, Management of Care*

Application Exercises Key

1. **A, B, C, D. CORRECT:** When taking action (implementation) the nurse should include in the discussion with the newly licensed nurses that risk factors for asthma include a family history of asthma and allergies, exposure to smoke, and low birth weight and obesity

   Ⓝ *NCLEX® Connection: Health Promotion and Maintenance, Health Promotion/Disease Prevention*

2. **B, C, E. CORRECT:** When recognizing cues (assessing), the nurse should expect findings of wheezing, retraction of the sternal muscles, and cough for a child who has asthma. Wheezing occurs because of bronchoconstriction of the airway which makes difficult for the child to move air into and out of the lungs.
   A. An oxygen saturation level of 96% is within the expected reference range. A child who is has an exacerbation of asthma will have a decrease oxygen saturation level.
   D. Bronchovesicular breath sounds are expected findings; however, a child who has an asthma exacerbation would have unexpected findings such as wheezing and rhonchi.

   Ⓝ *NCLEX® Connection: Physiological Adaptation, Illness Management*

3. A. Fluticasone/salmeterol is a combination of LABA and corticosteroid medications, and to use it for maintenance control of asthma.
   B. Montelukast is a leukotriene modifier, that affects the immune response to prevent bronchospasms and should be used for maintenance control of asthma.
   C. Prednisone is a glucocorticoid that is used to decrease inflammation and is used short-term for exacerbations of asthma
   D. **CORRECT:** When taking action (implementation), the nurse should instruct the adolescent to take albuterol which is a short acting beta 2 agonist (SABA) medication prior to exercise. SABAs are used for bronchodilation to provide immediate relief of bronchoconstriction.

   Ⓝ *NCLEX® Connection: Pharmacological and Parenteral Therapies, Medication Administration*

4. **A, C. CORRECT:** When taking action (implementation) to teach a child how to use a peak flow meter, the nurse should instruct the child to zero the meter before each use and to perform three attempts. These actions ensure that accurate results are achieved.
   B. After 3 attempts, the parent or child should record the highest value of the attempts and not the average.
   D. The child should breathe hard and fast, not long and slow.
   E. The child should stand upright, not to sit in a chair when feet on the floor when using the peak flow meter.

   Ⓝ *NCLEX® Connection: Reduction of Risk Potential, Therapeutic Procedures*

5. **B, C, D. CORRECT:** When generating solutions (planning) for a child who has an exacerbation of asthma, the nurse should plan to place the child in an upright position, monitor the child's oxygen saturation, and administer bronchodilators. Placing the child in an upright position promotes ventilation. Monitoring oxygen saturation allows the nurse to detect changes in the child's condition. Administering bronchodilators relieves bronchoconstriction and promotes ventilation.
   A, E. Chest percussion and the administration of dornase alfa are not indicated for the management of a child who has an exacerbation of asthma; however, these are indicated for a child who has cystic fibrosis

   Ⓝ *NCLEX® Connection: Physiological Adaptation, Medical emergencies*

Active Learning Scenario Key

Using the ATI Active Learning Template: System Disorder

TRIGGERS TO ASTHMA
- Allergens
  - Indoor: mold, cockroach antigen, dust, dust mites, animal dander
  - Outdoor: grasses, pollen, trees, shrubs, molds, spores, air pollution, weeds
  - Irritants: tobacco smoke, wood smoke, odors, sprays
- Exercise
- Cold air or changes in weather or temperature
- Environmental change (new home or school)
- Infections/colds
- Animals: dogs, cats, horses, rodents
- Medications: aspirin, NSAIDs, antibiotics, beta blockers
- Strong emotions: fear, anger, laughing, crying
- Conditions: GRED, tracheoesophageal fistula
- Foods: nuts, eggs, dairy products
- Endocrine factors: menses, pregnancy, thyroid disease

Ⓝ *NCLEX® Connection: Physiological Adaptation, Alterations in Body Systems*

CHAPTER 19 Cystic Fibrosis

Cystic fibrosis is a respiratory disorder that results from inheriting a mutated gene. It is characterized by mucus glands that secrete an increase in the quantity of thick, tenacious mucus, which leads to mechanical obstruction of organs (pancreas, lungs, liver, small intestine, and reproductive system); an increase in organic and enzymatic constituents in the saliva; an increase in the sodium and chloride content of sweat; and autonomic nervous system abnormalities.

ASSESSMENT

RISK FACTORS

- Both biological parents carry the recessive trait for cystic fibrosis.
- Non-Hispanic white American ethnicity.

EXPECTED FINDINGS

- Family history of cystic fibrosis
- Medical history of respiratory infections, growth failure
- Meconium ileus at birth manifested as distention of the abdomen, vomiting, and inability to pass stool. Meconium ileus is the earliest indication of cystic fibrosis in the newborn.

RESPIRATORY FINDINGS
- Stasis of mucus increases the risk for respiratory infections.
- Early manifestations
  - Wheezing, rhonchi
  - Dry, nonproductive cough
- Increased involvement
  - Dyspnea
  - Paroxysmal cough
  - Obstructive emphysema and atelectasis on chest x-ray
- Advanced involvement
  - Cyanosis
  - Barrel-shaped chest
  - Clubbing of fingers and toes
  - Multiple episodes of bronchitis or bronchopneumonia

GASTROINTESTINAL FINDINGS
- Large, frothy, bulky, greasy, foul-smelling stools (steatorrhea)
- Voracious appetite (early), loss of appetite (late)
- Failure to gain weight or weight loss
- Delayed growth patterns
- Distended abdomen (infant)
- Thin arms and legs (infant)
- Deficiency of fat-soluble vitamins
- Anemia
- Reflux
- Prolapse rectum (infant, child)
- Constipation

INTEGUMENTARY FINDINGS
Sweat, tears, and saliva have an excessively high content of sodium and chloride.

ENDOCRINE AND REPRODUCTIVE SYSTEM FINDINGS
- Viscous cervical mucus
- Decreased or absent sperm
- Decreased insulin production

LABORATORY TESTS

Blood specimen: Nutritional panel to detect a deficiency of fat-soluble vitamins (A, D, E, and K)

Sputum culture for detection of infection: *Pseudomonas aeruginosa, Haemophilus influenzae, Burkholderia cepacia, Staphlococcus aureus, Escherichia coli,* or *Klebsiella pneumoniae*

DIAGNOSTIC PROCEDURES

DNA testing: To isolate the mutation

Pulmonary function tests (PFTs): Evaluate the small airways

Chest x-ray: Can indicate diffuse atelectasis and obstructive emphysema

Abdominal x-ray: Detect meconium ileus

Stool analysis: For presence of fat and enzymes

Duodenal analysis: Analyze pancreatic trypsin levels (NG tube)

Sweat chloride test
- The child must be well hydrated to ensure accurate test results.
- A device that uses an electrical current stimulates sweat production. Q EBP
- Collection of sweat from two different sites for adequate sample.
- Expected reference range is chloride content less than 40 mEq/L and sodium content less than 70 mEq/L.

> Diagnostic confirmation of cystic fibrosis: Chloride greater than 40 mEq/L for infants less than 3 months of age and greater than 60 mEq/L for all others.

PATIENT-CENTERED CARE

NURSING CARE

- Assess lung sounds and respiratory status.
- Vital signs with oxygen saturation.
- Obtain IV access. Use of a peripherally inserted central catheter or IV port allows for home IV antibiotic therapy.
- Obtain sputum for culture and sensitivity.
- Provide support to the child and family.

Pulmonary management

- Assist in providing airway clearance therapy (ACT) to promote expectoration of pulmonary secretions. Usually prescribed twice a day in the morning and evening. Avoid ACT immediately before or after meals. Several methods of ACT are available.
  - Chest physiotherapy (CPT) with postural drainage as prescribed (manual or mechanical percussion).
  - Positive expiratory therapy (PEP) uses a device (a flutter mucus clearance device) to encourage the client to breathe with forceful exhalations.
  - Active-cycle-of-breathing techniques ("huffing" or forced expiration), are encouraged.
  - Autogenic drainage uses an electronic chest vibrator or handheld percussor along with breathing techniques.
  - High-frequency chest compression uses a mechanical chest device combined with nebulization therapy.
- Administer aerosol therapy as prescribed (bronchodilator, human deoxyribonuclease). Often recommended prior to ACT.
- Administer IV or aerosolized antibiotics.
- Encourage physical aerobic exercise.
- Provide oxygen as prescribed (assess for carbon dioxide retention).
- Monitor for hemoptysis or pneumothorax.

Gastrointestinal management

- Provide a well-balanced diet high in protein and calories.
- Give three meals a day with snacks.
- Encourage oral fluid intake.
- Administer pancreatic enzymes within 30 min of eating a meal or snack.
- Administer vitamin supplements: multivitamin; vitamins A, D, E, and K.
- Administer laxatives or stool softeners for constipation. Polyethylene-glycol electrolyte solution is administered orally or via nasogastric tube.
- Administer histamine-receptor antagonist and motility medications for GERD.
- Administer possible formula supplements in addition to breastfeedings or via gastric tube.
- Encourage to add salt to food during hot weather- (dehydration).
- Consult a dietitian. Child should receive regular nutritional evaluations.

Endocrine management

- Cystic fibrosis related diabetes (CFRD) necessitates monitoring of blood glucose levels and quarterly glycosylated hemoglobin (A1C) levels..
- Administer insulin. Oral glycemic medications are not effective for CFRD.

MEDICATIONS

Respiratory medications

Short-acting beta2 agonists (albuterol)

NURSING ACTIONS
- Monitor for tremors and tachycardia when the child is taking albuterol.
- Observe for dry mouth when the child is taking ipratropium.

CLIENT EDUCATION
- Teach how to properly use an MDI, PEP, or nebulizer.
- Rinse mouth after fluticasone propionate/salmeterol.

Dornase alfa (aerosol)
Decreases the viscosity of mucus and improves lung function

NURSING ACTIONS
- Monitor sputum thickness and ability of client to expectorate.
- Monitor the child for improvement in PFTs.

CLIENT EDUCATION
- Understand how to use a nebulizer.
- Administer once or twice a day.
- This medication can cause laryngitis.

Antibiotics

- Administer through IV or aerosol.
- Specific to treat pulmonary infection. Common medications include tobramycin, ticarcillin, or gentamicin. Q EBP

NURSING ACTIONS
- Assess for allergies.
- High doses may be prescribed. Collect blood specimens before and after some IV antibiotics to maintain therapeutic levels.

Pancreatic enzymes

Pancrelipase treats pancreatic insufficiency associated with cystic fibrosis.

NURSING ACTIONS
- Monitor stools for adequate dosing (1 to 2 stools/day).
- Monitor weight.
- Administer capsules with all meals and snacks.
- Child can swallow or sprinkle capsules on food. Do not sprinkle on hot foods or add to bottles or formula.
- Increase dosage of enzymes when eating high-fat foods.
- Capsule contents can be added to a small amount of formula or breast milk for an infant.

Vitamins

Daily multivitamin and fat-soluble vitamins A, E, D, and K

INTERPROFESSIONAL CARE

- Respiratory and physical therapy, social services, pulmonologist, pharmacist, pediatrician, infectious disease specialists, and dietitians may be involved in the care of the child who has cystic fibrosis.
- Adolescents who have advanced disease can be considered for lung transplants.

CLIENT EDUCATION

- Utilize information provided regarding access to medical equipment and medications.
- Understand equipment and medications prior to discharge.
- Teach ways to provide CPT and breathing exercises.
- Visit the provider regularly.
- Stay up-to-date on immunizations, including a yearly influenza vaccine and pneumococcal vaccine.
- Practice regular dental hygiene
- Understand the importance of diet and ways to increase calorie intake.
- Observe for indications of infection and notify the provider if necessary.
- Know methods to manage chronic illness in children.
- Change diapers frequently.
- Monitor for impairments of skin integrity.
- Perform regular physical activity. Encourage the child to rest prior to meals and before physiotherapy.
- Change positions frequently.
- Participate in a support group and use community resources.
- Identify specific needs based on the client's developmental level. For example, older adolescents are at a higher risk for depression due to the emotional and physical effects of cystic fibrosis.
- Provide home palliative care for the child or adolescent in the terminal stages of CF.

COMPLICATIONS

RESPIRATORY: Respiratory infections, respiratory colonizations, bronchial cysts, emphysema, pneumothorax, nasal polyps

GASTROINTESTINAL: Meconium ileus, prolapse of the rectum, intestinal obstruction, GERD

ENDOCRINE: Diabetes mellitus

Application Exercises

1. A nurse is performing an admission assessment for a child who has cystic fibrosis. Which of the following findings should the nurse expect? (Select all that apply.)
   A. Wheezing
   B. Clubbing of fingers and toes
   C. Barrel-shaped chest
   D. Thin, watery mucus
   E. Rapid growth spurts

2. A nurse is reviewing the diagnostic findings for a preschool age child who is suspected of having cystic fibrosis. Which of the following findings should the nurse identify as an indication of cystic fibrosis?
   A. Sweat chloride content 85 mEq/L
   B. Increased blood levels of fat-soluble vitamins
   C. 72 hr stool analysis sample indicating hard, packed stools
   D. Chest x-ray negative for atelectasis

3. A nurse is providing discharge teaching for a child who has cystic fibrosis. Which of the following instructions should the nurse include?
   A. Provide a low-calorie, low-protein diet.
   B. Administer pancreatic enzymes with meals and snacks.
   C. Implement a fluid restriction during times of infection.
   D. Restrict physical activity.

4. A nurse is admitting a child who has cystic fibrosis. Which of the following medications should the nurse expect to include in the plan of care? (Select all that apply.)
   A. Tobramycin
   B. Loperamide
   C. Vitamins A, D, E, K
   D. Albuterol
   E. Dornase alfa

5. Review the nursing interventions and medications. Match each intervention/medication to the body system the intervention/medication is intended to treat: Pulmonary, GI, or Endocrine.
   A. Chest physiotherapy
   B. Pancreatic enzymes
   C. Insulin
   D. Positive expiratory therapy
   E. Vitamins A, D, E, K
   F. Increase fluid intake
   G. Monitor blood glucose levels
   H. Albuterol

Active Learning Scenario

A nurse is caring for a child who has cystic fibrosis. What nursing interventions should the nurse expect to provide? Use the ATI Active Learning Template: System Disorder to complete this item.

NURSING CARE

- Describe at least three general nursing actions.
- Describe three nursing actions related to the management of pulmonary function.
- Describe two nursing actions related to gastrointestinal system management.
- Describe two nursing actions related to endocrine system management.

Active Learning Scenario Key

Using the ATI Active Learning Template: System Disorder
NURSING CARE

General Nursing Actions
- Assess lung sounds and respiratory status.
- Assess vital signs with oxygen saturation.
- Obtain IV access (peripherally inserted central catheter).
- Obtain sputum for culture and sensitivity.
- Provide support to the child and family.

Pulmonary Management
- Perform ACT as prescribed. Avoid immediately before and after meals.
- Administer aerosol therapy (bronchodilator, human deoxyribonuclease).
- Administer IV antibiotics (tobramycin, ticarcillin, or gentamicin).
- Encourage physical aerobic exercise.
- Provide oxygen as prescribed. (Assess for carbon dioxide retention.)

Gastrointestinal Management
- Consume a well balanced diet high in protein and calories.
- Eat three meals a day with snacks.
- Encourage oral fluid intake.
- Administer pancreatic enzymes within 30 min of eating.
- Take vitamin supplements: multivitamin, vitamins A, D, E, and K.
- Administer laxatives or stool softeners for constipation.
- Administer histamine-receptor antagonist and motility medications for GERD.
- Administer possible formula supplements in addition to breastfeeding or via a gastric tube.
- Consult a dietitian.

Endocrine Management
- Monitor blood glucose levels.
- Administer insulin as prescribed.

Ⓝ *NCLEX® Connection: Physiological Adaptation, Illness Management*

Application Exercises Key

1. A, B, C. **CORRECT:** When recognizing cues while assessing a child who has cystic fibrosis, the nurse should expect to find wheezing, clubbing of the fingers and toes, and a barrel-shaped chest.
   D. Thick, viscous mucus, not thin, watery mucus is an expected finding of cystic fibrosis.
   E. Delayed growth, not rapid growth spurts is an expected finding of cystic fibrosis.

   Ⓝ *NCLEX® Connection: Physiological Adaptation, Pathophysiology*

2. A. **CORRECT:** When analyzing diagnostic findings for a preschool age child who is suspected of having cystic fibrosis, the nurse should identify that a sweat chloride content of 85 mEq/L is above the expected reference range and is an indicator of cystic fibrosis. Children who have cystic fibrosis excrete an excessive amount of sodium and chloride in their sweat.
   B. Children who have cystic fibrosis are expected to have decreased, not increased, blood levels of fat-soluble vitamins.
   C. Children who have cystic fibrosis are expected to have large, bulky, frothy, greasy, foul-smelling stools (steatorrhea), not hard, packed stools.
   D. Children who have cystic fibrosis have mucus plugs. Administering a bronchodilator is an

   Ⓝ *NCLEX® Connection: Reduction of Risk Potential, Diagnostic Tests*

3. A. Children who have cystic fibrosis should eat a high-calorie, high-protein diet to allow for proper growth.
   B. **CORRECT:** When talking action and implementing discharge teaching for a child who has cystic fibrosis, the nurse should include in the teaching to administer pancreatic enzymes within 30 minutes of every meal and snack.
   C. Children who have cystic fibrosis should increase fluids to assist in thinning thick mucus.
   D. Children who have cystic fibrosis should engage in daily aerobic activity to assist with lung expansion and to stimulate mucus expectoration.

   Ⓝ *NCLEX® Connection: Physiological Adaptation, Alterations in Body Systems*

4. A, C, D, E. **CORRECT:** When generating solutions for the child who has cystic fibrosis, the nurse should plan to administer tobramycin, vitamins A, D, E, and K, albuterol, and dornase alfa. Tobramycin is administered to treat pulmonary infections. Supplementation of water-miscible forms of fat-soluble vitamins is included because children who have cystic fibrosis have difficulty absorbing fat. Albuterol and dornase alfa are administered to facilitate clearing of mucous plugs from the airway.
   B. Children who have cystic fibrosis have constipation and are expected to have a laxative or stool softener as part of the plan of care. Loperamide is an antidiarrheal medication.

   Ⓝ *NCLEX® Connection: Pharmacological and Parenteral Therapies, Expected Actions/Outcomes*

5. **PULMONDARY:** A,D,H; **GI:** E,F,B; **ENDOCRINE:** C,G

   Ⓝ *NCLEX® Connection: Physiological Adaptation, Alterations in Body Systems*

When reviewing the following chapters, keep in mind the relevant topics and tasks of the NCLEX outline, in particular:

Safety and Infection Control

ACCIDENT/ERROR/INJURY PREVENTION: Assess client for allergies and intervene as needed (e.g., food, latex, environmental allergies).

Pharmacological and Parenteral Therapies

ADVERSE EFFECTS/CONTRAINDICATIONS/SIDE EFFECTS/ INTERACTIONS: Provide information to the client on common side effects/adverse effects/potential interactions of medications and inform the client when to notify the primary health care provider.

MEDICATION ADMINISTRATION
Review pertinent data prior to medication administration.

Administer and document medications given by parenteral route.

Reduction of Risk Potential

SYSTEM-SPECIFIC ASSESSMENT: Assess the client for abnormal peripheral pulses after a procedure or treatment.

Physiological Adaptation

HEMODYNAMICS: Provide client with strategies to manage decreased cardiac output.

MEDICAL EMERGENCIES: Explain emergency interventions to a client.

UNIT 2   SYSTEM DISORDERS
SECTION: CARDIOVASCULAR AND HEMATOLOGIC DISORDERS

CHAPTER 20 *Cardiovascular Disorders*

Heart disease can be congenital or acquired.

Anatomic abnormalities present at birth can lead to congenital heart disease (CHD) most commonly, heart failure, and hypoxemia.

Heart failure occurs when the heart is unable to meet the metabolic and physical demands of the body due to inadequate blood flow.

Hyperlipidemia has increased due to poor diet and decreased activity levels in children. Children who have hyperlipidemia are at a greater risk for childhood obesity and for developing heart disease as an adult.

Congenital Heart Disease

ASSESSMENT

RISK FACTORS

MATERNAL FACTORS
- Infection
- Alcohol or other substance use disorder during pregnancy
- Diabetes mellitus

GENETIC FACTORS
- History of congenital heart disease in other family members
- Syndromes (Trisomy 21 [Down syndrome])
- Presence of other congenital anomalies or chromosomal abnormalities

EXPECTED FINDINGS

Defects that increase pulmonary blood flow

Defects with increased pulmonary blood flow allow blood to shift from the high pressure left side of the heart to the right, lower pressure side of the heart.
- Increased pulmonary blood volume on the right side of the heart increases pulmonary blood flow.
- These defects include manifestations and findings of heart failure.

Ventricular septal defect (VSD) (20.1)
A hole in the septum between the right and left ventricle that results in increased pulmonary blood flow (left-to-right shunt)
- Loud, harsh murmur auscultated at the left sternal border
- Heart failure
- Many VSDs close spontaneously early in life

Atrial septal defect (ASD)
A hole in the septum between the right and left atria that results in increased pulmonary blood flow (left-to-right shunt)
- Systolic murmur and a fixed split second heart sound may be present
- Heart failure
- Asymptomatic (possibly)

Patent ductus arteriosus (PDA)
A condition in which the normal fetal circulation conduit between the pulmonary artery and the aorta fails to close and results in increased pulmonary blood flow (left-to-right shunt)
- Systolic murmur (machine hum)
- Wide pulse pressure
- Bounding pulses
- Asymptomatic (possibly)
- Heart failure
- Rales

OBSTRUCTIVE DEFECTS

Obstructive defects include those where blood flow exiting the heart meets an area of narrowing (stenosis), which causes obstruction of blood flow.
- The pressure that occurs before the defect is increased (ventricle) and the pressure that occurs after the defect is decreased. This results in a decrease in cardiac output.
- These children can present with manifestations of heart failure. ○EBP

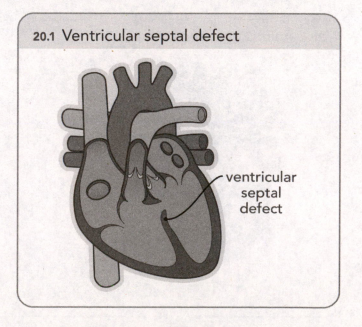

20.1 Ventricular septal defect

ventricular septal defect

Pulmonary stenosis (20.2)

A narrowing of the pulmonary valve or pulmonary artery that results in obstruction of blood flow from the ventricles
- Systolic ejection murmur
- Asymptomatic (possibly)
- Cyanosis varies with defect, worse with severe narrowing
- Cardiomegaly
- Heart failure

Aortic stenosis

A narrowing of the aortic valve
- **Infants:** Faint pulses, hypotension, tachycardia, poor feeding tolerance
- **Children:** Intolerance to exercise, dizziness, chest pain, possible ejection murmur

Coarctation of the aorta (20.3)

A narrowing of the lumen of the aorta, usually at or near the ductus arteriosus, that results in obstruction of blood flow from the ventricle
- Elevated blood pressure in the arms
- Bounding pulses in the upper extremities
- Decreased blood pressure in the lower extremities
- Cool skin of lower extremities
- Weak or absent femoral pulses
- Heart failure in infants
- Dizziness, headaches, fainting, or nosebleeds in older children

Defects that decrease pulmonary blood flow

- Defects that decrease pulmonary blood flow have an obstruction of pulmonary blood flow and an anatomic defect (ASD or VSD) between the right and left sides of the heart.
- In these defects, there is a right to left shift allowing deoxygenated blood to enter the systemic circulation.
- Hypercyanotic spells (blue, or "Tet," spells) manifest as acute cyanosis and hyperpnea.

Tricuspid atresia

A complete closure of the tricuspid valve that results in mixed blood flow. An atrial septal opening needs to be present to allow blood to enter the left atrium.
- Infants: Cyanosis, dyspnea, tachycardia
- Older children: Hypoxemia, clubbing of fingers

Tetralogy of Fallot (20.4)

Four defects that result in mixed blood flow: Pulmonary stenosis, ventricular septal defect, overriding aorta, right ventricular hypertrophy
- Cyanosis at birth: progressive cyanosis over the first year of life
- Systolic murmur
- Episodes of acute cyanosis and hypoxia (blue or "Tet" spells)

Mixed defects

Transposition of the great arteries

A condition in which the aorta is connected to the right ventricle instead of the left, and the pulmonary artery is connected to the left ventricle instead of the right. A septal defect or a PDA must exist in order to oxygenate the blood.
- Murmur depending on presence of associated defects
- Severe to less cyanosis depending on the size of the associated defect
- Cardiomegaly
- Heart failure

Truncus arteriosus

Failure of septum formation, resulting in a single vessel that comes off of the ventricles
- Heart failure
- Murmur
- Variable cyanosis
- Delayed growth
- Lethargy
- Fatigue
- Poor feeding habits

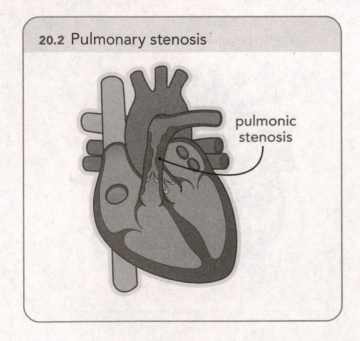

20.2 Pulmonary stenosis

pulmonic stenosis

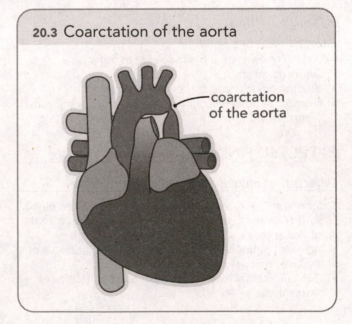

20.3 Coarctation of the aorta

coarctation of the aorta

Hypoplastic left heart syndrome

Left side of the heart is underdeveloped. An ASD or patent foramen ovale allows for oxygenation of the blood.

- Mild cyanosis
- Heart failure
- Lethargy
- Cold hands and feet
- Once PDA closes, progression of cyanosis and decreased cardiac output result in eventual cardiac collapse

PATIENT-CENTERED CARE

THERAPEUTIC PROCEDURES

Ventricular septal defect

NONSURGICAL PROCEDURE/THERAPIES
- Closure during cardiac catheterization
- Careful observations for spontaneous closure
- Diuretics

SURGICAL PROCEDURES
- Pulmonary artery banding
- Complete repair with patch (increased risk for heart block)

Atrial septal defect

NONSURGICAL PROCEDURES/THERAPIES
- Closure during cardiac catheterization
- Diuretics
- Low dose aspirin 6 months after procedure

SURGICAL PROCEDURE:
- Patch closure
- Cardiopulmonary bypass

Patent ductus arteriosus

NONSURGICAL PROCEDURES/THERAPIES
- Administration of indomethacin (to allow for closure)
- Insertion of coils to occlude PDA during cardiac catheterization
- Administration of diuretics (furosemide)
- Provide extra calories for infants Q EBP

SURGICAL PROCEDURE: Thoracoscopic repair (ligate vessels)

Pulmonary stenosis

NONSURGICAL PROCEDURES/THERAPIES: Balloon angioplasty with cardiac catheterization

SURGICAL PROCEDURES
- Infants: Brock procedure
- Children: pulmonary valvotomy

Aortic stenosis

NONSURGICAL PROCEDURES/THERAPIES
- Balloon dilation with cardiac catheterization
- Administer beta blockers, calcium channel blockers

SURGICAL PROCEDURES
- Norwood procedure
- Aortic valvotomy

Coarctation of the aorta

NONSURGICAL PROCEDURES/THERAPIES
- Infants and children: Balloon angioplasty
- Adolescents: Placement of stents

SURGICAL PROCEDURE: Repair of defect recommended for infants less than 6 months of age

Tricuspid atresia

SURGICAL PROCEDURES: Surgery in 3 stages: shunt placement, Glenn procedure, modified Fontan procedure

Tetralogy of Fallot

SURGICAL PROCEDURES
- Shunt placement until able to undergo primary repair
- Complete repair within the first year of life

Transposition of the great arteries

SURGICAL PROCEDURE/THERAPIES
- Surgery to switch the arteries within the first 2 weeks of life.
- IV prostaglandin E (keep ducts open).

Truncus arteriosus

SURGICAL PROCEDURE: Surgical repair within the first month of life

Hypoplastic left heart syndrome

SURGICAL PROCEDURES: Surgery in three stages starting shortly after birth: Norwood procedure, Glenn shunt, and Fontan procedure

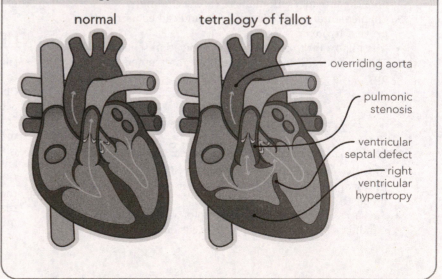

20.4 Tetralogy of Fallot

normal   tetralogy of fallot

- overriding aorta
- pulmonic stenosis
- ventricular septal defect
- right ventricular hypertropy

Pulmonary Artery Hypertension

Pulmonary artery hypertension (PAH) is high blood pressure in the arteries of the lungs that is a progressive and eventually fatal disease. There is no cure for pulmonary hypertension.

ASSESSMENT

RISK FACTORS

Although anyone can develop PAH, there can be a genetic link in children who have family who have PAH.

EXPECTED FINDINGS

- Dyspnea with exercise
- Chest pain
- Syncope

DIAGNOSTIC PROCEDURES

- Radiography (chest x-ray)
- Electrocardiogram
- Echocardiography
- Cardiac catheterization

PATIENT-CENTERED CARE

NURSING CARE

- Support the child and family regarding diagnosis and decisions of treatment options.
- Prepare the child and family for possible lung transplantation.

CLIENT EDUCATION Qpcc

- High altitude can cause hypoxia and should be avoided if possible. However, for those who live in high altitude area the provider will manage care accordingly.
- Supplemental oxygen is available and can be used to prevent hypoxia.
- It is important to adhere to the medication schedule.
- The prostacyclin infusion cannot be interrupted for any reason.

Infective (bacterial) endocarditis

- Infective endocarditis is an infection of the inner lining of the heart and the valves that can enter the bloodstream.
- Causative organisms include Streptococcus viridans, Candida albicans, and Staphylococcus aureus.

ASSESSMENT

RISK FACTORS

- Congenital or acquired heart disease
- Indwelling catheters

EXPECTED FINDINGS

- Fever, malaise, new murmur, myalgias, arthralgias, diaphoresis, weight loss, splinter hemorrhages under fingernails
- Neonates: Feeding problems, respiratory distress, tachycardia, heart failure, septicemia

LABORATORY TESTS

- CBC
- Erythrocyte sedimentation rate (ESR): elevated
- Urinalysis
- Blood cultures (positive for diagnosis)

DIAGNOSTIC PROCEDURES

- Electrocardiogram (ECG; vegetations present)
- Echocardiogram

PATIENT-CENTERED CARE

NURSING CARE

- Administer antibiotics parenterally for an extended length of time (2 to 8 weeks) usually via a peripherally inserted central catheter.
- Maintain a high level of oral care.
- Advise the guardians to notify their child's dentist of existing cardiac problems to ensure preventative treatment.

MEDICATIONS

High-dose anti-infectives are given for 2 to 8 weeks IV.

CLIENT EDUCATION Qpcc

- High risk children require prophylactic antibiotics prior to dental and surgical procedures.
- Observe for manifestations and findings of infection.
- Schedule follow-up appointments.
- Follow the American Heart Association's recommendations for infective endocarditis prophylaxis. Only high-risk clients should receive prophylactic antibiotic therapy.
- High-risk clients should receive prophylactic antibiotic therapy prior to dental procedures, surgical procedures that involve the respiratory tract, and procedures on infected skin or musculoskeletal tissue.

- The high-risk group requiring prophylaxis treatment includes children who have artificial heart valves; previous diagnosis of infective endocarditis; unrepaired cyanotic congenital heart disease; repaired congenital heart disease using prosthetic material or device during the first 6 months of the procedure; and residual defects after congenital heart disease repair.
- Observe for manifestations of endocarditis (low-grade fever, malaise, decreased appetite with weight loss).
- Children can require long-term antibiotics at home.

COMPLICATIONS

- Heart failure
- Myocardial infarction
- Embolism

Cardiomyopathy

Cardiomyopathy refers to abnormalities of the myocardium which interfere with its ability to contract effectively. Can lead to heart failure.

CLASSIFICATIONS

Dilated (DCM): Most common.

Hypertrophic (HCM): Autosomal genetic increase in heart muscle mass leads to abnormal diastolic function

Restrictive: Rare; prevents filling of the ventricles and causes a decrease in diastolic volume

ASSESSMENT

RISK FACTORS

Genetic factors, infection, deficiency states, metabolic conditions, collagen diseases, drug toxicity, dysrhythmias

EXPECTED FINDINGS

- Tachycardia and dysrhythmias
- Dyspnea
- Hepatosplenomegaly
- Fatigue and poor growth
- DCM: Palpations, syncope, infant poor feeding-respiratory distress
- HCM: Chest pain, syncope, dyspnea

PATIENT-CENTERED CARE

THERAPEUTIC MEASURES

- Beta blockers, calcium channel blockers, ACE inhibitors, anticoagulants
- Heart transplant

DIAGNOSTIC PROCEDURES

- Radiography (chest x-ray)
- ECG
- Echocardiogram
- Cardiac catheterization

COMPLICATIONS

- Infection
- Embolic complications (restrictive)

Shock

Cardiogenic shock results from impaired cardiac function that leads to a decrease in cardiac output.

Anaphylactic shock results from a hypersensitivity to a foreign substance that leads to massive vasodilation and capillary leak and can occur in response to an allergy to latex or drugs, insect stings, or blood transfusions.

ASSESSMENT

RISK FACTORS

- Cardiogenic shock can be seen in children following cardiac surgery and with acute dysrhythmias, congestive heart failure, trauma, or cardiomyopathy.
- Anaphylaxis can be seen in children who have allergies, asthma, or a family history of anaphylaxis.

EXPECTED FINDINGS

- Dyspnea
- Breath sounds with crackles
- Grunting
- Hypotension
- Tachycardia
- Weak peripheral pulses

MANIFESTATIONS OF HEART FAILURE

- **Impaired myocardial function:** Sweating, tachycardia, fatigue, pallor, cool extremities with weak pulses, hypotension, gallop rhythm, cardiomegaly
- **Pulmonary congestion:** Tachypnea, dyspnea, retractions, nasal flaring, grunting, wheezing, cyanosis, cough, orthopnea, exercise intolerance
- **Systemic venous congestion:** Hepatomegaly, peripheral edema, ascites, neck vein distention, periorbital edema, weight gain

MANIFESTATIONS OF HYPOXEMIA: Cyanosis, poor weight gain, tachypnea, dyspnea, clubbing, polycythemia **(20.5)**

MANIFESTATIONS OF ANAPHYLAXIS: Urticaria, periorbital or perioral angioedema, stridor, bronchospasm

LABORATORY TESTS

- ABGs including pH
- Hemoglobin, hematocrit, and blood electrolytes

DIAGNOSTIC PROCEDURES

ECG monitoring

To identify cardiac dysrhythmias

NURSING ACTIONS
- Assist with the application of electrodes.
- Assist with maintaining the child in a quiet position.

CLIENT EDUCATION: Tell the child that the test will not be painful.

Radiography (chest x-ray)

To determine heart size and blood flow

NURSING ACTIONS: Assist with positioning the child.

Echocardiography

To determine cardiac defects and heart function by use of ultrasound

NURSING ACTIONS: Assist with positioning the child.

Cardiac catheterization

An invasive test used for diagnosing, repairing some defects, and evaluating dysrhythmias. A radiopaque catheter is peripherally inserted and threaded into the heart with the use of fluoroscopy. A contrast medium (can be iodine-based) is injected, and images of the blood vessels and heart are taken as the medium is diluted and circulated throughout the body.

PREPROCEDURE NURSING ACTIONS
- Perform a nursing history and physical exam. Evidence of infection (a severe diaper rash) can necessitate canceling the procedure if femoral access is required.
- Check for allergies to iodine and shellfish. Qs
- Provide age-appropriate teaching.
- Describe how long the procedure will take, how the child will feel, and what care will be required after the procedure.

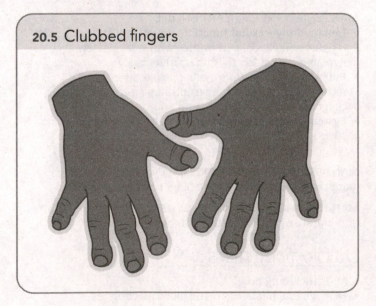

20.5 Clubbed fingers

- Provide for NPO status 4 to 6 hr prior to the procedure. (If the procedure is performed as outpatient, be sure the child and family are given instructions in advance.)
- Obtain baseline vital signs, including oxygen saturation.
- Locate and mark the dorsalis pedis and posterior tibial pulses on both extremities. Document the quality of the pulses.
- Administer pre-sedation as prescribed based on the child's age, height, weight, condition, and type of procedure being performed.

POSTPROCEDURE NURSING ACTIONS
- Provide for continuous cardiac monitoring and oxygen saturation to assess for bradycardia, dysrhythmias, hypotension, and hypoxemia.
- Assess heart and respiratory rate for 1 full minute.
- Assess pulses for equality and symmetry.
- Assess temperature and color of affected extremity. A cool extremity with skin that blanches (check surrounding skin tissue for changes in pigmentation as well) can indicate arterial obstruction.
- Assess insertion site (femoral or antecubital area) for bleeding or hematoma.
- Maintain clean dressing.
- Prevent bleeding by maintaining the affected extremity in a straight position for 4 to 8 hr.
- Monitor I&O for adequate urine output, hypovolemia, or dehydration.
- Monitor for hypoglycemia. IV fluids with dextrose can be necessary.
- Encourage oral intake, starting with clear liquids.
- Encourage the child to void to promote excretion of the contrast medium.

CLIENT EDUCATION
- Fluid intake can help with the removal of the dye from the body.
- Monitor the site for infection.
- Use mild analgesics for pain.
- Keep dressing clean and dry.
- No strenuous exercise.

PATIENT-CENTERED CARE

NURSING CARE
- Remain calm when providing care.
- Keep the child well-hydrated.
- Conserve the child's energy by providing frequent rest periods; clustering care; providing small, frequent meals; bathing PRN; and keeping crying to a minimum in cyanotic children.
- Perform daily weight and I&O to monitor fluid status and nutritional status.
- Monitor heart rate, blood pressure, blood electrolytes, and kidney function to assess for complications.
- Provide support and resources for parents to promote developmental growth in the child.
- Monitor family coping and provide support.
- Administer prescribed medications.

- Maintain fluid and electrolyte balance.
  - Administer potassium supplements if prescribed. These might not be indicated if the child is concurrently taking an ACE inhibitor.
  - Maintain sodium and fluid restrictions if prescribed.
- Decrease workload of the heart.
  - Maintain bed rest.
  - Position in an infant seat or hold at a 45° angle. Keep safety restraints low and loose on the abdomen.
  - Allow the child to sleep with several pillows and encourage a semi-Fowler's or Fowler's position while awake.
- Provide adequate nutrition.
  - Plan to feed the infant using a feeding schedule of every 3 hr. The infant should be rested, which occurs soon after awakening.
  - Use a soft preemie nipple or a regular nipple with a slit to provide an enlarged opening.
  - Hold the infant in a semi-upright position.
  - Allow the infant to rest during feedings, taking approximately 30 min to complete the feeding.
  - Gavage feed the infant if they are unable to consume enough formula or breast milk.
  - Increase caloric density of formula gradually from 20 kcal/oz to 30 kcal/oz.
  - Encourage clients who are breastfeeding to alternate feedings with high-density formula or fortified breast milk.

- Increase tissue oxygenation.
  - Provide cool, humidified oxygen via an oxygen hood (or tent), mask, or nasal cannula.
  - Suction the airway as indicated.
  - Monitor oxygen saturation every 2 to 4 hr.

MEDICATIONS

Digoxin

Improves myocardial contractility

NURSING ACTIONS
- Determine the heart rate and withhold the medication if it is below the hold rate specified by the provider. Generally, medication is held for any infant who has a heart rate less than 110/min, a young child with a heart rate less than 90/min, and an older child with a heart rate of less than 70/min. Qs
- Monitor for toxicity as evidenced by bradycardia, dysrhythmias, nausea, vomiting, or anorexia.
- Plan to administer digoxin immune fab as an antidote for toxicity.
- Therapeutic blood levels can vary between conditions and clients. Consider manifestations and digoxin level when toxicity is suspected.

20.6 Case Study

Scenario Introduction

Thomas is a registered nurse on a cardiovascular unit who will be caring for Javier, who is an adolescent male that is scheduled for a cardiac catherization. Javier is accompanied by his mother, Mari.

Scene 1

Thomas: Javier, I am going to be preparing you for your procedure today. I will start by getting your vital signs and then do a physical exam, like listening to your heart and lungs and checking your pulses. Do either of you have any questions for me about what we will do today or what was discussed with you yesterday about the procedure?

Mari: No, not right now.

Javier: Me either.

Scene 2

Thomas: Now that we have completed your physical exam, I have a few questions. Javier, do you have any allergies to any medications or to iodine or shellfish?

Javier: I don't think so, but you may want to ask my mom.

Mari: No. Javier is not allergic to anything.

Thomas: Ok. Good. When was the last time he had anything to eat or drink?

Mari: Last night before bed.

Scene 3

Thomas: Has Javier had fever or any other manifestations of an infection recently?

Mari: No, he has not.

Thomas: Ok. Javier, now I am going to need to start an IV and mark the pulses on your feet with a marker. Have you ever had an IV before?

Javier: Yes. I have had a lot. I am pretty used to them by now.

Scenario Conclusion

Thomas has initiated Javier's IV and marked his pedal and posterior tibial pulses with a marker. Thomas has also ensured that Javier and his mother understand the procedure and that a signed consent form is in the medical record. Javier is transported to the cath lab for the procedure.

Case Study Exercises

1. The nurse in this scenario is caring for a school-aged child who had a cardiac catheterization using the femoral vein one hour ago. Which of the following actions should the nurse take?

   A. Remove pressure dressing from the insertion site.

   B. Palpate pulses distal to the insertion site.

   C. Place the child in a semi-fowlers position.

   D. Maintain the child on NPO status.

2. The nurse in this scenario is providing discharge teaching to the child's mother. Which of the following instructions should the nurse include in the teaching?

   A. "Your child may resume their normal level of activity in 24 hours."

   B. "You should administer acetaminophen to your child for discomfort at the insertion site."

   C. "Drainage and swelling are expected at the insertion site for the first week after the procedure."

   D. "It is expected for the extremity that was used for the procedure to be cool to the touch."

Captopril or enalapril

Angiotensin-converting enzyme (ACE) inhibitors reduce afterload by causing vasodilation, resulting in decreased pulmonary and systemic vascular resistance.

NURSING ACTIONS
- Monitor blood pressure before and after the medication is administered.
- Monitor for evidence of hyperkalemia.

CLIENT EDUCATION: Monitor blood pressure frequently.

Metoprolol or carvedilol

Beta-blockers decrease heart rate and blood pressure, and promote vasodilation.

NURSING ACTIONS
- Monitor blood pressure and pulse prior to administration.
- Monitor for adverse effects (dizziness, hypotension, and headache).

Furosemide or chlorothiazide

Potassium-wasting diuretics rid the body of excess fluid and sodium.

NURSING ACTIONS
- Encourage a diet high in potassium.
- Monitor I&O.
- Monitor for adverse effects (hypokalemia, nausea, vomiting, and dizziness).
- Monitor weight daily.

INTERPROFESSIONAL CARE

Dietitians should be consulted to assist the family with appropriate food choices.

CLIENT EDUCATION Qᴘᴄᴄ

Cardiac catheterization

- Monitor for possible complications (bleeding, infection, thrombosis).
- Limit activity for 24 hr.
- Encourage fluids.

Digoxin administration

- Take pulse prior to medication administration. Notify provider if pulse is lower than specified rate.
- Administer digoxin every 12 hr.
- Direct oral elixir toward the side and back of mouth when administering. Qs
- Give water following administration to prevent tooth decay if the child has teeth.
- If a dose is missed, do not give an extra dose or increase the next dose.
- If the child vomits, do not re-administer the dose.
- Observe for manifestations of digoxin toxicity (decreased heart rate, decreased appetite, nausea, vomiting). Notify the provider if these occur.
- Keep the medication in a locked cabinet.

Diuretic administration

- Offer small amounts of fluids in small cups or containers.
- Observe for adverse effects of diuretics, which can include nausea, vomiting, and diarrhea.
- Observe for manifestations of blood potassium level imbalances (muscle weakness, irritability, excessive drowsiness, and increased or decreased heart rate).
- Encourage the child to eat foods high in potassium (bran cereals, bananas, legumes, leafy vegetables, oranges, and orange juice.)

CLIENT EDUCATION
- Monitor weight daily.
- Report evidence of worsening heart failure (increased sweating and decreased urinary output [fewer wet diapers or less frequent toileting]).

COMPLICATIONS

Cardiac catheterization (potential)

- Nausea, vomiting
- Low-grade fever
- Loss of pulse in the catheterized extremity
- Transient dysrhythmias
- Acute hemorrhage from entry site
- Hypoglycemia: Monitor blood glucose levels

NURSING ACTIONS
- Apply direct continuous pressure at 2.5 cm (1 in) above the catheter entry site to localize pressure over the location of the vessel puncture.
- Position the child flat to reduce the gravitational effect on the rate of bleeding.
- Notify the provider immediately.
- Prepare for the possible administration of replacement fluids and/or medication to control emesis.

CLIENT EDUCATION
- Monitor for infection.
- Monitor for bleeding.

Hypoxemia

A hypercyanotic spell can result in severe hypoxemia, which leads to cerebral hypoxemia, and should be treated as an emergency.

NURSING ACTIONS: Immediately place the child in the knee-chest position, attempt to calm the child, and call for help.

Heart failure requiring transplant

Cardiomyopathy and congenital heart disease are causes of heart failure.

NURSING ACTIONS
- Maintain pharmacological support as ordered (oxygen, diuretics, digoxin, afterload reducers [ACE inhibitors]).
- Provide family and child support.

CLIENT EDUCATION
- Adhere to the medication regimen.
- Be aware of infection control precautions.

Rheumatic fever

Rheumatic fever is an inflammatory disease that occurs as a reaction to Group A beta-hemolytic streptococcus (GABHS) infection of the throat.

ASSESSMENT

RISK FACTORS

Rheumatic fever usually occurs within 2 to 6 weeks following an untreated or partially treated upper respiratory infection (strep throat) with GABHS.

EXPECTED FINDINGS

- History of recent upper respiratory infection
- Fever
- Tachycardia, cardiomegaly, new or changed heart murmur, muffled heart sounds, pericardial friction rub, and report of chest pain, which can indicate carditis
- Nontender, subcutaneous nodules over bony prominence
- Large joints (knees, elbows, ankles, wrists, shoulders) with painful swelling, indicating polyarthritis Qpcc
- Findings can be present for a few days and then disappear without treatment, frequently returning in another joint.
- Pink, nonpruritic macular rash on the trunk and inner surfaces of extremities that appears and disappears rapidly, indicating erythema marginatum
- CNS involvement (chorea) including involuntary, purposeless muscle movements; muscle weakness; involuntary facial movements; difficulty performing fine motor activities; labile emotions; and random, uncoordinated movements of the extremities
- Irritability, poor concentration, and behavioral problems

LABORATORY TESTS

Throat culture for GABHS: currently recommend screening all school-aged children who have sore throats

Blood antistreptolysin O titer: Elevated or rising titer, most reliable diagnostic test

C-reactive protein (CRP): Elevated in response to an inflammatory reaction

Erythrocyte sedimentation rate: Elevated in response to an inflammatory reaction

DIAGNOSTIC PROCEDURES

Radiography (chest x-ray)

To assess for cardiomegaly

Cardiac function

- ECG to reveal the presence of conduction disturbances and to evaluate the function of the heart and valves
- Echocardiography to document pericardial effusions

NURSING ACTIONS: Position the child correctly for the procedure.

CLIENT EDUCATION: Explain the need for decreased movement during the procedure.

Jones criteria

The diagnosis of rheumatic fever is made on the basis of modified Jones criteria. The child should demonstrate the presence of two major criteria or the presence of one major and two minor criteria following an acute infection with GABHS infection.

MAJOR CRITERIA
- Carditis
- Subcutaneous nodules
- Polyarthritis
- Rash (erythema marginatum)
- Chorea

MINOR CRITERIA
- Fever
- Arthralgia

PATIENT-CENTERED CARE

NURSING CARE

- Encourage bed rest during the acute illness.
- Administer antibiotic as prescribed.
- Encourage nutritionally balanced meals.
- Assess for chorea (nervousness, behavioral changes, decreased attention span).

MEDICATIONS

Antibiotic prophylaxis

Follow the prescribed prophylactic treatment regimen, which can include one of the following.
- Two daily oral doses of penicillin V
- Monthly IM injection of penicillin G
- Daily oral dose of sulfadiazine

The length of treatment varies according to residual heart disease, ranging from 5 years to indefinitely.

NURSING ACTIONS
- Assess for an allergic response (anaphylaxis, hives, rashes).
- Assess for nausea, vomiting, or diarrhea.

CLIENT EDUCATION: Encourage compliance with medication regimen.

CLIENT EDUCATION Q̇pcc

- Promote rest during the acute phase.
- Provide information and reassurance related to the development of chorea and its self-limiting nature.
- Consume a diet of well-balanced meals.
- Seek medical care if infection recurrence is suspected.
- Child may need valve repair or replacement surgery.
- Follow up with cardiologist regularly.

COMPLICATIONS

Carditis and heart disease, atrial fibrillation, embolism

Dyslipidemia

Dyslipidemia refers to disorders of lipid metabolism that can result in abnormalities in the lipid profile. Cholesterol is part of the lipoprotein complex in blood.

Triglycerides come from two sources: Naturally made in the body from carbohydrates, and the end product of fat ingestion.

Total cholesterol: The sum of all forms of cholesterol

High density lipoprotein (HDL) cholesterol: "Good" cholesterol, having low level of cholesterol and triglycerides and high level of protein

Low density lipoprotein (LDL) cholesterol: "Bad" cholesterol, having a high level of cholesterol, low level of triglycerides, and moderate levels of protein

ASSESSMENT

RISK FACTORS

- Family history
- Genetic
- Obesity
- Lack of exercise
- History of health condition: diabetes, hypertension
- Congenital heart disease and transplant recipients
- Cancer survivors
- History of Kawasaki disease with coronary artery aneurysms
- Chronic inflammatory diseases
- Medications: birth control pills, diuretics, beta-blockers

LABORATORY TESTS

Lipid profile: fasting for 12 hr prior to test

Fasting blood glucose

PATIENT-CENTERED CARE

NURSING CARE

- Assist in screening clients who are at risk. Recommend two screenings between 2 to 8 years and the results of both tests are averaged.
- Assess clients for febrile illness 3 weeks prior to screening. (Illness will alter results.)

CLIENT EDUCATION Q̇pcc

- Keep a diet history for review by the dietitian.
- Diet to lower cholesterol: low fat, whole grains, fruit and vegetables.
- Use olive oil and canola oil.
- Recommend physical activity for children and adolescents for at least 60 min/day; young child can be performed in smaller increments throughout the day.

MEDICATION

Cholestyramine and colestipol

- Used in clients who do not respond to conventional treatment
- Used in children 10 years and older who have LDL 190 mg/dL or higher, or 160 mg/dL in clients who have risk factors

NURSING ACTIONS
- Powdered medication mixed in 4 to 6 oz water or juice, then administered immediately.
- Monitor for adverse effects: Constipation, abdominal pain, flatulence, nausea and abdominal bloating.
- Monitor laboratory findings: Liver function tests, CBC, creatinine kinase, and fasting lipid profile at 4- and 8-week intervals and with any dosage change.

CLIENT EDUCATION
- Understand how to administer medications.
- Observe for adverse effects of medications.
- Discontinue medication if experiencing dark urine or muscle aches, and notify the provider.
- Take multivitamin supplements while taking this medication.

HMG-CoA reductase inhibitors (statins)

NURSING ACTIONS
- Monitor for liver function, creatine kinase (CK) prior to start of therapy and during therapy.
- Can cause rhabdomyolysis (dark urine and muscle aches)
- Most effective in older children and adolescents.

CLIENT EDUCATION: Take in the evening.

INTERPROFESSIONAL CARE

Dietary counseling

COMPLICATIONS

Atherosclerosis and coronary heart disease

NURSING ACTIONS: Identify children who are at risk and promote early screening.

CLIENT EDUCATION: Practice healthy eating habits.

Kawasaki disease

Acute systemic vasculitis, resolves in less than 8 weeks. Also known as "mucocutaneous lymph node syndrome."

ASSESSMENT

RISK FACTORS

Etiology unknown

EXPECTED FINDINGS

Acute phase

Onset of high fever, lasting 5 days to 2 weeks, that is unresponsive to antipyretics.
- Irritability
- Red eyes without drainage
- Bright red, chapped lips
- Strawberry tongue with white coating or red bumps on the posterior aspect
- Red oral mucous membranes with inflammation including the pharynx
- Swelling of hand and feet with red palms and soles
- Nonblistering rash
- Bilateral joint pain
- Enlarged lymph nodes
- Desquamation of the perineum
- Cervical lymphadenopathy
- Cardiac manifestations: Myocarditis, decreased left ventricular function, pericardial effusion, and mitral regurgitation

Subacute phase

Resolution of fever and gradual subsiding of other manifestations
- Irritability
- Peeling skin around the nails, on the palms and soles
- Temporary arthritis

Convalescent

No manifestations seen except altered laboratory findings. Resolution in about 6 to 8 weeks from onset.

LABORATORY TESTS

CBC, CRP, ESR, blood albumin, elevated liver enzymes, lumbar puncture to assess for aseptic meningitis and inflammation

DIAGNOSTIC PROCEDURES

Radiography (chest x-ray)

Echocardiogram to evaluate heart size and functioning of the ventricles and valves. A follow up study is recommended 4 to 6 weeks after treatment.

PATIENT-CENTERED CARE

NURSING CARE

- Monitor vital signs and cardiac status. Maintain cardiac monitoring.
- Assess for heart failure (decreased urine output, gallop heart rhythm, tachycardia, respiratory distress).
- Monitor I&O.
- Obtain daily weight.
- Administer IV fluids to prevent dehydration.
- Offer clear liquids and soft, non-acidic foods.
- Administer IV gamma globulin according to facility policy.
- Administer aspirin as prescribed.
- Provide care to promote comfort due to findings.
  - Perform oral hygiene. Apply lip balm as needed.
  - Apply cool cloths to skin.
  - Apply skin lotions to maintain hydration.
  - Provide for a calm, quiet environment.
  - Promote rest by clustering care.

MEDICATION

Gamma globulin

NURSING ACTIONS
- Administer via IV infusion.
- High dosage: 2 g/kg over 8 to 12 hr.
- Ideally, administer within the first 10 days of illness.
- Repeat for clients who remain febrile.
- Monitor vital signs.
- Assess for allergic reaction.

Aspirin

HIGH DOSE: 80 to 100 mg/kg/day divided every 6 hr.

ONCE AFEBRILE: 3 to 5 mg/kg/day to continue until platelet count returns to expected range which can be approximately 6 to 8 weeks.

> If coronary abnormalities develop, continue aspirin therapy indefinitely.

CLIENT EDUCATION Qpcc

- Understand disease progression.
- Maintain follow-up appointments.
- The irritability can last 2 months.
- Arthritic manifestations can last several weeks.
- Skin manifestations are painless but the skin could be tender.
- Perform passive ROM exercises in the bathtub.
- Avoid live immunizations for 11 months.
- Notify the provider of any fever.

CARE AFTER DISCHARGE

- Avoid smoking.
- Maintain a heart healthy diet.
- Screen for heart disease as child ages.
  - Blood cholesterol testing
  - Blood pressure monitoring
  - Periodic imaging of the heart

COMPLICATIONS

Coronary artery dilation or aneurysm formation

- Most common in the subacute phase
- Echocardiogram to monitor for changes
- Administer anticoagulation medications as prescribed (enoxaparin)

Application Exercises

1. A nurse is assessing an infant who has coarctation of the aorta. Which of the following findings should the nurse expect? (Select all that apply.)
   A. Weak femoral pulses
   B. Cool skin of lower extremities
   C. Severe cyanosis
   D. Clubbing of the fingers
   E. Low blood pressure

2. A nurse is caring for an infant who has the following clinical manifestations: systolic murmur, wide pulse pressure, bounding pulses, and rales when auscultating the lungs. Which of the following congenital heart conditions should the nurse suspect?
   A. Tetralogy of Fallot
   B. Patent ductus arteriosus
   C. Ventricular septal defect
   D. Pulmonary stenosis

3. A nurse is providing education to the parent of a child who has infective endocarditis. Which of the following statements by the parent indicates understanding of the teaching?
   A. "My child will need IV antibiotics for the next 7 days."
   B. "I will need to let our dentist know about my child's diagnosis."
   C. "My child will need to avoid high altitudes until the infection is gone."
   D. "Some children with this diagnosis eventually require a lung transplant."

4. A nurse is assessing an infant who has heart failure. Which of the following findings should the nurse expect to find? (Select all that apply.)
   A. Bradycardia
   B. Cool extremities
   C. Peripheral edema
   D. Increased urinary output
   E. Nasal flaring

5. A nurse is caring for a school-aged child who has heart failure. The nurse has assessed the child and found the clinical manifestations listed below. Sort the clinical manifestations into the following systems categoriesg: Myocardial, Pulmonary, or Vascular.
   A. Ascites
   B. Hepatomegaly
   C. Nasal flaring
   D. Orthopnea
   E. Pallor
   F. Retractions
   G. Tachycardia
   H. Tachypnea
   I. Weak pulses
   J. Weight gain

6. A nurse is caring for a 2-year-old child who has a heart defect and is scheduled for cardiac catheterization. Which of the following actions should the nurse take?
   A. Place on NPO status for 12 hr prior to the procedure.
   B. Check for iodine or shellfish allergies prior to the procedure.
   C. Elevate the affected extremity following the procedure.
   D. Limit fluid intake following the procedure.

7. A nurse is providing teaching to the caregiver of an infant who has a prescription for digoxin. Which of the following instructions should the nurse include?
   A. "Do not offer your baby fluids after giving the medication."
   B. "Digoxin increases your baby's heart rate."
   C. "Give the correct dose of medication at regularly scheduled times."
   D. "If your baby vomits a dose, you should repeat the dose to ensure that the correct amount is received."

8. A nurse is caring for a child who is suspected of having rheumatic fever. Which of the following findings should the nurse expect? (Select all that apply.)
   A. Erythema marginatum (rash)
   B. Continuous joint pain of the digits
   C. Tender, subcutaneous nodules
   D. Decreased erythrocyte sedimentation rate
   E. Elevated C-reactive protein

1. A, B, E. **CORRECT:** When recognizing cues while assessing an infant who has coarctation of the aorta, the nurse should expect the infant to have weak femoral pulses, cool skin on the lower extremities, and decreased blood pressure in the lower extremities. These clinical manifestations are caused by narrowing of the lumen of the aorta which causes and obstruction of blood flow from the ventricle.
   C. A child who has coarctation of the aorta exhibits adequate oxygenation of blood. Severe cyanosis is not present.
   D. Clubbing of the fingers is a manifestation of chronic hypoxemia and will not be observed in an infant who has coarctation of the aorta.

   Ⓝ *NCLEX® Connection: Physiological Adaptation, Pathophysiology*

2. A. The newborn who has tetralogy of Fallot has clinical manifestations that include cyanosis, hypoxia, and a systolic murmur.
   B. **CORRECT:** The newborn who has a patent ductus arteriosus has clinical manifestations that include a systolic murmur, wide pulse pressures, bounding pulses, and rales when auscultating the lungs.
   C. Newborns who have a ventricular septal defect have clinical manifestations that include a loud, harsh murmur at the left sternal boarder. Manifestations of heart failure may be present.
   D. Newborns who have pulmonary stenosis have clinical manifestations that include a systolic murmur, cardiomegaly, and varying degrees of cyanosis dependent on the degree of the defect. Manifestations of heart failure may be present.

3. A. "My child will need IV antibiotics for the next 7 days" is an incorrect statement because the child will require antibiotics for 2 to 8 weeks following the diagnosis, not 7 days.
   B. **CORRECT:** When evaluating the outcomes of teaching to the parents, the nurse should recognize that the following statement indicates understanding of the teaching, "I will need to let our dentist know about my child's diagnosis." Children who have had a diagnosis of infective endocarditis require prophylactic antibiotic therapy prior to dental procedures.
   C. "My child will need to avoid high altitudes until the infection is gone" is an incorrect statement because the child who has PAH should avoid high altitudes, not the child who has infective endocarditis.
   D. "Some children with this diagnosis eventually require a lung transplant" is an incorrect statement because the child who has PAH may eventually require a lung transplant, not the child who has infective endocarditis.

4. B, C, E. **CORRECT:** When recognizing cues for the infant who has heart failure, the nurse should recognize that cool extremities, peripheral edema, and nasal flaring are manifestations of heart failure. Cool extremities occur due to the hearts inability to adequately circulate oxygenated blood. Peripheral edema occurs because the heart is unable to adequately circulate blood through the body and back to the heart. Nasal flaring occurs due to inadequate oxygenation of blood.
   A. The nurse should expect the infant who has heart failure to be tachycardic, not bradycardic.
   D. The nurse should expect the infant who has heart failure to have decreased urinary output, not increased urinary output.

5. **MYOCARDIAL:** E, H, I;
   PULMONARY: D, C, F, G;
   VASCULAR: A, B, J

   The child who has congestive heart failure has impaired myocardial function which manifests as sweating, tachycardia, fatigue, pallor, cool extremities with weak pulses, hypotension, gallop rhythm, and cardiomegaly. Heart failure also causes pulmonary congestion manifested by tachypnea, dyspnea, retractions, nasal flaring, grunting, wheezing, cyanosis, cough, orthopnea, and exercise intolerance. As cardiac output decreases blood begins to pool in the vascular space leading to systemic venous congestion. Manifestations of systemic venous congestion include hepatomegaly, peripheral edema, ascites, neck vein distention, periorbital edema, and weight gain.

   Ⓝ *NCLEX® Connection: Physiological Adaptation, Alterations in Body Systems*

6. A. The child should remain NPO 4 to 6 hr prior to the procedure, not for 12 hours.
   B. **CORRECT:** When taking action while caring for a child who has a heart defect and is scheduled for cardiac catheterization, the nurse should check for iodine or shellfish allergies prior to the procedure.
   C. The affected extremity should be maintained in a straight position following the procedure, not elevated.
   D. Fluids should be encouraged, not limited, after the procedure to maintain adequate urine output and promote excretion of the dye.

   Ⓝ *NCLEX® Connection: Reduction of Risk Potential, Diagnostic Tests*

7. A. The nurse should include in the instructions that Digoxin can be given without regard to food or fluids, however, if the child has teeth, give water after administration to prevent tooth decay.
   B. The nurse should include in the instructions that Digoxin slows the heart rate by increasing contractility of the heart. Digoxin does not increase the heart rate.
   C. **CORRECT:** When taking action and providing teaching to the caregiver of an infant who has a prescription for digoxin, the nurse should instruct the caregiver to administer the correct amount of digoxin at regularly scheduled times to maintain therapeutic blood levels.
   D. The nurse should include in the instructions that it is not recommended to repeat digoxin following an episode of emesis because it is impossible to determine how much medication was lost.

   Ⓝ *NCLEX® Connection: Pharmacological and Parenteral Therapies, Medication Administration*

8. A, E. **CORRECT:** When recognizing cues while caring for the child who is suspected of having rheumatic fever, the nurse should expect to find an erythema marginatum (rash) and an elevated C-reactive protein.
   B. A client who has rheumatic fever exhibits migratory joint pain of the large joints, not continuous joint pain of the fingers.
   C. A client who has rheumatic fever exhibits nontender subcutaneous nodules of bony prominences, not tender subcutaneous nodules.
   D. Rheumatic fever is caused by Group A beta-hemolytic streptococcus, which results in an elevated erythrocyte sedimentation rate, not a decreased erythrocyte sedimentation rate.

   Ⓝ *NCLEX® Connection: Physiological Adaptation, Pathophysiology*

Case Study Exercises Key

1. A. The nurse should not remove the pressure dressing at the insertion site one hour after the procedure. The pressure dressing should remain in place for at least 24 hours after the procedure to help prevent post-procedure bleeding.
   B. **CORRECT:** When caring for a child who has had a cardiac catherization using the femoral vein, the nurse should implement interventions to promote and maintain the child's recovery as well as identify any complications that the child may experience. Therefore, the nurse should palpate pulses distal to the insertion site each time the vital signs are assessed. Weak pulses in the affected extremity may indicate impaired circulation in the extremity.
   C. The nurse should not place the child in a semi-fowlers position one hour after the procedure. The child should remain in a supine position with the affected extremity in a straight position for 4 to 8 hours after the procedure to help prevent post-procedure bleeding.
   D. The nurse should not maintain the child on NPO status. The child should begin taking fluids as soon as possible after the procedure to help prevent dehydration and to assist with removing the dye from the body.

2. A. When providing discharge education to the guardian of a child who has had a cardiac catherization, the nurse should inform the guardian that the child should avoid strenuous activity for several days following the procedure.
   B. **CORRECT:** When providing discharge education to the guardian of a child who has had a cardiac catherization, the nurse should inform the guardian that they can administer a mild analgesic such as acetaminophen or ibuprofen to the child for discomfort at the insertion site.
   C. When providing discharge education to the guardian of a child who has had a cardiac catherization, the nurse should inform the guardian that drainage and swelling at the site are manifestations of infection and should be reported to the provider.
   D. When providing discharge education to the guardian of a child who has had a cardiac catherization, the nurse should inform the guardian that the child's extremities should both be warm to the touch. The nurse should instruct the guardian to report any changes in warmth or color to the provider as these findings may indicate impaired blood flow to the extremity.

Active Learning Scenario

A nurse is discussing care of a child who has Kawasaki disease with a newly hired nurse. What should be included in this discussion? Use the ATI Active Learning Template: System Disorder to complete this item.

EXPECTED FINDINGS: Identify for the acute, subacute, and convalescent phase.

NURSING CARE: List seven nursing actions for this client.

Active Learning Scenario Key

Using the ATI Active Learning Template: System Disorder
EXPECTED FINDINGS

Acute phase: onset of high fever that is unresponsive to antipyretics, with development of other manifestations
- Fever greater than 38.9° C (102° F) lasting 5 days to 2 weeks and unresponsive to antipyretics
- Irritability
- Red eyes without drainage
- Bright red, chapped lips
- Strawberry tongue with white coating or red bumps on the posterior aspect
- Red oral mucous membranes
- Swelling of hands and feet with red palms and soles
- Non-blistering rash
- Bilateral joint pain
- Enlarged lymph nodes
- Subacute phase: resolution of the fever and gradual subsiding of other manifestations
- Irritability
- Peeling skin around the nails, on the palms and soles

Convalescent phase: no manifestations seen except altered laboratory findings. Resolution in about 6 to 8 weeks from onset.

NURSING CARE
- Monitor vital signs, ECG, and cardiac status.
- Assess client for heart failure (decreased urine output, gallop heart rhythm, tachycardia, respiratory distress).
- Monitor I&O. Obtain daily weight.
- Administer IV fluids. Offer clear liquids and soft foods.
- Administer IV gamma globulin according to facility policy.
- Administer aspirin as prescribed.
- Provide care to include oral hygiene, cool cloths to extremities, application of skin lotion; providing for a quiet environment to promote rest; cluster nursing care.

  Ⓝ *NCLEX® Connection: Physiological Adaptation, Unexpected Response to Therapies*

CHAPTER 21 Hematologic Disorders

Blood disorders that can affect children include epistaxis, iron deficiency anemia, sickle cell anemia, and hemophilia.

Epistaxis

- Short, isolated occurrences of epistaxis (nosebleeds) are common in childhood.
- Although epistaxis is rarely an emergency, it causes anxiety for the child and the child's caregivers.

ASSESSMENT

RISK FACTORS

- Trauma (picking or rubbing the nose) can cause mucous membranes in the nose, which are vascular and fragile, to tear and bleed.
- Low humidity, allergic rhinitis, upper respiratory infection, blunt injury, or a foreign body in the nose can precipitate a nosebleed.
- Medications that affect clotting factors can increase bleeding.
- Epistaxis can be the result of underlying diseases (von Willebrand disease, hemophilia, idiopathic thrombocytopenia purpura, leukemia).

PHYSICAL ASSESSMENT FINDINGS
- Active bleeding from nose
- Restlessness and agitation

PATIENT-CENTERED CARE

NURSING CARE

- Maintain a calm demeanor with the child and family.
- Have the child sit up with the head tilted slightly forward to prevent aspiration of blood. Qs
- Apply pressure to the lower nose with the thumb and forefinger for at least 10 min.
- Do not pack cotton or tissue into the nostril or ask the child to blow their nose because this could displace the clot. Encourage the child to breathe through their mouth while pressure is being applied to their nose to control the bleeding.
- Apply ice across the bridge of the nose if bleeding continues.

CLIENT EDUCATION

- For recurrences, sit up and slightly forward so blood does not flow down the throat and cause coughing.
- Bleeding usually stops within 10 min.

Iron Deficiency Anemia

- Iron deficiency anemia is the most prevalent anemia worldwide.
- Adolescents are at risk due to poor diet, rapid growth, menses, strenuous activities, and obesity.
- The production of hemoglobin (Hgb) requires iron. Iron deficiency will result in decreased Hgb levels.
- Iron deficiency anemia usually results from an inadequate dietary supply of iron and is the most preventable mineral disturbance.

ASSESSMENT

RISK FACTORS

- Premature birth resulting in decreased iron stores
- Excessive intake of cows' milk in toddlers
  - Milk is not a good source of iron.
  - Milk takes the place of iron-rich solid foods.
- Malabsorption disorders
- Poor dietary intake of iron
- Increased iron requirements (blood loss)

Infants: GERD, pyloric stenosis

Older Child: GI polyps, colitis,

Adolescents: Menorrhagia

21.1 Expected Reference Ranges for Blood Diagnostic Procedures

PROCEDURE	REFERENCE RANGES
RBC	1–18 years: 4–5.5
	6 months – 1 year: 3.5 – 5.2
	2 – 6 months: 3.5 – 5
	2 – 8 weeks: 4 – 6
WBC	Child 2 years or younger: 6200 – 17000/mm³
	Child older than 2 years: 5 – 10000 mm³
Hgb	6 – 18 years: 10 – 15.5 g/dL
	6 months – 6 year: 9.5 – 14 g/dL
	2 – 6 months: 10 – 17 g/dl
HCT	6 – 18 years: 32 – 44%
	1 – 6 years: 30 – 40%
	6 months – 1 year: 29 – 43%
	2 – 6 months: 35 – 50%
	2 – 8 weeks: 39 – 59%
Reticulocyte Count	Child: 0.5 – 2%
	Infant: 0.5 – 3.1%
Total Iron Binding Capacity	250 – 460 mcg/dL
Transferrin	Child: 203 – 360 mg/dL
Total Bilirubin	0.3 – 1.0 mg/dL

EXPECTED FINDINGS

- Tachycardia
- Pallor
- Brittle, spoon-shaped fingernails
- Fatigue, irritability, and muscle weakness
- Systolic heart murmur
- Cravings for non-nutritive substances (ice, dirt, paper)

LABORATORY TESTS

CBC: Decreased RBC count, Hgb, and Hct

Hgb levels: Vary with age

RBC indices: Decreased, indicating microcytic/hypochromic RBCs
- **Mean corpuscular volume**: Average size of RBC
- **Mean corpuscular Hgb**: Average weight of RBC
- **Mean corpuscular hemoglobin concentration**: Amount of Hgb relative to size of cell

Reticulocyte count: Can be decreased (indicates bone marrow production of RBCs)

Total iron binding capacity: Elevated

Transferrin: 10% indicative of anemia

Stool analysis: Guaiac test

PATIENT-CENTERED CARE

NURSING CARE

- Provide iron supplements for preterm and low-birth-weight infants by the age of 2 months. Q_{EBP}
- Provide iron supplements to full term infants by the age of 4 to 6 months.
- Recommend iron-fortified formula for infants when solids are introduced.
- Modify the infant's diet to include high iron, and vitamin C.
- Monitor formula intake in infants.
  - Limit formula intake to 32 oz (960 mL) per day.
  - Encourage intake of iron-rich foods.
  - Provide iron-fortified cereal when solid foods are introduced.
  - Allow frequent rest periods.
- If packed RBCs are required, follow protocols for administration.

MEDICATIONS

Iron Supplements

NURSING ACTIONS
- Give 1 hr before or 2 hr after milk, tea, or antacid to prevent decreased absorption.
- Gastrointestinal (GI) upset (diarrhea, constipation, nausea) is common at the start of therapy. These will decrease over time.
- If tolerated, administer iron supplements on an empty stomach. Give with meals and start with reduced dose and gradually increase if GI distress occurs.

- Give with vitamin C to increase absorption.
- Use a straw with liquid preparation to prevent staining of teeth.
- Use a Z-track into deep muscle for parenteral injections. Do not massage after injection.

CLIENT EDUCATION
- Expect stools to turn a tarry green color if dose is adequate.
- Brush teeth after oral dose to minimize or prevent staining.

SEVERE ANEMIA THERAPY

IV Administration Ferrous Sulfate

- Very painful infusion
- Requires close monitoring of the child during administration

Blood Transfusion

PRBC preferred

Supplemental Oxygen

Used for severe hypoxia

CLIENT EDUCATION

- Diarrhea, constipation, or nausea can occur at the start of therapy, but these adverse effects are usually self-limiting.
- Understand appropriate iron administration.
- Increase fiber and fluids if constipation develops.
- To prevent toxicity, store no more than 1 month's supply in a child-proof bottle out of reach of children.
- Allow adequate time for the child to rest.
- The length of treatment will be determined by the child's response to the treatment. If Hgb levels are not increased after 1 month of therapy, further evaluation is warranted.
- Return for follow-up laboratory tests to determine the effectiveness of treatment.
- Schedule universal anemia screens at 12 months of age.

Dietary sources of iron

- Infants: Iron-fortified cereals and formula or exclusive breastfeeding
- Older children: Dried beans and lentils; peanut butter; green, leafy vegetables; iron-fortified breads and flour; poultry; and red meat

COMPLICATIONS

DEVELOPMENTAL DELAY

NURSING ACTIONS
- Assess level of functioning.
- Improve nutritional intake.
- Refer to appropriate developmental services.

CLIENT EDUCATION: Provide support to the family.

Sickle Cell Anemia

Sickle cell disease (SCD) is a group of diseases in which abnormal sickle hemoglobin S (HbS) replaces normal adult hemoglobin (Hgb A).

Sickle cell anemia (SCA) is the homozygous and most common form of SCD.

- Manifestations and complications of SCA are the result of RBC sickling, which leads to increased blood viscosity, obstruction of blood flow, and tissue hypoxia. Manifestations of SCA are not usually apparent until later in infancy due to the presence of fetal Hgb.
- Tissue hypoxia causes tissue ischemia, which results in pain.
- Increased destruction of RBCs occurs.

Sickle cell trait: Child has the genes but is asymptomatic.

Sickle cell crisis is the acute exacerbation of SCA.

ASSESSMENT

RISK FACTORS

- SCD is an autosomal recessive genetic disorder.
- SCA primarily affects African Americans. Other forms of SCD can affect individuals of Mediterranean, Indian, or Middle Eastern descent.
- Children who have the sickle cell trait do not manifest the disease but can pass the trait to their offspring.

EXPECTED FINDINGS

- Family history of sickle cell anemia or sickle cell trait
- Reports of pain
- Shortness of breath, fatigue
- Pallor, pale mucous membranes
- Jaundice
- Hands and feet cool to touch
- Dizziness
- Headache

VASO-OCCLUSIVE CRISIS (PAINFUL EPISODE)

Acute (related to dehydration and decreased oxygen)

Severe pain, usually in bones, joints, and abdomen
Swollen joints, hands, and feet

- Abdominal pain
- Hematuria
- Obstructive jaundice
- Visual disturbances

Chronic

- Increased risk of respiratory infections and osteomyelitis
- Retinal detachment and blindness
- Systolic murmurs
- Renal failure and enuresis
- Liver cirrhosis; hepatomegaly
- Seizures
- Skeletal deformities; shoulder or hip avascular necrosis

SEQUESTRATION

- Excessive pooling of blood primarily in the spleen (splenomegaly), and sometimes in the liver (hepatomegaly)
- Reduced circulating blood volume results in hypovolemia and can progress to shock
- Hypovolemic shock: irritability, tachycardia, pallor, decreased urinary output, tachypnea, cool extremities, thready pulse, hypotension

APLASTIC CRISIS

- Extreme anemia as a result of a temporary decreased RBC production
- Typically triggered by an infection with a virus

Hyperhemolytic crisis

Increased rate of RBC destruction leading to anemia, jaundice, and/or reticulocytosis

LABORATORY TESTS

Screening for SCA in newborns is mandatory in all 50 US states and territories.

CBC to detect anemia.

Sickle-turbidity screening tool detects the presence of HbS but will not differentiate the trait from the disease.

Hemoglobin electrophoresis separates the various forms of Hgb and is the definitive diagnosis of sickle cell anemia or sickle cell trait.

Sickle-cell crisis

Hgb: decreased

WBC count: elevated

Bilirubin and reticulocyte levels: elevated

Peripheral blood smear reveals sickled cells

DIAGNOSTIC PROCEDURES

Transcranial Doppler (TCD) test

- Used to assess intracranial vascular flow and detect the risk for cerebrovascular accident (CVA). Qs
- A TCD is performed annually on children ages 2 to 16 years who have SCD.

PATIENT-CENTERED CARE

NURSING CARE

- Promote rest to decrease oxygen consumption.
- Administer oxygen as prescribed if hypoxia is present.
  - Provide intense hydration therapy while maintaining fluid and electrolyte balance.
  - Monitor I&O.
  - Give oral fluids.
  - Administer IV fluids with electrolyte replacement.
  - Use caution with potassium replacement.
- Administer blood products, usually packed RBCs, and exchange transfusions per facility protocol. Observe for manifestations of hypervolemia and transfusion reaction.
- Treat and prevent infection.
  - Administer antibiotics.
  - Perform frequent hand hygiene.
  - Give oral prophylactic penicillin. QEBP
  - Administer pneumococcal conjugate vaccine, meningococcal vaccine, and Haemophilus influenzae type B vaccine.
- Monitor and report laboratory results.

PAIN MANAGEMENT

- Use an interprofessional approach.
- Treat mild to moderate pain with acetaminophen or ibuprofen. Manage severe pain with opioid analgesics.
- Apply comfort measures (warm packs to painful joints).
- Schedule administration of analgesics to prevent pain.

MEDICATIONS

Opioids

Codeine, morphine sulfate, oxycodone, hydromorphone, and methadone provide analgesia for pain management.

NURSING ACTIONS
- Administer orally (immediate- or sustained-release) or IV (for severe pain).
- Administer on a regular schedule to maintain control or prevent pain if possible.
- Use patient-controlled analgesia if appropriate.

CLIENT EDUCATION
- Avoid activities that require mental alertness. Qs
- Analgesics can be necessary in high doses, and addiction is rare.

ANTINEOPLASTICS

Hydroxyurea not FDA approved for SCA but used widely to increase oxygenation to the cells.

Nursing Actions

- Administer PO
- Monitor nutrition intake

CLIENT EDUCATION: Antineoplastics can cause anorexia.

THERAPEUTIC PROCEDURES

Exchange transfusions: Replaces the sickled blood cells with normal blood cells.

Hematopoietic stem cell transplant: Permanent solution for SCD. High risk of neurologic complications.

CLIENT EDUCATION

- Provide emotional support and refer to social services if appropriate.
- Observe for manifestations of crisis and infection and notify the provider promptly.
- Promote rest and provide adequate nutrition for the child.
- Practice good hand hygiene and avoid individuals who have colds/infections/viruses.
- Adhere to fluid intake requirements (i.e. how many bottles or glasses of fluid should be consumed daily) to prevent dehydration.
- Consider genetic counseling.
- Maintain up-to-date immunizations.
- Wear a medical identification wristband or medical identification tags.
- Attend school regularly and avoid contact sports.

COMPLICATIONS

Stroke

Sickled cells can occlude blood vessels.

NURSING ACTIONS
Assess and report manifestations.
- Seizures
- Abnormal behavior
- Weakness of, or inability to move an extremity
- Slurred speech
- Visual changes
- Vomiting
- Severe headache

CLIENT EDUCATION: Blood transfusions are usually performed monthly to prevent a repeat stroke.

Acute chest syndrome

- Can be life-threatening
- Common in adolescents
- Increased risk for pneumonia due to decreased oxygen to lung tissue

NURSING ACTIONS

Assess and report manifestations.
- Chest, back, or abdominal pain
- Fever of 38.5° C (101.3° F) or higher
- Cough
- Tachypnea
- Dyspnea, wheezing
- Retractions
- Decreased oxygen saturations

CLIENT EDUCATION
- May need blood transfusion
- Take antibiotics as prescribed

Infections
- Risk for infections (streptococcus pneumoniae, H. influenzae)
- Spleen decreases in size
- Increased risk for septicemia

Other complications

- Kidney scarring
- Visual acuity decreased
- Priapism (males)

Hemophilia

Hemophilia is a group of bleeding disorders characterized by difficulty controlling bleeding. Deficiencies in the clotting factors.
- Bleeding time is extended due to lack of a factor required for blood to clot. Bleeding is internal or external.
- Bleeding tendencies are sometimes recognized during infancy following circumcision but might not become apparent until the infant becomes more active and prone to injuries during the toddler years.
- Hemophilia varies in severity based on the percentage of clotting factor a child's body contains. For example, a child who has mild hemophilia can have up to 40% of the normal factor VIII in his body, while a child who has severe hemophilia has very little factor VIII.
- Both hemophilia A and B are X–linked recessive disorders.

Hemophilia A

- Deficiency of factor VIII
- Referred to as classic hemophilia
- Accounts for 80% of cases

Hemophilia B

- Deficiency of factor IX
- Referred to as Christmas disease

Von Willebrand

Inherited lack of the von willebrand factor protein characterized by the inability of the platelets to aggregate

ASSESSMENT

EXPECTED FINDINGS

Episodes of bleeding, excessive bleeding, reports of joint pain and stiffness, impaired mobility, easy bruising, and activity intolerance

PHYSICAL ASSESSMENT FINDINGS
- Active bleeding, which includes bleeding gums, epistaxis, hematuria, and/or tarry stools
- Hematomas and/or bruising, even with minor injuries
- Hemarthrosis as evidenced by joint pain, stiffness, warmth, swelling, redness, loss of range of motion, and deformities
- Headache, slurred speech, and a decreased level of consciousness

LABORATORY TESTS

- Prolonged partial thromboplastin time (aPTT)
- Factor-specific assays to determine deficiency
- Platelets and prothrombin time are within expected reference ranges
- Whole blood clotting time is within expected range or prolonged

DIAGNOSTIC PROCEDURES

DNA testing: Detects classic hemophilia trait in females

PATIENT-CENTERED CARE

NURSING CARE

Management of bleeding in the hospital
- Administer injections via the subcutaneous route instead of the intramuscular route whenever possible.
- Avoid unnecessary skin punctures and use surgical aseptic technique.
- Venipunctures are preferred over finger or heel sticks for blood sampling.
- Monitor urine, stool, and nasogastric fluid for occult blood.
- Do not administer aspirin or any products that contain aspirin.
- Acetaminophen is an acceptable substitute for aspirin.
- Control localized bleeding.
  - Administer factor replacement.
  - Observe for adverse effects, which include headache, flushing, low sodium, and alterations in heart rate and blood pressure.
  - Encourage the child to rest and immobilize the affected joints.
  - Elevate and apply ice to the affected joints.

MEDICATIONS

1-deamino-8-d-arginine vasopressin (DDAVP)

DDAVP is a synthetic form of vasopressin that increases plasma factor VIII (antihemophilic factor).
- Effective for mild, but not severe, hemophilia
- Not effective for hemophilia B, which involves a factor IX deficiency

NURSING ACTIONS: Can be given prior to dental or surgical procedures

Factor VIII, products that contain factor VIII, pooled plasma, and recombinant products

Used to prevent and treat hemorrhage

NURSING ACTIONS: Administer by IV infusion.

CLIENT EDUCATION
- Treatment can require numerous doses.
- Periodic administration has proven effective for preventing bleeding complications.

Corticosteroids

Used to treat hematuria, acute episodes of hemarthrosis, and chronic synovitis

NURSING ACTIONS: Monitor for infection and bleeding.

CLIENT EDUCATION: Maintain good hand hygiene and avoid individuals with colds/infection/viruses.

E-aminocaproic acid (EACA)

Inhibits clot destruction.

Nonsteroidal anti-inflammatory agents

Used with caution to treat chronic synovitis.

NURSING ACTIONS: Monitor for infection.

CLIENT EDUCATION
- Administer cautiously due to potential inhibition of platelet function.
- Take the medication with food.

INTERPROFESSIONAL CARE

An interprofessional approach includes the pediatrician, hematologist, orthopedist, nurse, nurse practitioner, physical therapist, school nurse, and social worker.

CLIENT EDUCATION

- Prevent bleeding at home. Qs
  - Environment should be made as safe as possible to prevent injury.
  - Provide a safe home and a play environment.
  - Set activity restrictions to avoid injury. Acceptable activities include low-contact sports (bowling, fishing, swimming, golf). While participating in these activities, children should wear protective equipment.
  - Use soft-bristled toothbrushes.
- Perform regular exercise and physical therapy after active bleeding is controlled.
- Maintain up-to-date immunizations.
- Wear medical identification.
- Observe for manifestations of internal bleeding and hemarthrosis.
- Control bleeding episodes using the RICE (rest, ice, compression, elevation) method.
- Participate in a support group.
- Administer factor replacement
- Adhere to active ROM; passive ROM contraindicated with acute episodes due to risk of damage to the capsule of the joints.

COMPLICATIONS

UNCONTROLLED BLEEDING

Intracranial hemorrhage, airway obstruction from bleeding in mouth, neck, or chest

NURSING ACTIONS
- Monitor vital signs for evidence of impending shock.
- Take measures to control bleeding.
- Administer appropriate factor replacement during bleeding episodes to treat excessive bleeding or hemarthrosis.
- Administer a blood transfusion as prescribed.
- Conduct a neurologic assessment for evidence of intracranial bleed.
- Provide prophylaxis treatment. Regimens include infusion of factor VIII concentrate:
  - Prior to joint bleed.
  - Three times a week or every other day after the first joint bleed.

CLIENT EDUCATION: Report manifestations of bleeding.

JOINT DEFORMITY

- Most often elbows, knees, and ankles.
- Repeated episodes of hemarthrosis (bleeding into joint spaces) lead to impaired range of motion, pain, tenderness, and swelling, which can develop into joint deformities.

NURSING ACTIONS
- Take appropriate measures to rest, immobilize, elevate, and apply ice to the affected joints during active bleeding.
- Encourage active range of motion after active bleeding is controlled.
- Encourage maintenance of ideal weight to minimize stress on joints.
- Encourage maintenance of regular exercise and physical therapy.

Application Exercises

1. A nurse is providing teaching about the management of epistaxis to an adolescent. Which of the following positions should the nurse instruct the adolescent to take when experiencing a nosebleed?

   A. Sit up and lean forward.

   B. Sit up and tilt the head up.

   C. Lie in a supine position.

   D. Lie in a prone position.

2. A nurse is providing teaching about epistaxis to the parent of a school-age child. Which of the following should the nurse include as an action to take when managing an episode of epistaxis? (Select all that apply.)

   A. Press the nares together for at least 10 min.

   B. Breathe through the nose until bleeding stops.

   C. Pack cotton or tissue into the naris that is bleeding.

   D. Apply a warm cloth across the bridge of the nose.

   E. Insert petroleum into the naris after the bleeding stops.

3. A nurse is providing teaching to the parent of a child who has a new prescription for liquid oral iron supplements. Which of the following statements by the parent indicates an understanding of the teaching?

   A. "I should take my child to the emergency department if his stools become dark."

   B. "My child should avoid eating citrus fruits while taking the supplements."

   C. "I should give the iron with milk to help prevent an upset stomach."

   D. "My child should take the supplement through a straw."

4. A nurse is preparing to administer iron dextran IM to a school-age child who has iron deficiency anemia. Which of the following actions by the nurse is appropriate?

   A. Administer the dose in the deltoid muscle.

   B. Use the Z-track method when administering the dose.

   C. Avoid injecting more than 2 mL with each dose.

   D. Massage the injection site for 1 min after administering the dose.

5. A nurse is caring for an infant whose screening test reveals a potential diagnosis of sickle cell disease. Which of the following tests should the nurse expect the provider to prescribe to distinguish whether the infant has sickle cell disease or sickle cell trait?

   A. Sickle solubility test

   B. Hemoglobin electrophoresis

   C. Complete blood count

   D. Transcranial Doppler

Active Learning Scenario

A nurse is caring for a child who has a new diagnosis of hemophilia A. Use the ATI Active Learning Template: System Disorder to complete this item.

EXPECTED FINDINGS: List two physical assessment findings associated with hemophilia.

CLIENT EDUCATION: List three concepts to include in the teaching with the family and child.

Active Learning Scenario Key

Using the ATI Active Learning Template: System Disorder

EXPECTED FINDINGS
- Active bleeding (possibly from the gums, epistaxis, hematuria, and/or GI tract)
- Hematomas and bruising occur easily even with minor injuries
- Joint pain and stiffness, warmth, swelling, redness, loss of range of motion of the joints
- Cerebral bleeding can cause headaches, slurred speech, and decreased level of consciousness

CLIENT EDUCATION
- Prevent bleeding at home.
- Provide a safe home and a play environment that is free of clutter.
- Place padding on corners of furniture.
- Set activity restrictions to avoid injury. Stress importance of wearing protective equipment during activities.
- Caution with contact sports.
- Recommend the use of soft-bristled toothbrushes or oral water irrigations.
- Encourage regular exercise and physical therapy when not actively bleeding.
- Encourage recommended immunizations remain up-to-date.
- Teach the importance of wearing a medical identification.
- Teach manifestations of internal bleeding and hemarthrosis
- Inform of the RICE (rest, ice, compression, elevation) method to control active bleeding.

(N) *NCLEX® Connection: Physiological Adaptation, Alterations in Body Systems*

Application Exercises Key

1. A. **CORRECT:** When taking action and providing teaching about the management of epistaxis to an adolescent the nurse should instruct the adolescent to sit up and lean to lean forward to prevent aspiration when experiencing a nosebleed.
   B. Sitting up and tilting the head up could cause aspiration of blood and is not the correct position when experiencing a nosebleed.
   C. Lying in a supine position could cause aspiration of blood and is not the correct position when experiencing a nosebleed.
   D. Lying in a prone position could cause aspiration of blood and is not the correct position when experiencing a nosebleed.

   (N) *NCLEX® Connection: Reduction of Risk Potential, Therapeutic Procedures*

2. A, D. **CORRECT:** When taking action and providing teaching about epistaxis to the parent of a school-age child the nurse should instruct the parent to press the nares together for at least 10 min and to apply an ice pack to the bridge of the nose.
   B. The child should breathe through the mouth, not the nose, until the bleeding stops.
   C. Packing cotton or tissue into the naris is not a correct action when managing an episode of epistaxis.
   E. Inserting petroleum into the naris after the bleeding stops is not a correct action when managing an episode of epistaxis.

   (N) *NCLEX® Connection: Reduction of Risk Potential, Therapeutic Procedures*

3. A. A child's stools will become a tarry-green color if the iron supplement dose is adequate.
   B. Vitamin C increases absorption of the iron and should be encouraged while taking the supplement.
   C. Milk prevents absorption of the iron. The supplement should be given 1 hr before or 2 hr after consuming milk.
   D. **CORRECT:** When evaluating the effectiveness of teaching, the nurse should identify that the statement, "My child should take the supplement through a straw" indicates understanding of the teaching.

   (N) *NCLEX® Connection: Pharmacological and Parenteral Therapies, Medication Administration*

4. A. The nurse should administer the injection into a large muscle mass such as the ventrogluteal.
   B. **CORRECT:** When generating solutions for the IM administration of iron dextran to a school-age child, the nurse should plan to use the Z-track injection method for administration.
   C. The nurse should avoid injecting more than 1 mL with each dose.
   D. To reduce irritation and skin staining, the nurse should not massage the injection site after administering the dose.

   (N) *NCLEX® Connection: Pharmacological and Parenteral Therapies, Medication Administration*

5. A. The sickle solubility test is a screening tool that detects the presence of abnormal hemoglobin but does not distinguish between the trait and the disease.
   B. **CORRECT:** When caring for an infant whose screening reveals a potential diagnosis of sickle cell disease, the nurse should expect the provider to prescribe a hemoglobin electrophoresis test to distinguish whether the infant has sickle cell disease of sickle cell trait.
   C. A complete blood count tests for anemia. It indicates the average size of the red blood cells, and the amount of hemoglobin in the red blood cells. It will not distinguish between sickle cell disease and sickle cell trait.
   D. The transcranial Doppler is performed to assess intracranial vascular flow and detect the risk for cerebrovascular accident. It will not distinguish between sickle cell disease and sickle cell trait.

   (N) *NCLEX® Connection: Reduction of Risk Potential, Diagnostic Tests*

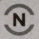
When reviewing the following chapters, keep in mind the relevant topics and tasks of the NCLEX outline, in particular:

Basic Care and Comfort

ELIMINATION: Assess and manage client who has an alteration in elimination.

NUTRITION AND ORAL HYDRATION: Manage the client's nutritional intake.

Reduction of Risk Potential

DIAGNOSTIC TESTS: Perform diagnostic testing.

SYSTEM-SPECIFIC ASSESSMENT: Perform focused assessment.

THERAPEUTIC PROCEDURES: Provide preoperative and postoperative education.

Physiological Adaptation

ALTERATIONS IN BODY SYSTEMS: Identify signs, symptoms, and incubation periods of infectious diseases.

FLUID AND ELECTROLYTE IMBALANCES: Manage the care of the client who has a fluid and electrolyte imbalance.

ILLNESS MANAGEMENT: Implement interventions to manage the client's recovery from an illness.

CHAPTER 22 ## Acute Infectious Gastrointestinal Disorders

Diarrhea can be mild to severe, and acute or chronic. It can result in mild to severe dehydration.

Acute diarrhea is a sudden increase in frequency and change in consistency of stool. It is usually secondary to an infectious agent in the GI tract, upper respiratory infection, urinary tract infection, antibiotic use, or laxative use. Self-resolution occurs in less than 14 days if dehydration does not occur. Acute infectious diarrhea is caused by a variety of viral, bacterial, or parasitic pathogens.

Chronic diarrhea is an increase in frequency and change of consistency of stools for more than 14 days. It is caused by chronic conditions (malabsorption syndrome, food allergies, or inflammatory bowel disease). Chronic nonspecific diarrhea has no identified cause.

Dehydration is a body fluid disturbance that occurs when water is lost form the body resulting in hypernatremia. Dehydration can be cause by fluid losses through the skin, respiratory, urinary, or GI tract).

ASSESSMENT

RISK FACTORS

Lack of normal elimination pattern, lack of clean water, poor hygiene, crowded living environments, poor sanitation, and nutritional deficiency Ⓠsᴅᴏʜ

EXPECTED FINDINGS

- Reports of fatigue, malaise, change in behavior, change in stool pattern, poor appetite, weight loss, and pain.
- Assess for manifestations of dehydration.

Rotavirus

Viral infection

MANIFESTATIONS
- Most common cause of diarrhea in children younger than 5 years
- Affects children of all ages
- Fever
- Onset of watery stools
- Diarrhea for 5 to 7 days
- Vomiting for approximately 2 days

TRANSMISSION: fecal–oral

INCUBATION PERIOD: 48 hr

Yersinia enterocolitis

Bacterial infection

MANIFESTATIONS
- Mucoid, possibly bloody diarrhea
- Abdominal pain, fever, and vomiting

TRANSMISSION: pets and food

INCUBATION PERIOD: 1 to 3 weeks

Escherichia coli

Bacterial infection

MANIFESTATIONS
- Watery diarrhea for 1 to 2 days, followed by abdominal cramping and bloody diarrhea
- Could lead to hemolytic uremic syndrome

TRANSMISSION: depends on strain of E. coli

INCUBATION PERIOD: 3 to 4 days

Salmonella nontyphoidal groups

Bacterial infection

MANIFESTATIONS
- Mild to severe nausea, vomiting, abdominal cramping, bloody diarrhea, and fever (can be afebrile in infants)
- Diarrhea can last 2 to 3 weeks
- Possible headache, confusion, drowsiness, and seizures
- Can lead to meningitis or septicemia

TRANSMISSION: person to person, undercooked meats and poultry

INCUBATION PERIOD: 6 to 72 hr

Clostridium difficile

Bacterial infection

Infection can occur from overgrowth of *C. difficile* following antibiotic therapy.

MANIFESTATIONS
- Mild, watery diarrhea for a few days
- Possible less severe manifestations in children than adults
- Possible leukocytosis, hypoalbuminemia, and high fever in certain children
- Possible pseudomembranous colitis

TRANSMISSION: contact with colonized spores.

INCUBATION PERIOD: nonspecified

Clostridium botulinum

Bacterial infection

MANIFESTATIONS
- Manifestations depend on strain
- Abdominal pain, cramping, and diarrhea
- Possible respiratory or CNS problems

TRANSMISSION: contaminated food products

INCUBATION PERIOD: 12 to 26 hr

Shigella groups: Shigellosis

Bacterial infection

MANIFESTATIONS
- Sick appearance
- Fever, fatigue, and anorexia
- Cramping abdomen followed by watery or bloody diarrhea lasting 5 to 10 days

TRANSMISSION: contaminated food or water

INCUBATION PERIOD: 1 to 7 days

Noroviruses: Caliciviruses

Viral infection

MANIFESTATIONS
- Abdominal cramps, nausea and vomiting, malaise, watery diarrhea
- Lasts 2 to 3 days

TRANSMISSION: contaminated water

INCUBATION PERIOD: 12 to 48 hr

Staphylococcus

Bacterial infection

MANIFESTATIONS: Diarrhea, nausea, and vomiting

TRANSMISSION: inadequately cooked or refrigerated food

INCUBATION PERIOD: 1 to 8 hr

Enterobius vermicularis (pinworm)

Helminthic infection

MANIFESTATIONS: Perianal itching, enuresis, sleeplessness, restlessness, and irritability due to itching

TRANSMISSION: fecal–oral

Ingested or inhaled eggs hatch in the upper intestine, and mature. After mating, worms migrate out of the intestine and lay eggs. Eggs can survive for 2 to 3 weeks on surfaces.

Giardia lamblia: parasitic pathogen

MANIFESTATIONS
- Children 5 years of age or younger
  - Diarrhea
  - Vomiting
  - Anorexia
- Older children
  - Abdominal cramps
  - Intermittent loose, malodorous, pale, greasy stools

TRANSMISSION: person to person, food, animals

The nonmotile stage of protozoa can survive in the environment for months.

LABORATORY TESTS

- CBC with differential to determine anemia and/or infection.
- Hct, Hgb, BUN, creatinine, and urine-specific gravity levels are usually elevated with dehydration.
- Stool specimen analysis
  - Occult blood
  - Cultures
- Urinalysis if dehydration is suspected.

DIAGNOSTIC PROCEDURES

Tape test

Performed to check for *Enterobius vermicularis*.

CLIENT EDUCATION
- Parents should place transparent tape over the child's anus at bedtime, preferably after the child is asleep. The caregiver should remove the tape just prior to the child awaking, if possible, prior to the child toileting or bathing.
- The specimen should be brought to the laboratory for microscopic evaluation for the presence of pinworm ova..
- Parents should use good hand hygiene during this procedure.

Infectious gastroenteritis

Rotavirus: Enzyme immunoassay (stool sample)

E. coli: Sorbitol-MacConkey agar (stool sample)

Salmonella: Gram-stained stool culture

C. difficile: Stool culture

C. botulinum: Blood and stool culture

Staphylococcus: Identification of organism in stool, blood, food, or aspirate

G. lamblia: Enzyme immunoassay (stool sample)

Shigellosis: Stool culture

Caliciviruses: Enzyme-linked immunoassay (ELISA, stool sample)

Yersinia enterocolitis: Identification of organism in stool culture, ELISA

PATIENT-CENTERED CARE

NURSING CARE

- Obtain baseline height and weight.
- Obtain the child's weight at the same time each day.
- Avoid taking a rectal temperature.
- Assess and monitor I&O (urine and stool).
- Initiate IV fluids as ordered.
- Administer antibiotic as prescribed (*Shigella*, *C. difficile*, and *G. lamblia*).
- Avoid antibiotics (*E. coli*, *Salmonella*).
- Avoid antimotility agents (*E. coli*, *Salmonella*, *Shigella*).

Oral rehydration therapy

- Start replacement with an oral replacement solution (ORS) of 75 to 90 mEq of sodium/L at 40 to 50 mL/kg over 4 hr. ⓠEBP
- Determine the need for further rehydration after initial replacement.
- Initiate maintenance therapy per facility protocol.
  - Give ORS alternately with intake of other liquids (breast milk, formula, milk).
  - Give infants water, breast milk, or lactose-free formula if supplementary fluid is needed.
  - Older children may resume their regular diets for additional intake.
- Replace each diarrheal stool with 10 mL/kg of ORS for ongoing diarrhea.

MEDICATIONS

Metronidazole and tinidazole

Indicated for *C. difficile* and *G. lamblia*

NURSING ACTIONS
- Monitor for allergies.
- Monitor for GI upset.

CLIENT EDUCATION: Take the medication as prescribed and report any GI disturbances.

Mebendazole, albendazole, and pyrantel pamoate

Indicated for *Enterobius vermicularis*

NURSING ACTIONS
- Administer in a single dose that can need to be repeated in 2 weeks.
- Administer mebendazole for children older than 2 years of age.

CLIENT EDUCATION: Entire family should be treated at the same time.

CLIENT EDUCATION

- Parents should inform the child's school or day care of the infection/infestation. The child should stay home during the incubation period.
- Teach the family to use commercially prepared ORS when the child experiences diarrhea. Foods and fluids to avoid include
  - Fruit juices, carbonated sodas, and gelatin, which all have high carbohydrate content, low electrolyte content, and a high osmolality
  - Caffeine, due to its mild diuretic effect
  - Chicken or beef broth, which has too much sodium and not enough carbohydrates
- Perform prevention measures, including immunization for rotavirus.
- Provide frequent skin care to prevent skin breakdown.
- Teach the family how to prevent the spread of infectious diseases.
  - Change bed linens and underwear daily for several days. Avoid shaking linens to prevent the spread of disease.
  - Keep the child's toys away from other children. Cleanse toys and child care areas thoroughly to prevent further spread or reinfestation.
  - Shower frequently.
  - Avoid undercooked or under-refrigerated food.
  - Perform proper hand hygiene after toileting and after changing diapers.
  - Do not share dishes and utensils. Wash them in hot, soapy water or in the dishwasher.
  - Clip nails and discourage nail biting and thumb sucking.
  - Clean toilet areas.

COMPLICATIONS

Dehydration

- Pure water loss
- Results in hypernatremia

LEVELS OF DEHYDRATION

- **Mild**
  - WEIGHT LOSS
    - 3% to 5% in infants
    - 3% to 4% in children
  - MANIFESTATIONS
    - Behavior, mucous membranes, anterior fontanel, pulse, and blood pressure within expected findings
    - Capillary refill greater than 2 seconds
    - Possible slight thirst
- **Moderate**
  - WEIGHT LOSS
    - 6% to 9% in infants
    - 6% to 8% in children
  - MANIFESTATIONS
    - Capillary refill between 2 and 4 seconds
    - Possible thirst and irritability
    - Pulse slightly increased with normal to orthostatic blood pressure
    - Dry mucous membranes and decreased tears and skin turgor
    - Slight tachypnea
    - Normal to sunken anterior fontanel on infants
- **Severe**
  - WEIGHT LOSS
    - Greater than 10% in infants
    - 10% in children
  - MANIFESTATIONS
    - Capillary refill greater than 4 seconds
    - Tachycardia present, and orthostatic blood pressure can progress to shock
    - Extreme thirst
    - Very dry mucous membranes and tented skin
    - Hyperpnea
    - No tearing with sunken eyeballs
    - Sunken anterior fontanel
    - Oliguria or anuria

NURSING ACTIONS

- Oral rehydration is attempted first for mild and moderate cases of dehydration.
  - **Mild:** 50 mL/kg rehydration fluid within 4 hr
  - **Moderate:** 100 mL/kg rehydration fluid within 4 hr
  - **Replacement of diarrhea losses** with 10 mL/kg each stool
- Administer parenteral fluid therapy as prescribed.
  - Initiate when a child is unable to drink enough oral fluids to correct fluid losses, and those with severe dehydration or continued vomiting.
  - Isotonic solution at 20 mL/kg IV bolus.
  - Monitor for manifestations of increased intracranial pressure.
  - Administer maintenance IV fluids as prescribed.
  - Avoid potassium replacement until kidney function is verified.
- Assess capillary refill.
- Assess vital signs.
- Monitor weight. Q EBP
- Maintain accurate I&O.

CLIENT EDUCATION

- Increase oral fluids.
- Resume normal diet as soon as possible.
- Monitor how many times the child voids.

Active Learning Scenario

A nurse is teaching the caregiver of a child who has an acute gastrointestinal infection. What information should the nurse include in the teaching? Use the ATI Active Learning Template: System Disorder to complete this item.

CLIENT EDUCATION: Describe at least 10 points to review regarding care after discharge.

Active Learning Scenario Key

Using the ATI Active Learning Template: System Disorder

CLIENT EDUCATION

- Have the parents inform the child's school or day care center of the infection/infestation. The child should stay home during the incubation period.
- Use commercially prepared oral rehydration therapy when the child experiences diarrhea. Foods and fluids to avoid include the following:
  - Fruit juices, carbonated sodas, and gelatin, which have high carbohydrate content, low electrolyte content, and high osmolality
  - Caffeine, due to its mild diuretic effect
  - Chicken or beef broth, which have high sodium content and inadequate carbohydrates
- Follow prevention measures, including immunization for rotavirus and methods to prevent further spread of the disease.
- Provide frequent skin care to prevent skin breakdown.
- Teach the family how to avoid the spread of infectious diseases.
- Change bed linens and underwear daily for several days. Avoid shaking linens to prevent the spread of disease.
- Cleanse toys and child care areas thoroughly to prevent further spread or reinfestation.
- Shower frequently.
- Avoid undercooked or under-refrigerated food.
- Perform proper hand hygiene after toileting and after changing diapers.
- Do not share dishes and utensils. Wash them in hot, soapy water or in the dishwasher.
- Clip nails, and discourage nail-biting and thumb-sucking.
- Clean toilet areas.

Ⓝ *NCLEX® Connection: Physiological Adaptation, Illness Management*

Application Exercises

1. A nurse is assessing a child who has a rotavirus infection. Which of the following findings should the nurse expect? (Select all that apply.)

   A. Fever

   B. Vomiting

   C. Watery stools

   D. Bloody stools

   E. Confusion

2. A nurse is teaching a group of parents about *Salmonella*. Which of the following information should the nurse include in the teaching? (Select all that apply.)

   A. Incubation period is nonspecific.

   B. It is a bacterial infection.

   C. Bloody diarrhea is common.

   D. Transmission can be from house pets.

   E. Antibiotics are used for treatment.

3. A nurse is teaching a group of caregivers about *E. coli*. Which of the following information should the nurse include in the teaching? (Select all that apply.)

   A. Severe abdominal cramping occurs.

   B. Watery diarrhea is present for more than 5 days.

   C. It can lead to hemolytic uremic syndrome.

   D. It is a foodborne pathogen.

   E. Antibiotics are given for treatment.

4. A nurse is caring for a child who is suspected to have *Enterobius vermicularis*. Which of the following actions should the nurse take?

   A. Perform a tape test.

   B. Collect stool specimen for culture.

   C. Test the stool for occult blood.

   D. Initiate IV fluids.

5. A nurse is caring for a child who has had watery diarrhea for the past 3 days. Which of the following is an action for the nurse to take?

   A. Offer chicken broth.

   B. Initiate oral rehydration therapy.

   C. Start hypertonic IV solution.

   D. Keep NPO until the diarrhea subsides.

Application Exercises Key

1. A, B, C. **CORRECT:** When recognizing cues during the assessment of a child who has rotavirus, the nurse should identify that fever, vomiting, and watery stools are manifestation of rotavirus.
   D. Bloody stools are a manifestation of *E. coli*.
   E. Confusion is a manifestation of *Salmonella*.

   Ⓝ *NCLEX® Connection: Physiological Adaptation, Alterations in Body Systems*

2. B, C, D. **CORRECT:** When taking action and teaching a group of parents about Salmonella, the nurse should include that Salmonella is classified as a bacterial infection and can be transmitted to children from household pets (cats, dogs, hamsters, and turtles). The nurse should also include that manifestations of Salmonella include bloody diarrhea, nausea, vomiting, and abdominal cramping.
   A. The incubation period of Salmonella is 6 to 72 hr.
   E. Salmonella is a bacterial infection. Antibiotics are not prescribed unless complications occur.

   Ⓝ *NCLEX® Connection: Physiological Adaptation, Illness Management*

3. A, C, D. **CORRECT:** When taking action and teaching a group of caregivers about E. coli, the nurse should include that manifestations of E. coli include severe abdominal cramping. The nurse should also include the E. coli is a bacterial infection that can lead to hemolytic uremic syndrome.
   B. Watery diarrhea lasts 1 to 2 days, then advances to bloody diarrhea.
   E. Antibiotics can worsen an *E. coli* infection. They are not recommended.

   Ⓝ *NCLEX® Connection: Physiological Adaptation, Illness Management*

4. A. **CORRECT:** When taking action during the care of a child who is suspected of having Enterobius vermicularis the nurse should perform a tape test as part of the diagnostic process.
   B. Stool cultures are obtained to diagnose *Salmonella* or *C. difficile* infection.
   C. A manifestation of *E. coli* is bloody stools.
   D. IV fluids are initiated for children who are dehydrated.

   Ⓝ *NCLEX® Connection: Reduction of Risk Potential, Diagnostic Tests*

5. A. Chicken broth is avoided for children who have diarrhea because of its increased sodium and inadequate carbohydrates.
   B. **CORRECT:** When taking action during the care of a child who has had watery diarrhea for the past 3 days, the nurse should initiate oral rehydration therapy to replace lost electrolytes.
   C. Isotonic IV solutions are recommended for children who experience severe dehydration.
   D. Children who experience diarrhea are at risk for dehydration. Keeping them NPO is contraindicated.

   Ⓝ *NCLEX® Connection: Physiological Adaptation, Fluid and Electrolyte Imbalances*

CHAPTER 23

Gastrointestinal Structural and Inflammatory Disorders

Gastrointestinal structural disorders include cleft lip and palate, gastroesophageal reflux disease, hypertrophic pyloric stenosis, Hirschsprung's disease, and intussusception.

Inflammatory disorders include appendicitis and Meckel's diverticulum.

Cleft lip and palate

- Cleft lip (CL) results from the incomplete fusion of the oral cavity during intrauterine life. Cleft palate (CP) results from the incomplete fusion of the palates during intrauterine life.
- Although a CL and CP can occur together, either defect can appear alone. The defects can be unilateral (one-sided) or bilateral (two-sided). **(23.1)**

ASSESSMENT

RISK FACTORS

- Genetic syndromes
- Combination of maternal and environmental factors
- Family history of cleft lip or palate
- Exposure to alcohol, cigarette smoke, anticonvulsants, retinoids, or steroids during pregnancy
- Folate deficiency during pregnancy; folic acid supplements during pregnancy can prevent clefting

EXPECTED FINDINGS

PHYSICAL ASSESSMENT FINDINGS

- Cleft lip is a visible separation from the upper lip toward the nose.
- Cleft palate is a visible or palpable opening of the palate connecting the mouth and the nasal cavity.

PATIENT-CENTERED CARE

NURSING CARE

- Support and encourage parents in the general care of their child.
- Promote parent-infant bonding.
- Promote healthy self-esteem throughout the child's development.

THERAPEUTIC PROCEDURES

Cleft lip
- Repair is typically done between 2 to 3 months of age.
- Additional surgeries are usually required to the lip and nose in severe defects to improve aesthetic outcome.

Cleft palate
- Repair is typically done between 6 to 12 months of age.
- Most require additional surgeries to improve speech quality and aesthetic outcome.

PREOPERATIVE NURSING ACTIONS
- Inspect the lip and palate, using a gloved finger to palpate the palate.
- Assess ability to suck.
- Obtain baseline weight.
- Observe interaction between the family and infant.
- Determine emotional needs of the family and provide support. Qpcc
- Refer parents to appropriate support groups.
- Consult with social services to provide needed services (financial, insurance) for the family and infant.
- Instruct parents about proper feeding and care.
- Assess ability to feed.
- Initiate strategies for successful feeding.
  - **For isolated cleft lip**
    - Encourage breast feeding.
    - Use a wide-based nipple for bottle feeding.
    - Squeeze the infant's cheeks together during feeding to decrease the gap.
  - **For cleft palate or cleft lip and palate**
    - Position the infant upright while cradling the head during feeding.
    - Use a specialized bottle with a one-way valve and a specially cut nipple.
    - Burp the infant frequently.
    - Syringe feeding can be necessary for the infant who is unsuccessful with other methods.

POSTOPERATIVE NURSING ACTIONS
- Perform standard postoperative care, including assessment of vital signs, oxygen saturation, and pain management using an age-appropriate tool. Qs
- Keep the infant pain-free to decrease crying and stress on repair.
- Administer analgesics as prescribed.
- Assess operative sites for manifestations of crusting, bleeding, and infection.
- Avoid having the infant suck on a nipple or pacifier.
- Avoid spoons, forks, and other objects the infant might bring to the mouth that could damage the incision site.
- Monitor I&O and weigh daily.
- Observe the family's interaction with the infant.
- Determine emotional needs of the family and provide support.

- **For cleft lip**
  - Monitor the integrity of the postoperative protective device to ensure proper positioning.
  - Position the infant on the back and upright, or on the side during the immediate postoperative period to maintain the integrity of the repair.
  - Apply elbow restraints to keep the infant from injuring the repair site. Restraints should be removed periodically to assess skin, allow limb movement, and provide for comfort.
  - Use sterile 0.9% sodium chloride, sterile water diluted hydrogen peroxide to clean the incision site. Apply antibiotic ointment if prescribed.
  - Gently aspirate secretions of mouth and nasopharynx to prevent respiratory complications.
- **For cleft palate**
  - Change the infant's position frequently to facilitate drainage and breathing.
  - Place the infant in side-lying position to facilitate drainage of secretions and prevent aspiration.
  - Maintain IV fluids until the infant is able to eat and drink.
  - The infant is usually NPO for 4 hr then allowed liquids only for the first 3 to 4 days, then progressed to a soft diet.
  - Avoid placing a straw, tongue depressor, hard pacifier, rigid utensils, hard-tipped sippy cups, or suction catheters in the infant's mouth after cleft palate repair.
  - Elbow restraints can be used to prevent the infant from injuring the repair.
  - Close observation for manifestations of airway obstruction, hemorrhage, and laryngeal spasm.
  - Use a face mask to deliver oxygen.

CLIENT EDUCATION
- Provide instructions on the proper use of the restraints.
- Provide guidelines for postoperative diet and feeding techniques.
- Provide education on proper care of operative site.

INTERPROFESSIONAL CARE

Care of the child who has CL and CP requires care from members of various disciplines (plastic surgeon, orthodontist, otolaryngologist, speech-language pathologist, pediatrician, nursing, audiologist, social worker and psychologist).

COMPLICATIONS

Ear infections and hearing loss

Related to altered structure and recurrent otitis media

NURSING ACTIONS
- Feed the infant in an upright position.
- Monitor temperature.

CLIENT EDUCATION
- Observe for manifestations of ear infections and seek treatment early.
- Insertion of pressure-equalizing tubes to facilitate fluid drainage from the ears and prevent middle ear effusion and otitis media can be required.

Speech and language impairment

More common with cleft palate

NURSING ACTIONS: Refer parents to a speech therapist for intervention as early as possible.

Dental problems

Teeth might not erupt normally, and orthodontia is usually necessary later in life.

CLIENT EDUCATION
- Promote healthy dental hygiene.
- Seek early dental care.

Gastrointestinal reflux disease

- Gastroesophageal reflux (GER) occurs when gastric contents reflux back up into the esophagus, making esophageal mucosa vulnerable to injury from gastric acid.
- Gastroesophageal reflux disease (GERD) is tissue damage from GER.
- GER is self-limiting and usually resolves by 1 year of age.

ASSESSMENT

RISK FACTORS

GER: Prematurity, bronchopulmonary dysplasia, neurologic impairments, asthma, cystic fibrosis, cerebral palsy, scoliosis

GERD: Neurologic impairments, hiatal hernia, morbid obesity

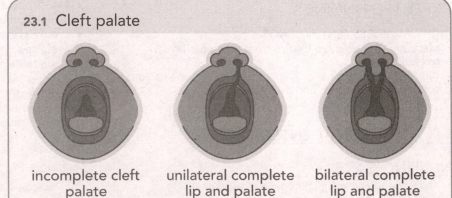

23.1 Cleft palate

incomplete cleft palate

unilateral complete lip and palate

bilateral complete lip and palate

EXPECTED FINDINGS

INFANTS

- Spitting up or forceful vomiting, irritability, excessive crying, blood in vomitus, arching of back, stiffening
- Respiratory problems
- Failure to thrive
- Apnea

CHILDREN: Heartburn, abdominal pain, difficulty swallowing, chronic cough, noncardiac chest pain

DIAGNOSTIC PROCEDURES

- Upper GI endoscopy to detect GI structural abnormalities
- 24-hr intraesophageal pH study to measures the amount of gastric acid reflux into the esophagus
- Endoscopy with biopsy to detect esophagitis and strictures
- Scintigraphy to identify the cause of gastric content aspiration

PATIENT-CENTERED CARE

NURSING CARE

GER

- Depends on the severity of the findings
- Offer small, frequent meals.
- Thicken infants formula with 1 tsp to 1 tbsp rice cereal per 1 oz formula.
- Avoid foods that cause reflux (caffeine, citrus, peppermint, spicy or fried foods).
- Assist with weight control.
- Position the child with the head elevated after meals.
- Place infants supine to sleep, rather than prone, side-lying, or sitting upright. Qs

GERD: Initiate interventions for GER, plus administering a proton pump inhibitor (omeprazole, esomeprazole, pantoprazole and rabeprazole), or an H_2-receptor antagonist (cimetidine or famotidine).

THERAPEUTIC PROCEDURES

Nissen fundoplication

- Laparoscopic surgical procedure that wraps the fundus of the stomach around the distal esophagus to decrease reflux.
- Used for clients who have severe cases of GERD

COMPLICATIONS

Recurrent pneumonia, weight loss, and failure to thrive
Repeated reflux of stomach contents can lead to erosion of the esophagus or pneumonia if stomach contents are aspirated.

NURSING ACTIONS

- Evaluate the prescribed treatment plan.
- Monitor for manifestations of pneumonia and failure to thrive.

CLIENT EDUCATION

- Reinforce the plan of care with the family.
- Observe for manifestations for pneumonia.

Hypertrophic pyloric stenosis

- Hypertrophic pyloric stenosis is the thickening of the pyloric sphincter, which creates an obstruction.
- Usually occurs the first few weeks of life.

ASSESSMENT

RISK FACTORS

Genetic predisposition

EXPECTED FINDINGS

- Vomiting that often occurs following a feeding, but can occur up to several hours following a feeding and becomes projectile as obstruction worsens.
- Nonbilious vomitus can be blood-tinged.
- Constant hunger.
- Olive-shaped mass in the right upper quadrant of the abdomen and possible peristaltic wave that moves from left to right when lying supine.
- Failure to gain weight and manifestations of dehydration (pallor, cool lips, dry skin and mucous membranes, decreased skin turgor, diminished urinary output, concentrated urine, thirst, rapid pulse, sunken eyes).

LABORATORY TESTS

Blood electrolytes

DIAGNOSTIC PROCEDURES

Ultrasound reveals an elongated mass surrounding an elongated pyloric canal.

PATIENT-CENTERED CARE

NURSING CARE

Prepare the child for surgery.

THERAPEUTIC PROCEDURES

Pyloromyotomy

Performed by laparoscope

PREOPERATIVE NURSING ACTIONS
- IV fluids for correction of dehydration and electrolyte imbalances
- Nasogastric (NG) tube for decompression
- NPO
- I&O
- Daily weights

POSTOPERATIVE NURSING ACTIONS
- Obtain routine postoperative vital signs.
- Provide IV fluids.
- Monitor daily weights and I&O.
- Administer analgesics for pain.
- Assess for manifestations of infection.
- Start clear liquids 4 to 6 hr after surgery. Advance to breast milk or formula as tolerated 24 hr after surgery.
- Document tolerance to feedings.

Hirschsprung's disease

Hirschsprung's disease (congenital aganglionic megacolon) is a structural anomaly of the GI tract caused by lack of ganglionic cells in segments of the colon resulting in decreased motility and mechanical obstruction.

ASSESSMENT

RISK FACTORS

Family history of Hirschsprung's disease

EXPECTED FINDINGS

Newborn
- Failure to pass meconium within 24 to 48 hr after birth
- Episodes of vomiting bile
- Refusal to eat
- Abdominal distention

Infant
- Failure to thrive
- Constipation
- Vomiting
- Episodes of diarrhea and vomiting

Child
- Undernourished, anemic appearance
- Abdominal distention
- Visible peristalsis
- Palpable fecal mass
- Constipation
- Foul-smelling, ribbonlike stool

LABORATORY TESTS

- Blood electrolytes
- CBC

DIAGNOSTIC PROCEDURES

Rectal biopsy to confirm the absence of ganglion cells

PATIENT-CENTERED CARE

NURSING CARE

- Prepare family and client for surgery.
- Assist family with improving nutritional status until surgery.
  - High-protein, high-calorie, low-fiber diet
  - Total parenteral nutrition in some cases

THERAPEUTIC PROCEDURES

- Surgical removal of the aganglionic section of the bowel.
- Temporary colostomy can be required.

PREOPERATIVE NURSING ACTIONS
- Prepare the child and family for surgery using developmentally appropriate techniques.
- Administer electrolyte and fluid replacement.
- Monitor for enterocolitis.
- Bowel prep with saline enemas and oral antibiotics.

POSTOPERATIVE NURSING ACTIONS
- Assess respiratory status and maintain airway.
- Provide supplemental oxygen.
- Obtain vital signs.
- Administer analgesics for pain.
- Assess surgical site for bleeding or other abnormalities.
- Provide Foley catheter care.
- Assess bowel sounds and bowel function.
- Provide ostomy care if appropriate.
- Make appropriate referrals.

CLIENT EDUCATION
- Perform ostomy care if indicated.
- Practice incisional care and to monitor for infection.
- Observe for manifestations of dehydration.

COMPLICATIONS

Enterocolitis (inflammation of the bowel)

Treatment focuses on resolving inflammation, preventing bowel perforation, maintaining hydration, initiating antibiotic therapy, and performing surgery for colostomy or ileostomy if there is extensive bowel involvement.

NURSING ACTIONS

- Monitor vital signs.
- Assess abdominal girth.
  - Measure girth with a paper tape at the level of the umbilicus or at the widest point of the abdomen.
  - Mark the area with a pen to ensure continuity of future measurements.
- Monitor for manifestations of sepsis, peritonitis, or shock caused by enterocolitis.
- Monitor and manage fluid, electrolyte, and blood product replacement.
- Administer antibiotics as prescribed.

Anal stricture and incontinence

- Bowel-retraining therapy
- Can require further procedures (dilatation)

Intussusception

- Proximal segment of the bowel telescopes into a more distal segment, resulting in lymphatic and venous obstruction causing edema in the area. With progression, ischemia and increased mucus into the intestine will occur.
- Common in infants and children ages 3 months to 6 years

ASSESSMENT

EXPECTED FINDINGS

- Sudden episodic abdominal pain
- Screaming with drawing knees to chest during episodes of pain
- Abdominal mass (sausage-shaped)
- Stools mixed with blood and mucus that resemble the consistency of red currant jelly
- Vomiting
- Fever
- Tender, distended abdomen

DIAGNOSTIC PROCEDURES

Ultrasound

PATIENT-CENTERED CARE

NURSING CARE

- Stabilize the child prior to the procedure.
  - IV fluids to correct and prevent dehydration
  - Nasogastric (NG) tube for decompression
- Teach the family and child about the nonsurgical procedure.

THERAPEUTIC PROCEDURES

Air enema

- With or without contrast
- Performed by a radiologist

Hydrostatic enema

- Ultrasound guided
- No radiation required

COMPLICATIONS

Reoccurring intussusception

Surgery is required for reoccurring cases.

Appendicitis

- Inflammation of the vermiform appendix caused from an obstruction of the lumen of the appendix.
- Average client age is 10 years.

ASSESSMENT

EXPECTED FINDINGS

- Abdominal pain in the right lower quadrant
- Rigid abdomen
- Decreased or absent bowel sounds
- Fever
- Diarrhea or constipation
- Lethargy
- Tachycardia
- Rapid, shallow breathing
- Anorexia
- Possible vomiting

LABORATORY TESTS

- CBC
- Urinalysis

DIAGNOSTIC PROCEDURES

Computed tomography scan shows an enlarged diameter of appendix, as well as thickening of the appendiceal wall.

PATIENT-CENTERED CARE

NURSING CARE

- Prepare the child and family for surgery using developmentally appropriate techniques.
- Avoid applying heat to the abdomen.
- Avoid enemas or laxatives. Qs

THERAPEUTIC PROCEDURES

Removal of the nonruptured appendix

Laparoscopic surgery

PREOPERATIVE NURSING ACTIONS

- Administer IV fluid replacement as prescribed.
- Administer IV antibiotic.

POSTOPERATIVE NURSING ACTIONS

- Assess respiratory status and maintain airway.
- Provide supplemental oxygen as prescribed.
- Obtain vital signs.
- Administer analgesics for pain as prescribed.
- Assess surgical site for bleeding or any other abnormalities.
- Assess bowel sounds and bowel function.

Removal of the ruptured appendix

Laparoscopic or open surgery

PREOPERATIVE NURSING ACTIONS

- Administer electrolyte and fluid replacement as prescribed.
- Place NG tube for decompression.
- Administer IV antibiotics.

POSTOPERATIVE NURSING ACTIONS

- Assess respiratory status, and maintain airway.
- Provide supplemental oxygen.
- Obtain vital signs.
- Administer analgesics for pain.
- Assess surgical site for bleeding or other abnormalities.
- Assess bowel sounds and bowel function.
- Administer IV fluids and antibiotics.
- Maintain NPO status.
- Maintain NG tube to low continuous suction.
- Provide wound irrigation care for open surgical sites with antibacterial solution or saline-soaked gauze.
- Provide drain care.
- Assess for peritonitis.
  - Fever
  - Sudden relief from pain after perforation, followed by a diffuse increase in pain
  - Irritability
  - Rigid abdomen
  - Abdominal distention
  - Tachycardia
  - Rapid, shallow breathing
  - Pallor
  - Chills

CLIENT EDUCATION

- Follow instructions for incision care.
- Observe for manifestations of infection.

COMPLICATIONS

Peritonitis (inflammation in the peritoneal cavity)

NURSING ACTIONS

- Assess for peritonitis.
- Provide pain management. Qpcc
  - Assess for pain using a developmentally appropriate tool.
  - Administer analgesics.
- Manage IV fluid therapy.
- Administer IV antibiotics for infection.
- Manage NG tube suction.
- Provide preoperative and postoperative nursing care.
- Provide surgical wound care with wound irrigation and/or dressings if delayed wound closure is necessary.
- Provide psychosocial support for the child and family.

CLIENT EDUCATION

- Preoperative care (the need to maintain NPO status and the need for pain medication).
- Postoperative care (early ambulation, advancement of diet, wound care, and monitoring for infection).

Meckel's diverticulum

Meckel's diverticulum is a complication resulting from failure of the omphalomesenteric duct to fuse during embryonic development.

ASSESSMENT

EXPECTED FINDINGS

- Rectal bleeding, usually painless
- Abdominal pain
- Bloody, mucus stools

LABORATORY TESTS

CBC and metabolic panel

DIAGNOSTIC EVALUATION

RADIONUCLIDE SCAN: Meckel's scan is the most effective diagnostic test.

PATIENT-CENTERED CARE

NURSING CARE

Prepare the child and family for surgery using developmentally appropriate techniques.

THERAPEUTIC PROCEDURES

Surgical removal of the diverticulum

PREOPERATIVE NURSING ACTIONS

- Provide blood transfusions to correct hypovolemia.
- Administer IV fluid and electrolyte replacement as prescribed.
- Provide oxygen as prescribed.
- Administer IV antibiotics.
- Maintain bed rest.
- Closely monitor blood loss in stools.

POSTOPERATIVE NURSING ACTIONS

- Assess respiratory status and maintain airway.
- Provide supplemental oxygen.
- Obtain vital signs.
- Administer analgesics for pain.
- Assess surgical site for bleeding or any other abnormalities.
- Assess bowel sounds and bowel function.
- Administer IV fluids and antibiotics.
- Maintain NPO status.
- Maintain NG tube to low continuous suction.

CLIENT EDUCATION: Observe for manifestations of infection.

COMPLICATIONS

GI hemorrhage and bowel obstruction (for untreated Meckel's diverticulum)

Active Learning Scenario

A nurse is caring for a child who is postoperative following an open appendectomy for a perforated appendix. Use the ATI Active Learning Template: System Disorder to complete this item.

NURSING CARE: List postoperative nursing interventions.

Application Exercises

1. A nurse is caring for an infant who has just returned from PACU following cleft lip and palate repair. Which of the following actions should the nurse take?
   - A. Remove the packing in the mouth.
   - B. Place the infant in an upright position.
   - C. Offer a pacifier with sucrose.
   - D. Assess the mouth with a tongue blade.

2. A nurse is teaching a parent of an infant about gastrointestinal reflux disease. Which of the following should the nurse include in the teaching? (Select all that apply.)
   - A. Offer frequent feedings.
   - B. Thicken formula with rice cereal.
   - C. Use a bottle with a one-way valve.
   - D. Position baby upright after feedings.
   - E. Use a wide-based nipple for feedings.

3. A nurse is caring for a child who has Hirschsprung's disease. Which of the following actions should the nurse take?
   - A. Encourage a high-fiber, low-protein, low-calorie diet.
   - B. Prepare the family for surgery.
   - C. Place an NG tube for decompression.
   - D. Initiate bed rest.

4. A nurse is caring for a child who has Meckel's diverticulum. Which of the following manifestations should the nurse expect? (Select all that apply.)
   - A. Abdominal pain
   - B. Fever
   - C. Mucus and blood in stools
   - D. Vomiting
   - E. Rapid, shallow breathing

5. A nurse on a pediatric unit is caring for a group of clients who have gastrointestinal disorders. Review the expected finding below and match them with the correct disorder: Hypertrophic Pyloric Stenosis, Intussusception, or Hirschsprung's Disease.
   - A. Foul-smelling, ribbon like stools
   - B. Sausage shaped abdominal mass
   - C. Constant hunger
   - D. Failure to pass meconium within 48 hours after birth
   - E. Sudeen, episodic abdominal pain
   - F. Projective vomiting
   - G. Bilious vomiting
   - H. Red, currant-jelly like stools
   - I. Olive shaped mass in the RUQ of the abdomen

1. A. The packing in the mouth should stay in place for 2 to 3 days.
   B. **CORRECT:** Place the infant in a side-lying position. When taking action during the care of an infant who has just returned from the PACU following a cleft lip and palate repair, the nurse should place the infant in a side-lying position to facilitate drainage and prevent aspiration.
   C. Objects in the mouth could injure the surgical site and should be avoided.
   D. Objects in the mouth could injure the surgical site and should be avoided.

   Ⓝ *NCLEX® Connection: Physiological Adaptation, Alterations in Body Systems*

2. A, B, D. **CORRECT:** When taking action while teaching the parent of a child who has gastrointestinal reflux disease, the nurse should instruct the parent to offer the infant frequent feedings, to thicken to formula with rice cereal, and to position the infant in an upright position after feedings. These actions assist in decreasing the number of vomiting episodes experienced by the infant.
   C. A bottle with a one-way valve is used for an infant who has cleft lip and palate.
   E. A wide-based nipple is used for an infant who has cleft lip and palate.

   Ⓝ *NCLEX® Connection: Basic Care and Comfort, Nutrition and Oral Hydration*

3. A. A client who has Hirschsprung's disease is encouraged to eat a low-fiber, high-protein, high-calorie diet.
   B. **CORRECT:** When taking action during the care of a child who has Hirschsprung's disease, the nurse should prepare the child and family for surgery. A child who has Hirschsprung's disease requires surgery to remove the affected segment of the intestine.
   C. A client who has Hirschsprung's disease is managed nutritionally. Placing an NG tube for decompression is not an appropriate action for the nurse to take.
   D. A client who has Meckel's diverticulum is placed on bed rest to prevent further bleeding.

   Ⓝ *NCLEX® Connection: Reduction of Risk Potential, Therapeutic Procedures*

4. A, C. **CORRECT:** When recognizing cues during the care of a child who had Meckel's diverticulum the nurse should expect the child to have abdominal pain and bloody, mucousy stools.
   B. Fever is a manifestation of appendicitis.
   D. Vomiting is a manifestation of appendicitis.
   E. Rapid, shallow breathing is a manifestation of appendicitis.

   Ⓝ *NCLEX® Connection: Physiological Adaptation, Pathophysiology*

5. **HIRSCHSPRUNG'S DISEASE:** A, D, G;
   INTUSSUSCEPTION: B, E, H;
   HYPERTROPHIC PYLORIC STENOSIS: C, F, I

   Infants who have hypertrophic pyloric stenosis vomit 30-60 minutes following feedings. As the obstruction worsens, vomiting becomes projectile. Due to the vomiting and inability to tolerate feedings, infants often display constant manifestations of hunger. The enlargement of the pyloric muscle often causes an olive shaped mass to be palpable in the right upper quadrant of the abdomen. Peristaltic waves moving from left to right may also be seen. The infant may also show signs of dehydration and poor weight gain.

   Infants and children who have an intussusception present with sudden, episodic abdominal pain, a sausage shaped abdominal mass, and red, currant-jelly like stools.

   Newborns who have Hirschsprung's disease fail to pass meconium with 24-48 hours after birth. Abdominal distention, refusal to eat, and episodes of bilious vomiting are also seen. The infant who has Hirschsprung's disease may present with failure to thrive, constipation, vomiting, and episodes of diarrhea and vomiting. Older children may have an undernourished, anemic appearance, abdominal distention, visible peristalsis, palpable fecal mass, constipation, and foul-smelling, ribbon-like stools

   Ⓝ *NCLEX® Connection: Physiological Adaptation, Alterations in Body Systems*

Active Learning Scenario Key

Using the ATI Active Learning Template: System Disorder

NURSING CARE

- Assess respiratory status and maintain airway.
- Provide supplemental oxygen as prescribed.
- Obtain vital signs.
- Administer analgesics for pain as prescribed.
- Assess surgical site for bleeding or any other abnormalities.
- Assess bowel sounds and bowel function.
- IV fluids and antibiotics as prescribed.
- Maintain NPO status.
- Maintain NG tube to low continuous suction.
- Provide wound care for open surgical sites with antibacterial solution or saline as prescribed.
- Provide drain care.
- Assess for peritonitis.

Ⓝ *NCLEX® Connection: Physiological Adaptation, Alterations in Body Systems*

When reviewing the following chapters, keep in mind the relevant topics and tasks of the NCLEX outline, in particular:

Health Promotion and Maintenance

AGING PROCESS: Provide care and education for the newborn, infant, and toddler client from birth through 2 years.

Reduction of Risk Potential

CHANGES/ABNORMALITIES IN VITAL SIGNS: Assess and respond to changes and/or trends in client vital signs.

LABORATORY VALUES: Notify primary health care provider about laboratory test results.

POTENTIAL FOR COMPLICATIONS OF DIAGNOSTIC TESTS/ TREATMENTS/PROCEDURES: Use precautions to prevent injury and/or complications associated with a procedure or diagnosis.

POTENTIAL FOR COMPLICATIONS FROM SURGICAL PROCEDURES AND HEALTH ALTERATIONS: Apply knowledge of pathophysiology to monitoring for complications.

Pharmacological and Parenteral Therapies

MEDICATION ADMINISTRATION: Educate client about medications.

Physiological Adaptation

ALTERATIONS IN BODY SYSTEMS
Monitor and maintain devices and equipment used for drainage.

Educate client about managing health problems

FLUID AND ELECTROLYTE IMBALANCES: Manage the care of the client with a fluid and electrolyte imbalance.

ILLNESS MANAGEMENT
Identify client data that needs to be reported immediately.

Educate client about managing illness.

PATHOPHYSIOLOGY: Identify pathophysiology related to an acute or chronic condition.

CHAPTER 24 Enuresis and Urinary Tract Infections

Enuresis is uncontrolled or unintentional urination that occurs after a child is beyond an age at which bladder control is achieved.

A urinary tract infection (UTI) is an infection in any portion of the urinary tract.

Enuresis

Inappropriate urination during the day or night at least twice a week for at least 3 successive months should be evaluated for children who have a developmental or chronological age of at least 5-years old.

Rule out other causes of incontinence (medication adverse effects, medical conditions) prior to diagnosis of enuresis.

Primary enuresis: A child has never been free of bed-wetting for any extended periods of time.

Secondary enuresis: A child who started bed-wetting after development of urinary control.

ASSESSMENT

RISK FACTORS

- Family history of enuresis
- Twin siblings
- Disorders associated with bladder dysfunction
- Assigned sex at birth: males
- Emotional events (new sibling, divorce)
- Behavioral disorders

EXPECTED FINDINGS

- History of alterations in toilet training, voiding behaviors, and bowel movement patterns Qpcc
- History of chronic or acute illness (UTI, diabetes mellitus, sickle cell disease, neurologic deficits)
- Fluid intake, especially in the evening
- Restlessness, urinary frequency and urgency

DIAGNOSTIC EVALUATION

- Physical examination by provider to evaluate for any physical causes of enuresis
- Functional bladder capacity screening: child is instructed to hold off urinating for as long as possible and then instructed to urinate into a container. The urine output is then measured. The expected bladder capacity (ounces) = child's age (up to 14 years of age) + 2.
- Record of enuresis pattern

PATIENT-CENTERED CARE

NURSING CARE

- Evaluate the child's self-esteem.
- Evaluate the child's coping strategies and available support systems.
- Evaluate the family's coping.
- Evaluate peer and family support groups.
- Educate the child and family regarding the management of enuresis. QEBP
  - Have the child urinate prior to bedtime.
  - Restrict fluids at least 2 hr prior to bedtime.
  - Avoid caffeinated drinks in the afternoon.
  - Use positive reinforcement. Avoid punishing, scolding, or teasing the child following an incident.
  - Assist the child/parents in keeping a calendar of wet and dry days.
  - Allow the child to assist with changing the bed linens and clothing following an incident.
  - Wake the child up at scheduled intervals during the night to void.
  - Administer prescribed medications.
  - Ensure stools are regular, soft, and formed.
  - Offer support to the child and the family.

THERAPEUTIC MEASURES

BEHAVIORAL THERAPY
Initial management for enuresis
- Reward system: the child's dry and wet nights are recorded, and the child is rewarded for the desired behavior
- Kegel/pelvic exercises: useful for daytime enuresis to strengthen bladder tone
- Retention control measures: the child consumes large amount of fluid and delays urination until no longer tolerable; to stretch the bladder
- Wake schedules: the child is awakened at scheduled intervals during the night to void; this method is effective at reducing the incidence of enuresis

CONDITIONING THERAPY

INVOLVES STIMULUS TRAINING
- Urine sensor alarms: a padded moisture wire sensor is placed inside the child's undergarments and buzzes/alarms to awaken the child when moisture is detected.

MEDICATIONS

Antidiuretic hormone

Desmopressin acetate: reduces the volume of urine.

NURSING ACTIONS
- Administer medication orally. Intranasal route is not recommended for management of enuresis in children because of the risk of hyponatremia and seizures.
- Monitor I&O.
- Monitor electrolytes.

CLIENT EDUCATION
- Restrict the child's fluid intake after dinner. Q EBP
- Administer the medication at bedtime.
- Possible adverse effects include headaches, nausea.

Tricyclic antidepressants

Imipramine hydrochloride: inhibits urination.

NURSING ACTIONS
- Monitor children for an increase in suicidality.
- Length of treatment is 4-6 months, with tapering gradually upon discontinuation.
- Monitor heart rate and blood pressure.

CLIENT EDUCATION
- Administer the mediation 1 hr before bedtime.
- Administer with food to decrease gastric adverse effects.
- Monitor child for decreased mood and suicidal tendencies.
- Avoid sun exposure.

Anticholinergics

Oxybutynin chloride: reduces bladder contractions.

NURSING ACTIONS: Monitor for effectiveness of therapy.

CLIENT EDUCATION: Observe for possible adverse effects such as dry mouth and constipation.

COMPLICATIONS

Emotional problems: low self-esteem, altered body image, social isolation, fears

NURSING ACTIONS
- Support the child and their guardians by listening to concerns and correcting misperceptions.
- Involve the child in the teaching and management.
- Make referrals to appropriate resources (support groups, counseling) as necessary.

CLIENT EDUCATION: Assist the child and their support to understand the emotional aspects of the disorder. Early interventions can alleviate long-term emotional issues.

Urinary Tract Infections

Bacteriuria: bacteria in the urine
- Asymptomatic bacteriuria: bacteriuria with no manifestations of UTI
- Symptomatic bacteriuria: bacteriuria with manifestations of UTI

Recurrent UTI: multiple occurrences of asymptomatic or symptomatic bacteriuria

Persistent UTI: bacteriuria that does not resolve with antibiotic therapy

Febrile UTI: symptomatic bacteriuria with fever
- Urosepsis: febrile UTI with systemic manifestations.

Cystitis: inflammation of the bladder

Urethritis: inflammation of the urethra

Pyelonephritis: inflammation of the upper urinary tract and the kidneys

ASSESSMENT

RISK FACTORS
- Urinary stasis
- Urinary tract anomalies
- Reflux within the urinary tract system
- Constipation
- Onset of toilet training
- Uncircumcised penis
- Assigned sex at birth: Females (urethra in close proximity to rectum)
- Bubble baths
- Sexual activity
- Catheterizations Q EBP

EXPECTED FINDINGS
- Children less than 2 years of age
  - Often have nonspecific findings Q PCC
  - Newborn: jaundice, tachypnea, cyanosis, hypothermia, fever
  - Poor feeding
  - Vomiting
  - Diarrhea
  - Irritability
  - Lethargy
  - Frequent urination
  - Fever
- Children greater than 2 years of age
  - Vomiting
  - Enuresis, frequent urination, dysuria
  - Blood in the urine
  - Constipation
  - Chills
  - Fever
  - Malodorous urine
  - Abdominal or flank pain

LABORATORY TESTS

Urinalysis and urine culture and sensitivity

- Sterile catheterization and suprapubic aspiration are the most accurate methods for obtaining urine for urinalysis and culture in children less than 2 years of age.
- Obtain a clean-catch urine sample from children who are able to cooperate.

NURSING ACTIONS

- To prevent a falsely low bacterial count, avoid having the child drink a large amount of fluid prior to obtaining a urine specimen.
- Send the specimen for culture to the laboratory without delay.
- Perform urinary dipstick for preliminary screening due to the length of time for culture results.
- Review findings indicative of UTI.
  - Urine culture: Positive for infecting organisms (Escherichia coli, Proteus, Pseudomonas, Klebsiella, Enterococcus, Staphylococcus aureus)
  - Microscopic examination/Gram stain: presumptive diagnosis for UTI; positive for pyuria and positive for bacteria
  - Urinalysis/dipstick
    - Appearance: cloudy, hazy, mucus, pus, +odor
    - pH: alkalemia
    - Protein: negative
    - Glucose: negative
    - Ketones: negative
    - Leukocytes: positive
    - Nitrites: positive
    - RBC: positive

DIAGNOSTIC PROCEDURES

Determine anatomic defects
- Ultrasonography
- Voiding cystourethrogram (VCUG)

NURSING ACTIONS

- Educate the child and their support about the procedure for the diagnostic test prescribed.
- Prepare the child if catheterization is necessary.
- Monitor the child after the procedure, according to facility protocol.

PATIENT-CENTERED CARE

NURSING CARE

- Encourage frequent voiding and complete emptying of the bladder.
- Encourage fluids.
- Monitor urine output.
- Prepare the child for diagnostic tests.
- Administer a mild analgesic (acetaminophen) for pain management.

MEDICATIONS

- Antibiotics based on findings of urine culture and sensitivity testing (penicillins, sulfonamide, cephalosporins, and nitrofurantoin).
- Antibiotics can be prescribed PO or IV depending on the severity.

NURSING ACTIONS: Monitor for potential allergic response.

CLIENT EDUCATION: Complete all prescribed antibiotics, even if manifestations are no longer present.

CLIENT EDUCATION

- Watch for manifestations of recurrence of UTIs (dysuria, frequency, urgency).
- Provide instruction to prevent recurrence. Ⓠ EBP
  - Wipe the perineal area from front to back.
  - For uncircumcised clients, ensure foreskin is retracted prior to performing hygiene and replaced afterward.
  - Change infant's diapers frequently.
  - Use cotton underwear.
  - Maintain adequate hydration with caffeine-free beverages.
  - Avoid bubble baths.
  - Void frequently.
  - Empty bladder completely.
  - Avoid constipation by increasing fiber intake.
  - If sexually active, void immediately after intercourse.
  - If child has a history of recurrent UTIs, the child will need a repeat urinalysis 7 days after treatment.

COMPLICATIONS

Progressive kidney injury

Pyelonephritis

Urosepsis

NURSING ACTIONS: Monitor for findings of UTIs.

CLIENT EDUCATION: Reinforce teaching about prevention, early identification, and treatment of UTIs.

Active Learning Scenario

A nurse educator is preparing an in-service for a group of newly hired pediatric nurse about caring for children who have enuresis. What should the educator include in the presentation? Learning Template: System Disorder to complete this item

ALTERATION IN HEALTH (DIAGNOSIS)

CLIENT EDUCATION: List at least 10 points to review.

Application Exercises

1. A nurse is providing teaching with the parents of a child who has enuresis about behavioral therapy management. Which of the following statement by a parent indicates understanding?

   A. "We should avoid waking our child up during the night to use the bathroom."

   B. "With behavioral therapy, we should scold our child when they have unexpected events."

   C. "We can reward our child when they have dry nights."

   D. "With behavioral therapy, we can purchase urine sensor alarms for our child."

2. A nurse is caring for child who has enuresis and has a prescription for desmopressin. Which of the following actions should the nurse take?

   A. Administer in the morning.

   B. Administer nasally.

   C. Monitor electrolytes.

   D. Encourage fluids after meals.

3. A nurse assessing a preschooler who is suspected of having a urinary tract infection. Which of the following findings should the nurse expect? (Select all that apply.)

   A. Chills

   B. Diarrhea

   C. Vomiting

   D. Fever

   E. Pale-colored urine

4. A nurse is planning care for a child who has a urinary tract infection. Which of the following interventions should the nurse take?

   A. Administer an antidiuretic.

   B. Restrict fluids.

   C. Evaluate the child's self-esteem.

   D. Encourage the child to void frequently.

5. A nurse is providing teaching with the guardian of a child who has a urinary tract infection. Which of the following instructions should the nurse include? (Select all that apply.)

   A. Wear nylon underpants.

   B. Avoid bubble baths.

   C. Empty bladder completely with each void.

   D. Watch for manifestations of infection.

   E. Increase fiber intake.

Application Exercises Key

1. D. **CORRECT:** The nurse should identify that the parents understand teaching when a parent makes a statement about the reward system of behavioral therapy for enuresis management. The parents should record their child's wet and dry nights and reward their child for positive behavior. This will motivate the child to continue to have more dry nights. The nurse should provide further teaching with the parent about the wake schedule because this is a form of behavioral management for enuresis in which the parents should awaken their child up at scheduled intervals throughout the night to use the bathroom which will decrease the incidence of enuresis. The parents should never scold their child. The nurse should provide further teaching with the parents to use positive reinforcement positive reinforcement to motive the child. The nurse should provide further teaching with the parents that urine sensor alarms are used as conditioning therapy for the management of enuresis.

   Ⓝ *NCLEX® Connection: Physiological Adaptation, Alterations in Body Systems*

2. C. **CORRECT:** The nurse should monitor the child's electrolytes while receiving desmopressin. Desmopressin is a synthetic antidiuretic hormone which reduces the volume of urine and can cause hyponatremia. Desmopressin is prescribed for oral administration at bedtime. The nasal route is no longer prescribed for children because of the adverse effects of hyponatremia and seizures. The nurse should limit the child's fluid intake 2 hours prior to bedtime to prevent the occurrence of enuresis.

   Ⓝ *NCLEX® Connection: Pharmacological and Parenteral Therapies, Expected Actions/Outcomes*

3. A, C, D. **CORRECT:** The nurse should expect the preschooler to have fever, chills, flank pain, urinary frequency, hematuria, and vomiting which are expected findings with a urinary tract infection. Diarrhea is an expected finding for UTI in a child who is less than 2 years of age.

4. D. **CORRECT:** The nurse should encourage the child to void frequently. This will assist the child with preventing urinary stasis and promote the excretion of bacteria through the urinary system. The nurse should not administer an antidiuretic because this is not indicated for the management of a child who has an UTI. The nurse should increase fluid intake to prevent the stasis of urine and constipation. The nurse should evaluate self-esteem for a child who has enuresis.

   Ⓝ *NCLEX® Connection: Physiological Adaptation, Illness Management*

5. B, C, D, E. **CORRECT:** The nurse should provide information with the guardian about prevention of UTI such as avoiding bubble baths, encouraging the child to empty their bladder completely with each void, and increasing fiber intake which will prevent constipation. The nurse should also provide teaching with the guardian about manifestations of urinary tract infection and to seek prompt management of their child's condition.

   Ⓝ *NCLEX® Connection: Physiological Adaptation, Illness Management*

Active Learning Scenario Key

Using the ATI Active Learning Template: System Disorder

ALTERATION IN HEALTH (DIAGNOSIS): Inappropriate urination must occur at least twice a week for at least 3 successive months, and the child must be at least 5 years of age before there's consideration about diagnosing enuresis

CLIENT EDUCATION
- Have the child empty the bladder prior to bedtime.
- Encourage fluids during the day, and restrict fluids 2 hr before bedtime.
- Avoid fruit and fruit drinks.
- Avoid caffeinated drinks.

- Use positive reinforcement. Avoid punishing, scolding, or teasing the child following an incident.
- Assist the child in keeping a calendar of wet and dry days.
- Have the child change bed linens and clothing following an incident.
- Wake the child at scheduled intervals during the night to void.
- Ensure the child takes all medications as prescribed.
- Use behavioral therapy techniques to manage enuresis such as the reward system, wake schedule, retention control, and reinforce Kegel/pelvic floor exercises.
- Use conditioning therapy such as the urine alarm sensor.

Ⓝ *NCLEX® Connection: Physiological Adaptation, Alterations in Body Systems*

CHAPTER 25   Structural Disorders of the Genitourinary Tract and Reproductive System

Various structural disorders can be evident at birth and can affect normal genitourinary and reproductive function.

Children become aware of and are very interested in the genital area, normality of genital function, and gender differences between 3 and 6 years of age. Due to this, repair of structural defects ideally should be done between 6 to 12 months of age, but before 3 years of age, to minimize impact on body image and to promote healthy development.

ASSESSMENT

RISK FACTORS

Can have a genetic link.

EXPECTED FINDINGS

OBSTRUCTIVE DEFECTS: Obstructive uropathy

- Hydronephrosis can be present if the ureteropelvic junction becomes obstructed and the renal pelvis and calyces become dilated, with potential detection during a fetal ultrasound.
- Partial obstructions can go undetected.
- Oligohydramnios can be a prenatal indicator of decreased kidney function or kidney obstruction in the fetus.
- Urinary tract infections
- Hypertension (secondary)
- Other possible findings: renal colic (severe pain in lower back), enuresis, urinary urgency, urge incontinence

PATIENT-CENTERED CARE

NURSING CARE

Nursing care should focus on education and support of the family and child. QPCC

- Evaluate the family's perception of the child's defect, family support, and coping.
- Assist guardians to identify ways to help the child maintain a positive self-image.
- Promote healthy growth and development.
- Assist child with maintaining self-image.

DEFECTS OF THE GENITOURINARY TRACT

Obstructive uropathy

Structural or functional obstruction in the urinary system

THERAPEUTIC PROCEDURE: Surgical procedures that divert the flow of urine to bypass the obstruction: insertion of a ureteral stent, cutaneous ureterostomy tubes, nephrostomy tubes

Chordee

Ventral curvature of the penis

THERAPEUTIC PROCEDURE: Surgical release of the fibrous band

Hypospadias

Urethral meatus that is unexpectedly located on the ventral aspect of the penile shaft, below or behind the glans penis, or perineal/scrotal junction.

- Possible chordee present

THERAPEUTIC PROCEDURE: Surgical repair at 6 to 12 months of age

Epispadias

Urethral meatus that is unexpectedly open or exposed on the dorsal aspect of the genitalia

MALE

- Urethra opened on dorsal surface of the penis
- Possible exstrophy of the bladder

FEMALE

- Wide urethra opening
- Possible exstrophy of the bladder

THERAPEUTIC PROCEDURE

- Surgery performed during the first year of life.

Bladder exstrophy

Eversion of the posterior bladder through the anterior bladder wall and lower abdominal wall.
- Exposed bladder, urethra, and ureteral orifices through the suprapubic area
- Findings: separation/widening of the pubic symphysis (diastasis), inguinal hernia, genital defects, anus positioned anteriorly, epispadias
- Male: undescended testes, short penis
- Female: bifid clitoris, short vagina, separated labia

NURSING ACTIONS
- Cover the exposed bladder with a plastic transparent dressing to provide moisture.
- Prepare the newborn for immediate surgery.
- Arrange for consult with enterostomal nurse if surgery is delayed.

THERAPEUTIC PROCEDURE
- Surgical repair immediately or within 3 months
- Reconstructive surgery for genital defects

Phimosis

Narrowing of the preputial opening of the foreskin which causes inability to retract the foreskin of the penis.
- Expected finding in infants and usually disappears as the child grows.

NURSING ACTION
- Proper hygiene for phimotic foreskin is external cleansing during routine bathing, the foreskin should not be forcibly retracted.

THERAPEUTIC PROCEDURE
- Topical steroids
- Circumcision

Cryptorchidism

Failure of one or both testes to descend into the scrotum.
- Inability to palpate testis or testes within the scrotum

THERAPEUTIC PROCEDURE
- Surgical orchiopexy
- Surgery performed at 6 and 24 months of age

Hydrocele

Collection of peritoneal fluid in the scrotum that causes painless swelling.
- Enlarged scrotal sac
- Can resolve spontaneously

THERAPEUTIC PROCEDURE: Surgical repair if not resolved in 1 year

Varicocele

Elongation, dilation, and tortuosity of the veins of the spermatic cord superior to the testicle.
- Possible discomfort during sexual intercourse
- Possible observation in variation of testicle size

THERAPEUTIC PROCEDURE: Varicocelectomy

Testicular torsion

Sudden twisting of the spermatic cord which results in the testis to hang free from its vascular structures.
- Acute pain (may also report abdominal pain), nausea, vomiting
- Scrotum warm and edematous, absent cremasteric reflex
- Inform parents that this is a medical emergency and prompt intervention is warranted Qs

THERAPEUTIC PROCEDURE: Manual detorsion can be attempted by a provider, followed by immediate surgery if unsuccessful.

Ambiguous genitalia

Erroneous or abnormal sexual differentiation
- Karyotyping is performed to determine the infant's chromosomal pattern and gonadal function tested. Adrenal function should also be tested because of the high-risk for adrenal insufficiency.
- Genetic counseling can help the family understand the cause.
- Involves several members of the interprofessional team: endocrinologist, social worker, urologist, surgeons, genetic counselors. Qᴛᴄ

NURSING ACTION
- Monitor labs and electrolytes

THERAPEUTIC PROCEDURE: Reconstructive Surgery

THERAPEUTIC PROCEDURES

Structural defects will be treated with surgical intervention. The goal of most structural defect repairs is to preserve or create normal urinary and sexual function. Early intervention will minimize emotional trauma.

PREOPERATIVE NURSING ACTIONS
- Provide education to the child and family related to the procedure and expectations for postoperative care.
- Provide emotional support to the child and family.
- Encourage parents to express concerns and fears related to the surgical procedure and outcomes.
- If NPO status is necessary, explain the parameters to the family and/or child.

POSTOPERATIVE NURSING ACTIONS
- Assess pain using a pain assessment tool.
- Administer pain medication. Anticholinergics may be administered to decrease spasms of the bladder.
- Monitor I&O.
- Monitor urinary catheters, drains, tubes, or stents.
- Provide wound and/or dressing care.
- Monitor for findings of infection (redness, warmth, drainage, or edema at surgical site, fever, lethargy, and foul-smelling urine).

CLIENT EDUCATION
- Perform measures to prevent infection including good hand hygiene, and care of wounds, drains, and urinary catheters and drainage bags.
- Do not provide tub baths for at least 1 week or as prescribed.
- Limit activity as prescribed.

COMPLICATIONS

Infection

NURSING ACTIONS
- Observe for findings of infection including fever, skin inflammation, foul urine odor, cloudy urine, and/or urinary frequency.

CLIENT EDUCATION
- Observe for findings of infection.
- Report any findings of infection immediately.

Emotional problems

Poor self-esteem, altered body image, social isolation, fears

NURSING ACTIONS
- Support the child and family by listening to concerns and correcting misperceptions.
- Use play therapy for toddlers and preschoolers.
- Encourage peer-to-peer social networking for older children.

CLIENT EDUCATION

Consider attending support groups. Q**PCC**

Active Learning Scenario

A nurse is teaching a newly licensed nurse about structural disorders of the genitourinary tract and reproductive system. What should the nurse include in the teaching? Use the ATI Active Learning Template: Basic Concept to complete this item.

RELATED CONTENT: Describe six structural disorders of the genitourinary tract and reproductive system.

Application Exercises

1. A nurse is caring for an infant who has obstructive uropathy. Which of the following findings should the nurse expect? (Select all that apply.)
   - A. Urethral meatus located on dorsum of the shaft of the genitalia
   - B. Urine culture positive for UTI
   - C. History of maternal oligohydramnios
   - D. Hematuria diaper changes
   - E. Kidney ultrasound that shows hydronephrosis

2. A nurse is assessing a male infant who has bladder exstrophy. Which of the following findings should the nurse expect? (Select all that apply.)
   - A. Epispadias
   - B. Hypospadias
   - C. Undescended testes
   - D. Widened pubic symptoms
   - E. Enlarged scrotal sac

3. A nurse is caring for an infant who has a hydrocele. Which of the following actions should the nurse take?
   - A. Prepare the child for surgery.
   - B. Explain to the parents that that condition generally self-resolves.
   - C. Retract the foreskin and cleanse several times daily.
   - D. Refer the parents for genetic counseling.

4. A nurse is caring for an infant who has ambiguous genitalia. Which of the following actions should the nurse take? (Select all that apply.)
   - A. Prepare the child for immediate surgery.
   - B. Obtain adrenal function laboratory testing.
   - C. Cover the infant's genitals with a sterile dressing.
   - D. Refer the parents for genetic counseling.
   - E. Teach the importance of chromosomal analysis with the infant's parents.

Active Learning Scenario Key

Using the ATI Active Learning Template: Basic Concept

RELATED CONTENT
- Obstructive uropathy: Structural or functional obstruction in the urinary system
- Chordee: Ventral curvature of the penis
- Bladder exstrophy: Eversion of the posterior bladder through the anterior bladder wall and lower abdominal wall
- Hypospadias: Urethral opening located just below the glans penis, behind the glans penis, or on the ventral surface of the penile shaft
- Epispadias: Urethral meatus that is unexpectedly open exposed on the dorsum of the genitalia
- Phimosis: Narrowing of the preputial opening of the foreskin
- Cryptorchidism: Failure of one or both testes to descend
- Hydrocele: Collection of peritoneal fluid in the scrotum
- Varicocele: Elongated, dilated, and tortuosity of the veins superior to the testicle
- Testicular torsion: Sudden twisting of the spermatic cord that cause the testicles to hang free from the vascular structures
- Ambiguous genitalia: Erroneous or abnormal sexual differentiation

Ⓝ *NCLEX® Connection: Physiological Adaptation, Pathophysiology*

Application Exercises Key

1. B, C, D, E. **CORRECT:** Obstructive uropathy can result in the impairment of urinary flow. UTI is an expected finding that obstructs the urinary tract because of the infection and inflammation. A history of maternal oligohydramnios is another expected finding which is low amniotic fluid during pregnancy which indicates that the fetus is not excreting urine. A history of this condition can lead to obstruction or kidney impairment after birth. Hematuria with diaper changes is another indicator of obstruction because of inflammation or infection. Hydronephrosis is an unexpected finding that can cause possible urinary obstruction which is the widening of the pelvis of the kidneys. The urethral meatus located on the dorsum of the shaft of the genitalia is a finding associated with epispadias.

   Ⓝ *NCLEX® Connection: Physiological Adaptation Alterations in Body Systems*

2. A, C, D. **CORRECT:** Bladder exstrophy is the eversion of the posterior bladder through the abdominal wall that is present at birth. Expected findings for a male infant include: epispadias, undescended testes, and widening of the pubic symphysis. Hypospadias is a condition in which the urethral meatus is unexpectedly located on the ventral aspect of the genitalia, and it is not a finding associated with bladder exstrophy. Hydrocele is a condition characterized by enlarged scrotal sac and is not a finding associated with bladder exstrophy

   Ⓝ *NCLEX® Connection: Physiological Adaptation Alterations in Body Systems*

3. B. **CORRECT:** Hydrocele is the collection of peritoneal fluid in the scrotum that resolves spontaneously without surgical intervention. Hydroceles are surgically repaired within 1 year if not spontaneously resolved on their own. Retracting the foreskin of the penis and cleansing several times a day is indicated for uncircumcised males or those with conditions such as phimosis. A hydrocele is not a genetic condition; therefore, genetic counseling is not indicated

   Ⓝ *NCLEX® Connection: Physiological Adaptation, Illness Management*

4. B, D, E. **CORRECT:** An infant with ambiguous genitalia has unexpected genitalia findings present at birth. The nurse should plan to obtain adrenal function studies because the infant is at risk for adrenal insufficiency. Genetic counseling and chromosomal analysis are recommended to determine the cause. The infant will possibly require reconstructive surgery; however, there is no immediate need. Covering the infant genitals with a sterile gauze is not indicated for this condition because there is no risk for infection or open areas.

   Ⓝ *NCLEX® Connection: Physiological Adaptation, Illness Management*

CHAPTER 26 *Kidney Disorders*

This chapter includes acute glomerulonephritis, nephrotic syndrome, hemolytic uremic syndrome (HUS), acute kidney injury (ARI), and chronic kidney disease (CRD).

Acute glomerulonephritis

- Benign inflammation of the glomeruli which causes intravascular coagulation that lasts about 1 to 2 weeks.
- Common features are oliguria, swelling, hypertension and circulatory congestion, proteinuria, and hematuria.
- Acute post-streptococcal glomerulonephritis (APSGN) is an antibody-antigen disease that occurs as a result of certain strains of the group A beta-hemolytic streptococcal infection and is most commonly seen in school aged children.

ASSESSMENT

RISK FACTORS

- Acute post-streptococcal glomerulonephritis
- Recent upper respiratory infection or streptococcal infection

EXPECTED FINDINGS

PHYSICAL ASSESSMENT FINDINGS
- Cloudy, tea-colored urine
- Decreased urine output
- Hematuria
- Proteinuria
- Irritability
- Ill appearance
- Lethargy
- Anorexia
- Vague reports of discomfort (headache, abdominal pain, dysuria)
- Periorbital edema
- Facial edema that is worse in the morning but then spreads to extremities and abdomen with progression of the day
- Mild to severe hypertension
- Low grade fever
- Vomiting
- Encephalopathy (headache, irritability, seizures)
- Genitalia and gonadal swelling

LABORATORY TESTS

Throat culture: to identify possible streptococcus infection (usually negative by the time of diagnosis)

Urinalysis: proteinuria, smoky or tea-colored urine, hematuria, increased specific gravity

Kidney function: elevated BUN and creatinine. Decreased glomerular filtration rates

Blood studies: decreased blood protein(hypoalbuminemia), decreased Hgb, Hct (anemia), elevated erythrocyte sedimentation rate (inflammation)

Antistreptolysin O (ASO) titer: positive indicator for the presence of streptococcal antibodies; other serologic testing to determine presence of previous streptococcal infection: Antihyaluronidase (AHase), Antideoxyribonuclease B (Anti-DNase B) Anti-streptokinase (ASKase), Antinicotyladenine dinucleotidase (ANADase)

Blood complement (C3): decreased initially; increases as recovery takes place; returns to normal at 8 to 10 weeks post glomerulonephritis

DIAGNOSTIC PROCEDURES

Kidney biopsy

Chest x-ray: evaluate cardiopulmonary function (heart enlargement, congestion of pulmonary system, and pleural effusions)

PATIENT-CENTERED CARE

NURSING CARE

- Children with a blood pressure within the expected reference range and adequate urine output can be managed at home with close monitoring.
- Monitor I&O.
- Monitor urine volume and character.
- Weigh the child on the same scale with the same amount of clothing daily.
- Monitor vital signs.
- Monitor neurologic status and observe for behavior changes, especially in children who have edema, hypertension, and gross hematuria. Implement seizure precautions if condition indicates.
- Encourage adequate nutritional intake. Regular diet is tolerable in mild cases.
  - Possible restriction of sodium and fluid.
  - Restrict foods high in potassium during periods of oliguria.
  - Restrict protein for severe azotemia.
- Manage fluid and dietary restrictions as prescribed. Fluids and sodium can be limited during periods of edema and hypertension.
- Assess tolerance for activity. Provide frequent rest periods and cluster care tasks.
- Provide for age-appropriate diversional activities.
- Monitor and prevent infection.

MEDICATIONS

Diuretics and antihypertensives

To remove accumulated fluid and manage hypertension. Diuretics are not beneficial if severe kidney failure is present.

NURSING ACTIONS
- Monitor blood pressure.
- Monitor I&O.
- Monitor for electrolyte imbalances (hypokalemia).
- Observe for adverse effects of medications.

CLIENT EDUCATION
- Dizziness can occur with the use of antihypertensives.
- Take the medication as prescribed and notify the provider if adverse effects occur. Continue the medication unless instructed otherwise.

Antibiotics

Treat streptococcal infections

Phosphate binders

Decreases the absorption of phosphate in the GI tract

Sodium polystyrene sulfonate

Corrects hyperkalemia

INTERPROFESSIONAL CARE

Obtain a dietary consult.

CLIENT EDUCATION

- Encourage the child to verbalize feelings related to body image.
- Educate the child regarding appropriate dietary management.
- Encourage adequate rest.
- Educate the family about the condition and the need for follow-up care.
- Teach the family how to monitor blood pressure and daily weight.
- Teach the family about administration and adverse effects of diuretics and antihypertensive medications.
- Encourage the child and family to avoid contact with others who might be ill.

COMPLICATIONS

- Hypertensive encephalopathy
- Circulatory overload
- Acute kidney injury

Nephrotic syndrome

- Alterations in the glomerular membrane allow proteins (especially albumin) to pass into the urine, resulting in decreased blood osmotic pressure, which leads to proteinuria, hyperlipidemia, hypoalbuminemia, and edema.
- There are 3 types of nephrotic syndrome: primary (direct glomeruli injury), secondary (related to systemic illness), or congenital (inherited disorder).
- Nephrotic syndrome is classified according to amount of membrane destruction: minimal change nephrotic syndrome (MCNS), focal glomerulosclerosis (FGS), and membranoproliferative (MPGN).
- MCNS is the most common that results in scant scarring of the glomeruli.

ASSESSMENT

RISK FACTORS

Minimal change nephrotic syndrome (MCNS)
- Increase incidence among preschoolers.
- Cause is unknown, but it can have a multifactorial etiology (metabolic, biochemical, or physiochemical disturbance in the basement membrane of the glomeruli).

EXPECTED FINDINGS

PHYSICAL ASSESSMENT FINDINGS
- Weight gain over a period of days or weeks
- Facial and periorbital edema: decreased throughout the day
- Ascites
- Edema to lower extremities and genitalia
- Muehrcke lines on fingernails (white lines parallel to the lunula)
- Pale skin color
- Anorexia
- Diarrhea
- Irritability
- Lethargy
- Dyspnea
- Vomiting
- Dark, frothy colored urine
- Decrease urinary output
- Blood pressure within expected reference range or slightly below. Hypertension can be rare finding in MCNS.

LABORATORY TESTS

Urinalysis/24-hr urine collection

- Proteinuria (massive): up to 15 grams of protein in a 24-hr specimen
- Hyaline casts
- Few RBCs
- Oval fat bodies
- Increased specific gravity

Blood chemistry

Hypoalbuminemia: reduced blood protein and albumin

Hyperlipidemia: elevated blood lipid levels

Hemoconcentration: elevated Hgb, Hct, and platelets

Possible hyponatremia: reduced sodium level

Glomerular filtration rate: normal or high

Total calcium: decreased

Erythrocyte sedimentation rate (ESR): increased

DIAGNOSTIC PROCEDURES

Kidney biopsy is indicated only if nephrotic syndrome is unresponsive to steroid therapy. Biopsy will show damage to the epithelial cells lining the basement membrane of the kidney.

MRI: Scarring of the kidneys' glomeruli

PATIENT-CENTERED CARE

NURSING CARE

Outcome of therapy and interventions is to decrease the excretion of protein by the kidneys.
- Provide rest.
- Maintain strict I&O. Weigh infant diapers for recording output.
- Monitor urine for protein.
- Monitor vital signs.
- Monitor daily weights; weigh the child on the same scale with the same amount of clothing.
- Monitor edema and measure abdominal girth daily. Measure at the widest area, usually at or above the umbilicus. Assess degree of pitting, color, and texture of skin.
- Elevate legs and feet to relieve edema.
- Monitor and prevent infection (increased risk for upper respiratory infection).
- Encourage nutritional intake within restriction guidelines. Salt can be restricted during the edematous phase.
- Cluster care to provide for rest periods.
- Assess skin for breakdown areas.
- Provide support to families and make appropriate referrals as needed. Relapses can cause physical, emotional, and financial stress for the client and family.

MEDICATIONS

Corticosteroid: prednisone

NURSING ACTIONS
- 60 mg/m²/day for 4 to 6 weeks followed by 40 mg/m² every other day for 2 to 5 months with taper. Ⓠ EBP
- Monitor for adverse effects (hirsutism, slowed linear growth, hypertension, GI bleeding, infection, and hyperglycemia).
- Administer with meals.

CLIENT EDUCATION
- Avoid large crowds (to decrease the risk of infection).
- Using corticosteroids can increase appetite, cause weight gain (especially in the face), and cause mood swings.
- Adhere to the medication regime.
- Observe for adverse effects and notify the provider if necessary.

DIURETIC: FUROSEMIDE

Eliminates excess fluid from the body

NURSING ACTIONS
- Encourage the child to eat foods that are high in potassium.
- Monitor blood electrolyte levels periodically (hypokalemia).

PLASMA EXPANDERS: 25% ALBUMIN

Increases plasma volume and decreases edema in severe cases

NURSING ACTIONS
- Administer per protocol.
- Monitor I&O.
- Monitor for anaphylaxis.

IMMUNOSUPPRESSANT: CYCLOPHOSPHAMIDE

Administer for children who cannot tolerate prednisone or who have repeated relapses of nephrotic syndrome, or to induce remission.

NURSING ACTIONS: Monitor for leukopenia.

INTERPROFESSIONAL CARE

- Obtain a dietary consult.
- Social worker, case manager, school counselor, school nurse: provide emotional support, ensure child's school needs are met, financial strain for family
- Nephrologist: manage condition

CLIENT EDUCATION

- Encourage the child to verbalize feelings related to body image.
- Manage diet appropriately.
- Take all immunizations as scheduled (pneumococcal). Use caution with live vaccines while taking steroids.
- Allow adequate rest.
- Follow-up with the provider as instructed for continued monitoring of the child's response to therapy.
- Strategies to decrease the risk of infection include good hand hygiene, up-to-date immunizations, avoidance of infected people.
- Monitor blood pressure, daily weight, and protein in urine. Notify the provider if manifestations worsen, which indicates relapse.
- Be aware of proper administration and adverse effects of medication.

COMPLICATIONS

SEPSIS/INFECTION
- Steroid therapy increases the risk for infection.
- Monitor for findings of infection.

CLIENT EDUCATION
- Even if the child improves, complete the full dose of antibiotic.
- To prevent infection, perform frequent hand hygiene.
- Contact the provider for any manifestations of infection.
- Keep the child away from potential infection sources.

Hemolytic uremic syndrome

- Hemolytic uremic syndrome (HUS) is an acute kidney condition characterized by acute kidney injury, hemolytic anemia, and thrombocytopenia.
- HUS represents one of the main causes of acute kidney injury in early childhood.
- The endothelial lining within the arterioles of the glomeruli becomes inflamed and causes the red blood cells clog the kidneys. This leads to the intravascular coagulation.
- Toxins enter the bloodstream and destroy red blood cells.

TYPES

Diarrhea–positive (D+) HUS: Responsible for 90% of cases; caused by ingestion of Shiga toxin producing Escherichia coli. There is an association with this condition with consuming undercooked meat (beef), exposure to contaminated water (swimming pools), and drinking unpasteurized apple juice.

Diarrhea–negative (D–) or atypical HUS: various causes; nonenteric infections, disturbances in the complement system, malignancies, or genetic disorders

ASSESSMENT

RISK FACTORS
- Peak incidence 6 months to 4 years.
- Predominantly in Caucasian people, and prevalent in South Africa, Argentina, and west coasts of North and South America.

EXPECTED FINDINGS

PHYSICAL ASSESSMENT FINDINGS
- Occurs after prodromal period of diarrhea and vomiting
- Occasionally occurs after varicella, measles, or a UTI
- Loss of appetite
- Irritable
- Lethargy
- Stupor
- Hallucinations
- Edema
- Pale skin color
- Bruising, purpura, petechiae, or rectal bleeding

- Anuric and hypertensive in severe form
- Urinary output can be reduced or increased with mild cases
- Fever

LABORATORY TESTS
- CBC: Decreased hemoglobin and hematocrit
- Urine: Positive for blood, protein, and casts
- Elevated BUN and blood creatinine
- Fibrin split products in blood and urine (thrombocytopenia)

PATIENT-CENTERED CARE

NURSING CARE

SUPPORTIVE MEASURES
- Monitor I&O.
- Obtain daily weights.
- Administer fluid replacement.
- Treat hypertension.
- Correct acidosis and electrolyte imbalances.
- Monitor CNS for seizure activity and stupor.
- Provide seizure precautions.
- Blood transfusions with fresh, washed packed cells for severe anemia: used with caution.
- For child anuric for 24 hr or having oliguria with uremia or hypertension and seizures.
  - Hemodialysis
  - Peritoneal dialysis
  - Continuous hemofiltration

NUTRITION
- Once vomiting and diarrhea resolves, enteral nutrition is initiated.
- Parenteral nutrition for children who have severe, persistent colitis and marked tissue catabolism.

MEDICATIONS
- No evidence that heparin, corticosteroids, or fibrinolytic agents are beneficial.
- Monoclonal antibodies (eculizumab) minimize the recurrence of D–HUS.

INTERPROFESSIONAL CARE

Obtain a dietary consult.

CLIENT EDUCATION
- Teach the family to avoid undercooked meat, especially ground beef. Internal temperature of meat should be at least 74° C (165° F).
- Avoid unpasteurized apple juice and unwashed raw vegetables.
- Avoid alfalfa sprouts.
- Avoid public pools.
- Do not use antimotility medications for diarrhea.
- Support the child and family regarding severity of the illness.

Acute kidney injury (AKI)

- AKI is the inability of the kidneys to excrete waste material, concentrate urine, and conserve electrolytes.
- The disorder is usually reversible and affects most of the systems of the body.
- Causes are classified as prerenal, intrinsic renal, and postrenal. Prerenal are most common cause of AKI.

ASSESSMENT

RISK FACTORS

Prerenal (caused by conditions that cause decrease kidney perfusion)
- Dehydration secondary to diarrheal disease or persistent vomiting
- Diabetes mellitus
- Surgical shock and trauma (including burns)
- Accidental poisoning
- Prolonged anesthesia

Intrinsic renal (caused by damage to the kidney structures: glomeruli, tubules, vasculature)
- Ingestion of nephrotoxic medications
- Hemolytic uremic syndrome, acute glomerulonephritis
- Ischemia

Postrenal(caused by obstruction of the urinary system): Kidney stones, tumors

EXPECTED FINDINGS

PHYSICAL ASSESSMENT FINDINGS
- Oliguria: (common finding) urinary output of less than 1 mL/kg/hr; with reversible AKI period decreased urinary output
- Abrupt diuresis: with return to normal urine volumes
- Edema
- Drowsiness
- Circulatory collapse
- Cardiac arrhythmia: from hyperkalemia (irregular, weak pulse, abdominal cramps, weakness)
- Seizures: from hyponatremia or hypocalcemia (tetany)
- Tachypnea: from metabolic acidosis
- CNS manifestations: from continued oliguria

LABORATORY/DIAGNOSTIC TESTS

Assess kidney function related to preexisting kidney disease.
- Electrolyte imbalance: hyperkalemia, hyponatremia, hypocalcemia, hyperphosphatemia
- Urine creatinine: decreased
- Glomerular filtration rate (GFR): decreased
- Metabolic acidosis
- Anemia (decreased Hgb, Hct)
- Azotemia
- Elevated blood creatinine
- Elevated BUN
- ECG for cardiac arrhythmias
- IVP and MRI evaluate kidney function

PATIENT-CENTERED CARE

NURSING CARE

- Treat underlying cause of AKI.
- Admit to pediatric intensive care unit.
- Monitor strict I&O.
- Assess fluid and electrolyte balance.
- Limit fluid intake.
- Obtain daily weights.
- Monitor vital signs for hypertension complication.
- Maintain neutral temperature.
- Provide replacement IV fluids slowly.
- Monitor central venous pressure.
- Insert urinary catheter if prescribed (monitor intake output or check urine retention).
- Limit activity.
- Assess for behavior changes or seizure activity.
- Implement seizure precautions if indicated.
- Assess for infection.
- Provide support for the child and family.

MEDICATIONS

Diuretics: furosemide to manage hypervolemia.

Hyperkalemia

- **Calcium gluconate** is administered IV every 2 to 4 min with continuous ECG monitoring to reduce blood potassium levels.
- **Sodium bicarbonate** is administered IV every 30 to 60 min, elevates blood pH and causes a transient fluid shift to reduce blood potassium levels by shifting potassium into the cells.
- **Glucose and insulin IV** causes glucose and potassium to move into cells. Insulin facilitates entry of glucose into cells and helps to reduce blood potassium levels by moving potassium into the cells.
- **Sodium polystyrene sulfonate** is administered orally or rectally to bind potassium and excrete it from the body.

Antihypertensives

- **Labetalol or sodium nitroprusside IV** (with close monitoring) hypertension if encephalopathy threat present.
- **Hydralazine, clonidine, or verapamil** can be given IV for hypertension in less urgent situations.
- **Captopril, hydralazine, minoxidil, propranolol, nifedipine, or furosemide** can be given orally for hypertension.

THERAPEUTIC PROCEDURES

- **Dialysis (Hemo or peritoneal)**: for management of continued oliguria, severe hyperkalemia, uremic syndrome, hypervolemia
- **Hemofiltration/ultrafiltration**: to remove excess wastes products from blood

NUTRITION

- Ingest concentrated foods without fluids.
- Maintain calories while minimizing tissue catabolism, metabolic acidosis, hyperkalemia, and uremia.
- When nourishment is via IV route, prevent fluid overload.

INTERPROFESSIONAL CARE

- Pediatric nephrologist
- Dietician
- Pharmacist
- Nurse case manager

CLIENT EDUCATION

- Get adequate rest.
- Adhere to the therapeutic regimen.
- Attend follow-up care.
- Monitor urinary output.

COMPLICATIONS

- Infection
- Anemia
- Fluid overload
- Hypertension

Chronic kidney disease (CKD)

- CKD or insufficiency begins when the diseased kidneys can no longer maintain the expected chemical structure of body fluids under expected conditions, and there is extensive irreversible damage to the nephrons.
- A variety of diseases and disorders can result in CKD.
- Classified in stages (1-5) according to the child's estimated glomerular filtration rate (eGFR). Stage 5 is most severe.

ASSESSMENT

RISK FACTORS

- Most common causes before 5 years of age are congenital, kidney, and urinary tract malformations and vesicoureteral reflux.
- Glomerular and hereditary kidney disease predominates in the 5- to 15-year-old age group.

EXPECTED FINDINGS

Physical Assessment Findings

- Loss of energy
- Increase fatigue on exertion
- Pale skin color
- Occasional elevated blood pressure
- Delayed growth
- Anorexia

- Nausea and vomiting
- Decrease interest in activities
- Decreased or increased urinary output and compensatory increase in fluid intake
- Uremic odor to breath
- Headache
- Muscle cramps
- Weight loss
- Puffiness to face
- Malaise
- Bone or joint pain
- Dry, itchy skin
- Bruising of skin
- Amenorrhea
- Circulatory overload manifested by hypertension, congestive heart failure and pulmonary edema
- Neurologic involvement (tremors, muscle twitching, confusion, seizures, coma)

LABORATORY/DIAGNOSTIC TESTS

- Glomerular filtration rate (eGFR): possibly decreased- determines the estimate of severity of kidney impairment
- Blood electrolytes: hyperkalemia, hypocalcemia, hyperphosphatemia, hyponatremia
- CBC: anemia
- Blood creatinine and BUN: elevated
- Arterial blood gases: metabolic acidosis

PATIENT-CENTERED CARE

NURSING CARE

- Provide rest.
- Monitor I&O. Initiate fluid restriction if edema present.
- Monitor vital signs.
- Monitor daily weights.
- Manage hypertension.
- Monitor for infection.
- Perform neurologic checks.
- Maintain sodium restriction.
- Encourage reduction of dietary phosphorus.
- Encourage parents to maintain dialysis schedule.
- Educate the family regarding medication compliance and adherence.
- Keep family informed of child's progress.

MEDICATIONS

- Thiazides or furosemide for hypertension
- Beta-blockers and vasodilators for severe hypertension
- Phosphorus binding agent to prevent retention of phosphorus
- Calcium supplements
- Vitamin D: active form
- Water-soluble vitamins
- Sodium bicarbonate and potassium citrate to alleviate acidosis
- Folic acid and recombinant human erythropoietin for anemia

- Recombinant growth hormone for children who have growth retardation
- Antimicrobials for infection
- Antiepileptic for seizures
- Diphenhydramine for pruritus
- Packed RBCs to correct anemia. Administer slowly.

THERAPEUTIC PROCEDURES

- Dialysis (Hemo or peritoneal): for management of continued oliguria, severe hyperkalemia, uremic syndrome, hypervolemia
- Hemofiltration/ultrafiltration: to remove excess wastes products from blood
- Transplantation: for stage 5 CKD in which a donated kidney from (parent, grandparent, sibling, or another donor), is surgically transplanted into child

NUTRITION

- Goal is to provide adequate calories and protein for growth.
- Restrict dietary phosphorus intake.
- Potassium is restricted if oliguria or anuria.
- Limit protein intake to the RDA for the child's age.
- Dietary sources of folic acid and iron.

INTERPROFESSIONAL CARE

- Pediatric nephrologist
- Dietician
- Pharmacist
- Case manager
- School nurse, counselor, teacher
- Social worker

CLIENT EDUCATION

- Increase rest.
- Adhere to therapeutic regimen.
- Encourage the child to remain active and attend school.
- Child should participate in meal planning according to dietary restrictions.
- Encourage child/family participation in support groups.
- Encourage child/family compliance with recommended immunization schedules.

COMPLICATIONS

- End-stage kidney disease
- Progressive deterioration
- Irreversible progress of kidney insufficiency
- Increased susceptibility to infections (pneumonia)

Application Exercises

1. A nurse is caring for a school-age child who has acute glomerulonephritis. Which of the following findings should the nurse report to the provider?

   A. BUN 8 mg/dL

   B. Blood creatinine 1.3 mg/dL

   C. Blood pressure 100/74 mm Hg

   D. Urine output 500 mL in 24 hr

2. A nurse is assessing a child who has nephrotic syndrome. Which of the following findings should the nurse expect? (Select all that apply.)

   A. Urine dipstick +2 protein

   B. Edema in the ankles

   C. Hyperlipidemia

   D. Polyuria

   E. Anorexia

3. A nurse admitting a child who has hemolytic uremic syndrome (HUS). Which of the following laboratory result findings should the nurse report to the provider?

   A. BUN 15 mg/dL

   B. Hgb 8 g/dL

   C. Hct 32%

   D. Platelet 300,000/mm³

4. A nurse is caring for a child who has an acute kidney injury. Which of the following actions should the nurse plan to take?

   A. Encourage fluid intake

   B. Obtain weight every other day

   C. Monitoring for hypokalemia

   D. Administer antihypertensive

5. A nurse is caring for a preschooler who has nephrotic syndrome. Which of the following findings should the nurse report to the provider?

   A. Blood protein 5.0 g/dL

   B. Hgb 14.5 g/dL

   C. Hct 40%

   D. Platelet 200,000 mm³

6. A nurse is assessing a child who has chronic kidney disease. Which of the following findings should the nurse expect?

   A. Flushed face

   B. Hyperactivity

   C. Weight gain

   D. Delayed growth

Active Learning Scenario

A nurse is teaching a parent of a child who has a new prescription for prednisone for nephrotic syndrome. Use the Active Learning Template: Medication to complete this item.

NURSING INTERVENTIONS: List three.

CLIENT EDUCATION: List four teaching points.

Active Learning Scenario Key

Using the Active Learning Template: Medication

NURSING INTERVENTIONS
- Administer 2 mg/kg/day for 6 weeks followed by 1.5 mg/kg every other day for 6 weeks.
- Monitor for adverse effects (hirsutism, slowed linear growth, hypertension, GI bleeding, infection, and hyperglycemia).
- Administer medication with meals.

CLIENT EDUCATION
- Avoid large crowds (to decrease the risk of infection).
- Using corticosteroids can increase appetite, cause weight gain (especially in the face), and cause mood swings.
- Adhere to the medication regimen.
- Monitor for adverse effects and notify the provider.

Ⓝ *NCLEX® Connection: Pharmacological and Parenteral Therapies, Medication Administration*

Application Exercises Key

1. A. A BUN of 8 mg/dL is within the expected reference range for a school-age child.
   B. **CORRECT:** Blood creatinine 1.3 mg/dL is above the expected reference range for school-age child, and should be reported to the provider.
   C. Blood pressure of 100/74 mm Hg is within the expected reference range for a school-age child.
   D. Urine output of 550 mL over 24 hr is within the expected reference range for a school-age child.

Ⓝ *NCLEX® Connection: Physiological Adaptation, Pathophysiology*

2. A. **CORRECT:** A client who has nephrotic syndrome will exhibit proteinuria of due to the kidneys' inability to filter urine.
   B. **CORRECT:** A client who has nephrotic syndrome will exhibit edema in the ankles due to the decreasing colloidal osmotic pressure in the capillaries.
   C. **CORRECT:** A client who has nephrotic syndrome will exhibit hyperlipidemia due to the increased hepatic synthesis of proteins and lipids.
   D. A client who has nephrotic syndrome will exhibit decreased urinary output.
   E. **CORRECT:** A client who has nephrotic syndrome will exhibit anorexia due to the edema of the intestinal mucosa.

Ⓝ *NCLEX® Connection: Physiological Adaptation, Pathophysiology*

3. A. A BUN of 15 mg/dL is within the expected reference range for a child who has HUS.
   B. **CORRECT:** An Hgb of 8 g/dL is below the expected reference range and could indicate anemia and should be reported to the provider.
   C. An Hct of 32% is within the expected reference range for a child who has HUS.
   D. A platelet count of 300,000/mm3 is within the expected reference range for a child who has HUS.

Ⓝ *NCLEX® Connection: Reduction of Risk Potential/ Laboratory Values*

4. D. **CORRECT:** A child who has an acute kidney injury is at risk for hypervolemia; therefore, the nurse should plan to limit the child fluid intake, implement strict intake and output and daily weights. These measures should provide an accurate assessment of fluid balance. The child is at risk for fluid imbalances due to decrease filtration and perfusion of the kidneys such as hyperkalemia and hyponatremia. The child is also at risk for hypertension, which is a complication of AKI, therefore, the nurse should monitor the child's vital signs frequently, and plan to administer antihypertensives such as beta blockers to manage hypertension.

5. A. **CORRECT:** Blood protein 5.0 g/dL is out of the expected reference range for a preschooler and should be reported to the provider.
   B. Hgb 14.5 g/dL is within the expected reference range for a preschooler.
   C. Hct 40% is within the expected reference range for a preschooler.
   D. Platelets 200,000 mm³ is within the expected reference range for a preschooler.

Ⓝ *NCLEX® Connection: Reduction of Risk Potential, Laboratory Values*

6. A. Expect the child to exhibit pallor, not flushing.
   B. Expect the child to be fatigued, not hyperactive.
   C. Expect the child to have weight loss from anorexia, nausea, and vomiting.
   D. **CORRECT:** Expect the child to exhibit delayed growth.

Ⓝ *NCLEX® Connection: Physiological Adaptation, Pathophysiology*

When reviewing the following chapters, keep in mind the relevant topics and tasks of the NCLEX outline, in particular:

Basic Care and Comfort

MOBILITY/IMMOBILITY: Maintain/correct the adjustment of client's traction device.

NONPHARMACOLOGICAL COMFORT INTERVENTIONS: Assess client need for pain management.

Pharmacological and Parenteral Therapies

ADVERSE EFFECTS/CONTRAINDICATIONS/SIDE EFFECTS/INTERACTIONS: Identify a contraindication to the administration of a medication to the client.

PHARMACOLOGICAL PAIN MANAGEMENT
Administer and document pharmacological pain management appropriate for client age and diagnoses.

Administer medications for pain management.

EXPECTED ACTIONS/OUTCOMES: Use clinical decision making/critical thinking when addressing expected effects/outcomes of medications.

Reduction of Risk Potential

POTENTIAL FOR COMPLICATIONS OF DIAGNOSTIC TESTS/ TREATMENTS/PROCEDURES: Use precautions to prevent injury and/or complications associated with a procedure or diagnosis.

SYSTEM-SPECIFIC ASSESSMENTS: Assess the client for abnormal peripheral pulses after a procedure or treatment.

THERAPEUTIC PROCEDURES
Apply knowledge of related nursing procedures and psychomotor skills when caring for clients undergoing therapeutic procedures.

Educate client about treatments and procedures.

Provide preoperative care.

DIAGNOSTIC TESTS: Apply knowledge of related nursing procedures and psychomotor skills when caring for clients undergoing diagnostic testing.

Physiological Adaptation

ALTERATIONS IN BODY SYSTEMS: Apply knowledge of nursing procedures, pathophysiology and psychomotor skills when caring for a client with an alteration in body systems.

UNIT 2   SYSTEM DISORDERS
SECTION: MUSCULOSKELETAL DISORDERS

CHAPTER 27 *Fractures*

A fracture occurs when the resistance between a bone and an applied stress yields to the stress, resulting in a disruption to the integrity of the bone. Bone healing and remodeling is faster in children than in adults, due to a thicker periosteum and good blood supply.

Epiphyseal plate injuries can result in altered bone growth. Radiographic evidence of previous fractures in various stages of healing or in infants can be the result of physical maltreatment or osteogenesis imperfecta.

ASSESSMENT

RISK FACTORS

- Obesity
- Poor nutrition
- Developmental characteristics, ordinary play activities, and recreation that place children at risk for injury (falls from climbing or running; trauma to bones from skateboarding, skiing, or playing soccer or basketball)

EXPECTED FINDINGS

PHYSICAL ASSESSMENT FINDINGS
- Pain
- Crepitus
- Deformity
- Edema
- Ecchymosis
- Decreased use of affected area

Common types of fractures in children

- **Plastic deformation (bend):** The bone is bent no more than 45° without breakage.
- **Buckle (torus):** Compression of the porous bone resulting in a bulge or raised area at the fracture site.
- **Greenstick:** Incomplete fracture of the bone.
- **Transverse:** Break is straight across the bone. Ⓠ EBP
- **Oblique:** Break is diagonal across the bone.
- **Spiral:** Break spirals around the bone.
- **Physeal (growth plate):** Injury to the end of the long bone on the growth plate.

27.1 Fractures

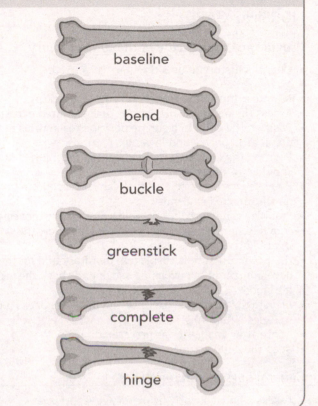

baseline

bend

buckle

greenstick

complete

hinge

- **Stress:** Small fractures/cracks in the bone due to repeated muscle contractions during weight bearing activities.
- **Complete:** Bone fragments are separated.
- **Incomplete:** Bone fragments are still attached.
- **Closed or simple:** The fracture occurs without a break in the skin.
- **Open or compound:** The fracture occurs with an open wound and bone protruding.
- **Complicated fracture:** The fracture results in injury to other organs and tissues.
- **Comminuted:** The fracture includes small fragments of bone that lie in surrounding tissue.

DIAGNOSTIC PROCEDURES

Radiograph

Used to confirm diagnosis and determine the positioning of the bone

NURSING ACTIONS: Instruct and assist the client to remain still during the procedure.

CLIENT EDUCATION
- Be aware of what to expect during the procedure.
- Provide emotional support.

PATIENT-CENTERED CARE

NURSING CARE

Provide emergency care at the time of injury

- Obtain a history of how the injury occurred.
- Maintain ABCs.
- Monitor vital signs, pain, and neurologic status.
- Assess the neurovascular status of the injured extremity.
- Position the child in a supine position for injuries to the distal arm, pelvis, and lower extremities.
- Position the child in a sitting position for injuries to the shoulder or upper arm.
- Remove jewelry or objects that can cause constriction on the affected extremity.
- Stabilize the injured area, avoid unnecessary movement.
- Provide splinting at the joint above and below the injured area.
- If a pelvic fracture is suspected, monitor child for the development of hypovolemic shock and check the urine for blood.
- Elevate the affected extremity and apply ice packs (not to exceed 20 min).
- Administer analgesics as prescribed.
- Keep the child warm.

General nursing interventions

- Assess pain frequently using an age-appropriate pain tool. Use appropriate pain management, both pharmacological and nonpharmacological.
- Monitor neurovascular status on a regular schedule. Report any change in status.
- Maintain proper alignment.
- Promote range of motion of fingers, toes, and unaffected extremities.
- Provide instructions to the child and family regarding activity restrictions.
- Reassure and provide comfort to the parents and child.

Neurovascular Assessment

- **Sensation:** Assess for numbness or tingling sensation of the extremity. Loss of sensation can indicate nerve damage.
- **Skin temperature:** Assess the extremity for temperature. It should be warm, not cool, to touch.
- **Skin color:** Assess the color of the affected extremity. Check distal to the injury and look for changes in pigmentation.
- **Capillary refill:** Press the nail beds of the affected extremity until blanching occurs. Blood return should be within 3 seconds.
- **Pulses:** Pulses should be palpable and strong. Pulses should also be equal to the pulses of the unaffected extremity.
- **Movement:** The client should be able to move the joints distal to the injury (fingers or toes).

MEDICATIONS

Analgesics

Administer analgesics for pain as prescribed.

Opioid analgesia

NURSING ACTIONS: Monitor for respiratory depression and constipation.

CLIENT EDUCATION: Be aware of the need for adequate pain relief.

Immunizations

Administer tetanus for open fractures.

Antibiotics

Administer for open fractures.

THERAPEUTIC PROCEDURES

Casting

Casts are applied to provide immobilization, maintain bone alignment, and manage fractures.

TYPES OF CASTS: long-leg, short-leg, bilateral long-leg, long-arm, short-arm, shoulder spica, 1 ½ spica, full spica, and single spica
- Plaster of Paris casts are heavy, not water-resistant, and can take 10 to 72 hr to dry. Synthetic fiberglass casts are light, water-resistant, and dry quickly (5 to 20 min).
- Prior to casting, the skin area should be observed for integrity, cleaned, and dried. Apply a stockinette or waterproof liner to the casted area. Bony prominences should be padded to prevent skin breakdown. The provider then applies the casting material.

NURSING ACTIONS
- Provide age-appropriate atraumatic care prior to cast application by showing the procedure to the child on a doll or toy.
- Assess and monitor neurovascular status.
- Elevate the casted area by using pillows during the first 24 to 48 hr to prevent swelling.
- Apply ice for the first 24 hr to decrease swelling.
- Turn and position the child every 2 hr so that dry air circulates around and under the cast for faster drying. This also will prevent pressure from changing the shape of the cast. Do not use heat lamps or warm hair dryers.
- Turn the child frequently while supporting all extremities and joints.
- Instruct the client to keep the affected extremity supported (with a sling) or elevated on a pillow when sitting.
- Monitor for drainage on the cast. Outline any drainage on the outside of the cast with a pen (and note date and time) so it can be monitored for any additional drainage.
- Assess the general skin condition and the area around the cast edges.

- Provide routine skin care and thorough perineal care to maintain skin integrity.
- For plaster casts, use palms of hands to avoid denting, and expose the cast to air to promote drying.
- Use moleskin to petal the edges over any rough area of the cast that can rub against the child's skin.
- Cover areas of the cast with plastic or waterproof tape to avoid soiling from urine or feces.
- Assist with proper crutch fitting and reinforce proper use.

CLIENT EDUCATION
- Teach the client and parents that when the cast is applied it will feel warm, but it will not burn the child.
- Teach the parents and child to report pain that is extremely severe or is not relieved 1 hr after the administration of pain medication.
- Teach the parents and child how to perform neurovascular checks and when to contact the provider.
- Give instructions for the proper use of crutches for lower-extremity casts.
- Reinforce skin and perineal care with a spica cast.
- Instruct the child not to place any foreign objects inside the cast to avoid trauma to the skin.
- Reinforce use of proper restraints when transporting the child in any vehicle.
- Teach the child and parents about cast removal and cast cutter.
- Notify provider immediately of any soft spots on the cast, change in sensation or increased pain.
- Cleanse with damp cloth if becomes soiled.
- Instruct the parents and child to soak the extremity in warm water after the cast has been removed.

Traction care

Traction is pulling an injured body part in one direction against a counterpull force in an opposite direction to immobilize a fracture, reduce a dislocation, maintain bone alignment, and provide muscle rest. The type of traction used depends on the fracture, age of the client, and associated injuries.
- **Skin traction** uses a pulling force that is applied by weights. Using tape and straps applied to the skin along with boots and/or cuffs, weights are attached by a rope to the extremity (Buck, Russell, Bryant traction).
- **Skeletal traction** uses a continuous pulling force that is applied directly to the skeletal structure and/or specific bone. It is used when more pulling force is needed than skin traction can withstand. A pin or rod is inserted through or into the bone. Force is applied through the use of weights attached by a pulley and rope. The weights are never to be removed by the nurse.
- **Halo traction (cervical traction)** uses a halo-type bar that encircles the head. Screws are inserted into the outer skull. The halo is attached to either bed traction or rods that are secured to a vest worn by the client.
- **Manual traction:** applied distal to injured area by the provider during casting or with closed reduction.

NURSING ACTIONS
- Maintain body alignment.
- Provide pharmacological and nonpharmacological interventions for the management of pain and muscle spasms.
- Notify the provider if the client experiences severe pain from muscle spasms that is unrelieved with medications or repositioning.
- Assess and monitor neurovascular status.
- Routinely monitor skin integrity and document findings. Qpcc
- Assess pin sites for pain, redness, swelling, drainage, or odor. Provide pin care per facility protocol.
- Assess for changes in elimination and maintain usual patterns of elimination.
- Ensure that all the hardware is tight and that the bed is in the correct position.

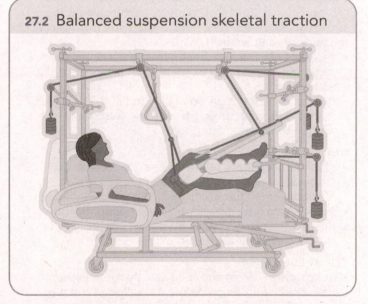

27.2 Balanced suspension skeletal traction

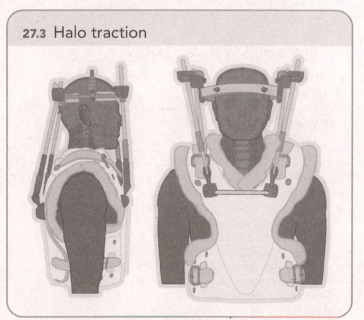

27.3 Halo traction

- Assess and maintain weights so that they hang freely, and the knots do not touch the pulley. Do not lift or remove weights unless prescribed and supervised by the provider.
- Consult with the provider for an overbed trapeze to assist the child to move in bed.
- Provide range of motion and encourage activity of nonimmobilized extremities to maintain mobility and prevent contractures.
- Encourage deep breathing and use of the incentive spirometry.
- Promote frequent position changing within restrictions of traction to prevent skin breakdown.
- Consult with provider for pressure reliving or foam mattress for the child's bed to prevent skin impairment.

Surgical interventions

Depending on the type of fracture, surgical intervention can be required. The most common fractures requiring surgery include supracondylar fractures and fractures of the humerus and femur.
- Surgical reduction is achieved by either a closed (no incision) or open (with incision) reduction with or without pinning.
- Distraction is the application of external fixator device to immobilize fractures, correct bone defects and provide bone lengthening.

NURSING ACTIONS
- Monitor for findings of infection at the incision site.
- Encourage mobilization as soon as prescribed.
- Medicate for pain as needed.
- Provide crutch training for lower-extremity fractures.
- Instruct the parents and child that weight-bearing to the affected extremity is limited.

CLIENT EDUCATION
- Instruct the parents and child about what to expect before and after the procedure, including NPO status.
- Monitoring site for infection.
- Medication for pain as necessary.

INTERPROFESSIONAL CARE

- Orthopedic specialists are generally consulted for fracture care in children.
- Notify social services in situations in which maltreatment is suspected.

CLIENT EDUCATION

CARE AFTER DISCHARGE
- Perform proper cast care, as well as pin care if indicated.
- Perform neurovascular checks and when to call or return to the provider.
- Use antipruritic medications if prescribed.
- Maintain physical restrictions as prescribed.
- Perform appropriate pain management.
- Report increasing pain, redness, inflammation, and/or fever to the provider.
- Perform follow-up care as instructed.

COMPLICATIONS

COMPARTMENT SYNDROME

CAUSES: tight dressing, skin traction, trauma, burns, surgery, hemorrhage, severe IV infiltration, or casting.
- Compression of nerves, blood vessels, and muscle inside a confined place, resulting in neuromuscular ischemia; most commonly occurring in relation to tibial fractures or fractures involving the forearm. Manifestations include severe pain, swelling, skin pallor, sensory deficits, motor weakness and absence of pulse in the affected extremity.
- If untreated, deformity of the extremity, paralysis and infection can result.

Volkmann contracture: a permanent contracture of the forearm and hand

FINDING (REMEMBER THE 5 P'S) Qs
- **Pain** that is unrelieved with elevation or analgesics; increases with passive movement.
- **Paresthesia** or numbness (early finding).
- **Pulselessness** distal to the fracture (late finding).
- **Paralysis** or an inability to move digits (nerve damage).
- **Pale**, cold skin and cyanosis to nail beds.

NURSING ACTIONS
- Assess the extremity every hour for the first 24 hr.
- The space between the skin and the cast should allow for one finger to be placed.
- Notify the provider if compartment syndrome is suspected.
- Avoid elevating the affected extremity.
- Loosen restrictive devices or dressings.
- Prepare the child for fasciotomy.

CLIENT EDUCATION: Report pain that is not relieved by analgesics, pain that continues to increase in intensity, numbness or tingling, or a change in color of the extremity.

Renal calculi

Occurs with non-weight-bearing injuries. Ensure adequate nutrition and hydration. Monitor urinary output.

Embolism

Fat embolism: Fat breaks away from the bone marrow of the injured one and enters the blood stream

Pulmonary embolism: Clot develops and forms at the injury site and travels to the lungs

NURSING ACTIONS
- Monitor for chest pain and difficulty breathing and notify provider.
- Encourage ambulation as indicated.
- Administer anticoagulants as prescribed.
- Provide active and passive range of motion.
- Elevate the child's head of bed.
- Administer oxygen as indicated.
- Apply sequential compression device sleeves as prescribed.

Osteomyelitis

Infection within the bone secondary to a bacterial infection from an outside source (with an open fracture [endogenous] or from a bloodborne bacterial source [hematogenous])

MANIFESTATIONS

- Irritability
- Fever
- Tachycardia
- Edema
- Pain is constant but increases with movement
- Not wanting to use the affected extremity
- Site of infection tender, swollen, and warm to touch

NURSING ACTIONS

- Assist in diagnostic procedures (obtaining skin, blood, and bone cultures).
- Assist with joint or bone biopsy.
- Administer IV and oral antibiotic therapy.
- Monitor hepatic, hematologic, and renal function.
- Monitor vital signs and intake and output.
- Monitor site for drainage.
- Monitor for the development of superinfection (candidiasis, C. difficile infection).
- Provide support for the affected extremity and position for comfort.
- Administer pain medication as prescribed.
- Consult with the parents and provider regarding home care needs.
- Consult physical therapy as prescribed.

CLIENT EDUCATION

- Educate the child and parents about the length of treatment that can be needed and long-term antibiotic therapy.
- Monitor hearing due to ototoxicity of some antibiotics.
- Limit movement of the affected limb and avoid bearing any weight until cleared by the provider.
- Provide for diversional activities consistent with the client's level of development.
- Ensure proper nutrition.

Application Exercises

1. A school nurse is planning an educational session for parents about fractures. Which of the following statements should the nurse make?

   A. "Children need a longer time to heal from a fracture than an adult."

   B. "Epiphyseal plate injuries can result in altered bone growth."

   C. "A greenstick fracture is a complete break in the bone."

   D. "Bones are unable to bend, so they break."

2. A nurse is caring for a child who has a fracture. Which of the following are manifestations of a fracture? (Select all that apply.)

   A. Crepitus

   B. Edema

   C. Pain

   D. Fever

   E. Ecchymosis

3. A nurse is caring for a child who sustained a fracture. Which of the following actions should the nurse take? (Select all that apply.)

   A. Place a heat pack on the site of injury.

   B. Elevate the affected limb.

   C. Assess neurovascular status frequently.

   D. Encourage ROM of the affected limb.

   E. Stabilize the injury.

4. A nurse is caring for a child who is in a plaster spica cast. Which of the following actions should the nurse take?

   A. Use a heat lamp to facilitate drying.

   B. Avoid turning the child until the cast is dry.

   C. Assist the client with crutch walking after the cast is dry.

   D. Apply moleskin to the edges of the cast.

5. A nurse is caring for a child who is in skeletal traction. Which of the following actions should the nurse take? (Select all that apply.)

   A. Remove the weights every 6 hours.

   B. Monitor pin sites frequently.

   C. Ensure weights hang freely.

   D. Ensure rope knot is in contact with pulley.

   E. Monitor skin integrity for impairment

Active Learning Scenario

A nurse is teaching about compartment syndrome to a group of nurses. Use the ATI Active Learning Template: System Disorder to complete this item.

EXPECTED FINDINGS: List five.

NURSING CARE: List three nursing actions.

CLIENT EDUCATION: List one teaching point.

Active Learning Scenario Key

Using the ATI Active Learning Template: System Disorder

EXPECTED FINDINGS
- Pain that is unrelieved with elevation or analgesics; increases with passive movement
- Paresthesia or numbness (early finding)
- Pulselessness distal to the fracture (late finding)
- Paralysis or an inability to move digits (nerve damage)
- Pale, cold skin and cyanosis to nail beds

NURSING CARE
- Assess the extremity every hour for the first 24 hr.
- The space between the skin and the cast should allow for one finger to be placed.
- Notify the provider if compartment syndrome is suspected.
- Avoid elevating the affected extremity.
- Loosen restrictive devices or dressings.
- Prepare the child for fasciotomy.

CLIENT EDUCATION: Report pain that is not relieved by analgesics, pain that continues to increase in intensity, numbness or tingling, or a change in color of the extremity.

(N) *NCLEX® Connection: Reduction of Risk Potential, Potential for Complications from Surgical Procedures and Health Alterations*

Application Exercises Key

1. A. The school nurse should also inform the parents that children heal from fractures quicker than adults because their bones have a thicker periosteum and adequate blood supply.
   B. **CORRECT:** The school nurse should inform the parents that epiphyseal plate injuries can result in altered bone growth because the site of injury influences longitudinal bone growth. It is imperative that these injuries are detected and managed early to prevent altered bone growth.
   C. A greenstick fracture is a partial break in the bone.
   D. Children's bones are soft and pliable and can bend up to a 45° prior to breaking.

   (N) *NCLEX® Connection: Physiological Adaptation, Pathophysiology*

2. A. **CORRECT:** A fracture can leave bone fragments that will exhibit a grating sound. Crepitus is a manifestation of a fracture.
   B. **CORRECT:** Swelling at the site occur related to the trauma. Edema is a manifestation of a fracture.
   C. **CORRECT:** A child who has a fracture will experience pain from the trauma.
   D. A child who has a fracture will not exhibit a fever related to the fracture.
   E. **CORRECT:** Bleeding under the skin can occur related to the trauma. Ecchymosis is a manifestation of a fracture.

   (N) *NCLEX® Connection: Physiological Adaptation, Pathophysiology*

3. A. Applying heat is not indicated for a fracture, instead the nurse should apply ice pack to the affected extremity to decrease swelling.
   B. **CORRECT:** Elevating the affected extremity will decrease swelling.
   C. **CORRECT:** Checking the neurovascular status frequently will provide information about circulation and perfusion to the extremity and allow the nurse to intervene for any unexpected findings.
   D. Encouraging ROM is not indicated because this can cause further injury.
   E. **CORRECT:** Stabilizing the affected extremity will promote comfort and prevent further injury.

   (N) *NCLEX® Connection: Physiological Adaptation, Illness Management*

4. A. A heat lamp is not used to dry the cast because this can result in burn injury; therefore, the nurse should use a cool fan to facilitate drying of plaster cast if needed.
   B. Turning the child frequently will prevent pressure injuries; therefore, the nurse should handle a wet cast with their palms of their hands to decrease indention and use pillows when turning and repositioning the child.
   C. Crutch walking is not indicated because the child is usually non-weight bearing until cast is removed.
   D. **CORRECT:** Applying moleskin to the edges of the cast will protect the child's skin from injury from friction of the cast.

   (N) *NCLEX® Connection: Reduction of Risk Potential, Therapeutic Procedures*

5. A. Removing the weights is performed by the provider.
   B. **CORRECT:** Assess the child's position frequently to ensure proper alignment is present. This avoids putting stress on the pinned areas and other areas of the body causing pain.
   C. **CORRECT:** The weights should hang freely to allow the prescribed traction force.
   D. The knot in the rope should not touch the pulley because this will influence the amount of traction.
   E. **CORRECT:** The child is at risk for skin impairment because of immobility, therefore, it is important for the nurse to monitor the skin frequently and turn and reposition the child frequently to prevent skin impairment.

   (N) *NCLEX® Connection: Basic Care and Comfort, Mobility/Immobility*

CHAPTER 28 # Musculoskeletal Congenital Disorders

Musculoskeletal congenital disorders might be identified at birth or might not be present until later in infancy, childhood, or adolescence. These disorders can involve a specific area of the child's body or affect the child's entire musculoskeletal system. Careful assessment and interprofessional management assist in promoting the child's growth, development, and mobility.

Clubfoot

- A complex deformity of the ankle and foot known as congenital talipes equinovarus.
- Can affect one or both feet, occur as an isolated defect, or in association with other disorders (cerebral palsy and spinal bifida).
- Categorized as positional (occurs from intrauterine crowding), syndromic (occurs in association with other syndromes), and congenital (idiopathic).

ASSESSMENT

RISK FACTORS: hereditary factors, occurs more commonly with boys

EXPECTED FINDINGS
- The affected foot (feet) is shorter and smaller with an empty heal pad and visible plantar crease visible at midfoot.
- If deformity is unilateral, calf atrophy is visible.
- Talipes varus: inversion (foot bending inward).
- Talipes valgus: eversion (foot bending outward).
- Talipes calcaneus: dorsiflexion (toes are higher than the heels).
- Talipes equinus ("horse foot"): plantar flexion (toes are lower than the heels).
- Talipes equinovarus: toes are facing inward and lower than the heel.

DIAGNOSTIC PROCEDURES: Prenatal ultrasound provides data for identification of the deformity.

PATIENT-CENTERED CARE

NURSING CARE
- Encourage parents to hold and cuddle the child.
- Encourage parents to meet the developmental needs of the child.
- Perform neurovascular and skin integrity checks.

THERAPEUTIC PROCEDURES

Casting
- Series of castings applied during the first month of life and continuing until maximum correction is accomplished (approximately 5 to 8 weeks).
- Weekly manipulation of the foot to stretch the muscles with subsequent placement of a long-leg cast. Q EBP
- Following casting, a heel cord tenotomy is usually performed followed by application of long leg cast for 3 weeks.
- After casting is complete, a Denis Browne bar and specialized sandals (abduction brace) are applied to maintain alignment and prevent recurrence.
- The abduction brace is worn at bedtime for approximately 3 to 5 years.

NURSING CARE
- Assess skin integrity and neurovascular status.
- Perform cast care.

CLIENT EDUCATION
- Proper cast care.
- Importance of regular cast changes.
- Change diapers frequently.
- Check for decrease circulation (pain, pallor, and coldness) and notify the provider.

INTERPROFESSIONAL COLLABORATION
- Orthopedic provider
- Physical therapist

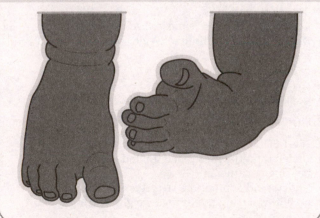

28.1 Clubfoot

COMPLICATIONS

Growth and development delays
- NURSING CARE: Monitor growth and development.
- CLIENT EDUCATION: Use strategies to enhance normal growth and development.

Effects of casting
- Skin breakdown
- Neurovascular alterations

Legg-Calve-Perthes Disease

Impaired circulation to femoral head that results in aseptic necrosis. Condition can be unilateral or bilateral with insidious onset. Stages include: synovitis, necrotic, fragmentation, reconstruction.

ASSESSMENT

RISK FACTORS
- Age: Affects children 2 to 12 years but more common between ages 4 to 8 years
- Gender: More common in boys
- Trauma, decreased circulation, inflammation to the femoral head

EXPECTED FINDINGS
- Intermittent painless limp
- Hip stiffness
- Limited ROM
- Hip, thigh, knee pain
- Shortening of the affected leg

DIAGNOSTIC PROCEDURES: Radiograph of the hip and pelvis, MRI

PATIENT-CENTERED CARE

NURSING CARE
- Treatment varies with the child's age and the condition of the femoral head.
- Administer NSAIDs as prescribed.
- Maintain rest and limited weight bearing (initial).
  - Abduction brace or casts
  - Physical therapy
  - Traction
- Advance to active range of motion as prescribed.

SURGICAL INTERVENTIONS: Osteotomy of the hip or femur

CLIENT EDUCATION
- Understand the prescribed limited weight bearing treatment.
- Understand appropriate strategies for learning and activities during the limited weight bearing periods. ◯PCC
- Understand the importance of attending school and performing other appropriate activities.

COMPLICATIONS

- Joint degeneration
- Permanent disability
- Chronic pain

Developmental dysplasia of the hip (DDH)

A variety of disorders resulting in abnormal development of the hip structures that can affect infants or children
- **Acetabular dysplasia**: delay in acetabular development (acetabular roof is shallow and oblique)
- **Subluxation**: incomplete dislocation of the hip (femoral head is partially out of the acetabulum but remains in contact)
- **Dislocation**: femoral head does not have contact with the acetabulum

ASSESSMENT

RISK FACTORS

- Birth order (firstborn)
- Female gender
- Family history
- Breech intrauterine position
- Improper swaddling
- Joint stability
- Oligohydramnios
- Large for gestational age
- Conditions: torticollis, metatarsus adductus, clubfoot

EXPECTED FINDINGS

INFANT
- Asymmetry and unequal number of skin folds on the posterior gluteal/thigh
- Limited hip abduction
- Shortening of the femur of affected side
- Audible clunking sound
- Widened perineum
- Positive Ortolani test performed by provider (hip is reduced by abduction)
- Positive Barlow test performed by provider (hip is dislocated by adduction)

CHILD
- One leg shorter than the other
- Walking on toes on one foot
- Walk with a limp
- Waddle gait, spine lordosis (bilateral dislocations)
- Trendelenburg sign positive

DIAGNOSTIC PROCEDURES

Screening test: Provider preforms physical exams and testing (Ortolani and Barlow) at each of the child's wellness visits to check for presence of DDH (up to 12 months of age)

Ultrasound: performed at 2 weeks for high-risk infants; selective testing for infants from 6 weeks to 6 months

X–ray: can diagnose DDH in infants older than 4 months of age

PATIENT-CENTERED CARE

NURSING CARE

- Treatment starts as soon as DDH is diagnosed and depends on the child's age and the extent of the dysplasia.
- Encourage parents to hold and cuddle the infant/child.
- Encourage parents to meet the developmental needs of the infant/child.

Newborn to 6 months

Abduction splint: (Pavlik harness: prevents hip flexion and adduction)
- Manage dislocation or persistent instability.
- Maintain harness placement for to 12 weeks.
- Harness typically worn 23 hours per day until the hip is stabilized (then worn during sleep for next 6 weeks).
- Straps may need readjustment by the provider at least every week.
- Check straps frequently at least 2 times each day.
- Perform neurovascular and skin integrity checks.
- Removing the harness is dependent on the parents.

CLIENT EDUCATION
- Do not adjust the harness straps.
- If removal is prescribed, instruct parents how to apply the harness. Qs
- Teach the family skin care (use an undershirt, wear knee socks, assess skin, gently massage skin under straps, avoid lotions and powders, place diaper under the straps).
- Assess skin under the straps.

COMPLICATIONS

- Osteonecrosis: Caused by improper fit and wear of harness. Ensure straps are adjusted by the provider.
- Impairment of skin integrity: Monitor skin frequently for redness under straps, avoid lotions or powders. Report unexpected findings promptly.

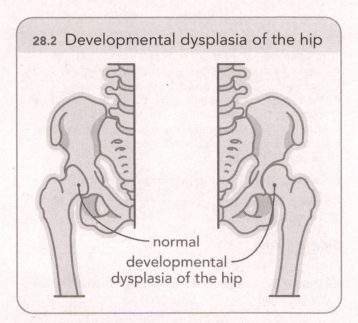

28.2 Developmental dysplasia of the hip

normal
developmental
dysplasia of the hip

6 months to 2 years

Surgical closed reduction with placement of hip spica cast
- Indicated when abduction splinting (Pavlik harness therapy) is unsuccessful.
- Closed surgical procedure under anesthesia in which the surgeon positions the femoral head back into the acetabulum; spica cast is applied to maintain position.

NURSING ACTIONS
- Prepare family and child for surgery.
- Perform neurovascular checks.
- CT/MRI scan after surgery to check reduction procedure.
- Manage postoperative pain.
- Perform skin care.
- Perform cast care.

CLIENT EDUCATION: Understand spica cast and home care management.

Hip spica cast (maintains external rotation of the hip): Changed frequently by the provider to accommodate growth

NURSING ACTIONS
- Assess and maintain the hip spica cast.
- Perform frequent neurovascular checks.
- Perform range of motion with the unaffected extremities.
- Perform frequent assessment of skin integrity, especially in the diaper area.
- Assess for pain control using an age-appropriate pain tool. Intervene as indicated. Qpcc
- Evaluate hydration status frequently.
- Assess elimination status daily.

CLIENT EDUCATION

- Understand proper positioning, turning, neurovascular assessments, and care of the cast.
- Note color and temperature of toes on casted extremity.
- Give sponge baths to avoid wetting the cast.
- Use a waterproof barrier around the genital opening of spica cast to prevent soiling with urine or feces.
- After discharge, use appropriate care and equipment (stroller, wagon, car seat; accommodate large cast) for maintaining mobility.

Open Reduction: If dislocation is non-reducible

Orthosis: Applied after spica casting, to maintain hip positioning

Older children

- Surgical reduction with presurgical traction
- Femoral osteotomy, reconstruction, and tenotomy are often needed

COMPLICATIONS

Postoperative complications: Atelectasis, ileus, infection

Effects of immobilization: Decreased muscle strength, bone demineralization, altered bowel motility

Effects of casting: Skin breakdown, neurovascular alterations

Osteogenesis imperfecta

An inherited connective tissue condition that results in bone fractures and deformity along with restricted growth. There are several types of osteogenesis imperfecta (OI). Type I is a mild and common form.

ASSESSMENT

RISK FACTORS: Parent who has (OI)

EXPECTED FINDINGS: Classic manifestations
- Multiple bone fractures (fragile bones and deformities)
- Blue sclera
- Early hearing loss
- Small, discolored teeth

DIAGNOSTIC PROCEDURES: Bone biopsy

NURSING ACTIONS
- Prepare the child and parents for any procedures.
- Provide frequent oral care.
- Obtain manual blood pressures.
- Assist with positioning the child to prevent fractures.

PATIENT-CENTERED CARE

NURSING CARE: Treatment is supportive.

MEDICATION: **Bisphosphonate therapy (pamidronate)**
- Increase bone density
- Prevent fractures

NURSING ACTIONS
- Administer IV.
- Monitor for adverse effects (hypokalemia, hypomagnesemia, hypocalcemia, hypophosphatemia, thrombocytopenia, neutropenia, dysrhythmias, kidney failure, general malaise).
- Monitor for respiratory infections.
- Vaccines containing live viruses are not recommended.

CLIENT EDUCATION
- Observe for adverse effects of therapy and call the provider if necessary.
- Understand oral and dental hygiene.
- Change position frequently and monitor for skin impairment.
- Adhere to the medication regime as prescribed.
- Assist with the application of braces and splints as prescribed.
- Assist child with meeting developmental milestones.
- Attend support groups.

INTERPROFESSIONAL COLLABORATION
- Orthopedic provider
- Dietician
- Pharmacist
- Physical therapist
- Infectious disease specialist
- Dentist
- Genetic specialist

SURGICAL INTERVENTIONS
- For severe cases
- Correct bone deformities, placement of rods
- Bone marrow transplant

Scoliosis

- Scoliosis is a complex deformity of the spine that also affects the ribs.
- Characterized by a lateral curvature of the spine and spinal rotation that causes rib asymmetry.
- Idiopathic or structural scoliosis is the most common form of scoliosis and can be seen in isolation or associated with other conditions.

ASSESSMENT

RISK FACTORS
- Genetic tendency
- Gender: more common in females
- Age: highest incidence between 8 to 15 years of age

EXPECTED FINDINGS
- Asymmetry in scapula, ribs, flanks, shoulders, and hips
- Improperly fitting clothing (one leg shorter than the other)

DIAGNOSTIC PROCEDURES

- Screen during preadolescence for boys and girls.
  - Observe the child, who should be wearing only underwear, from the back.
  - Have the child bend over at the waist with arms hanging down and observe for asymmetry of ribs and flank.
  - Measure spinal curvature with a scoliometer.
- Radiography
  - Use the Cobb technique to determine the degree of curvature.
  - Use the Risser scale to determine the skeletal maturity.
  - MRI and CT scans can be used.
  - Lung capacity: pulmonary function studies, chest x-ray

PATIENT-CENTERED CARE

NURSING CARE

Treatment depends on the degree, location, and type of curvature.

THERAPEUTIC PROCEDURES

Bracing: Customized braces slow the progression of the curve. Types of braces include Milwaukee, TLSO, Wilmington, and Charleston.

NURSING ACTIONS
- Assist with fitting the adolescent/child with a brace.
- Assess skin.
- Promote the adolescent's/child's positive self-image.

CLIENT EDUCATION
- Understand how to apply the brace.
- Wear brace for 23 hr per day only remove for personal hygiene (showering).

Surgical interventions

Spinal fusion with rod placement: Used for curvatures greater than 45°

PREOPERATIVE NURSING ACTIONS
- Inform and assist the parents and adolescent/child about autologous (self-donated) blood donations if indicated.
- Obtain routine laboratory studies, including a type and cross match for blood as prescribed.
- Orient the adolescent/child and family to the pediatric ICU.
- Inform the adolescent/child and family about what can be expected during the postoperative period (monitoring equipment, NG tube, chest tube, indwelling urinary catheter, breathing exercises, and self-administering analgesic pump).

POSTOPERATIVE NURSING ACTIONS
- Monitor the adolescent/child initially in the pediatric intensive care unit.
- Perform standard postoperative care to prevent complications.
- Monitor pain using an age-appropriate pain tool.

- Administer analgesia using a patient-controlled analgesic (PCA) pump as prescribed.
- Perform frequent neurovascular checks.
- Turn the adolescent/child frequently by log rolling to prevent damage to the spinal fusion.
- Assess skin for pressure areas, especially if a brace has been prescribed. Qs
- Provide skin care by keeping skin clean and dry.
- Monitor surgical and drain sites for indications of infection. Provide wound care as prescribed.
- Assess bowel sounds and monitor, observing for paralytic ileus.
- Monitor for decreases in Hgb and Hct. Observe for indications of bleeding.
- Administer blood transfusion as prescribed. The adolescent/child can have self-donated blood available for transfusion.
- Encourage mobility as soon as tolerated. Ambulation by 2nd or 3rd day.
- Assess for infection.
- Perform range of motion on unaffected extremities.
- Provide age-appropriate activities and opportunities to visit with peers and family during the hospital stay. Qpcc

CLIENT EDUCATION

PREOPERATIVE
- Reinforce teaching (use of incentive spirometer, turning, coughing, deep breathing) to prevent complications.
- Perform extensive preoperative teaching to educate the adolescent/child and family and to promote cooperation and participation in recovery.
- Demonstrate the use of a PCA pump if prescribed and age appropriate.
- Demonstrate log rolling that will be used after surgery.
- Demonstrate the respiratory therapy techniques that will be used postoperatively to reduce complications of anesthesia.
- Discuss medical terms that are unfamiliar to the adolescent/child and/or family.

POSTOPERATIVE
- Emphasize the importance of physical therapy and proper positioning of the spine.
- Encourage independence following surgery for the adolescent/child who has a brace.
- Encourage the adolescent/child to contact peers when able.
- Emphasize the necessity of follow-up care.

CARE AFTER DISCHARGE
- Reinforce the expected course of treatment and recovery.
- Suggest that the family arrange the environment to facilitate the adolescent's/child's ability to be as independent as possible (keep favorite items within reach).
- Emphasize the necessity of follow-up care.

COMPLICATIONS

Breathing difficulties (with severe curvatures)

Lowered self-esteem: Assist the adolescent/child with age-appropriate actions to promote positive self-esteem.

POSTOPERATIVE COMPLICATIONS
- Spinal cord or neurologic injury
- Pneumothorax (decreased mobility)
- Hypotension (blood loss)
- Atelectasis (decreased mobility)
- Ileus (decreased mobility)
- Infection (wound)

Superior mesenteric artery syndrome: Compression of the duodenum by the aorta and superior mesenteric artery that leads to an obstruction

NURSING ACTIONS
- Monitor and report findings of condition: nausea, severe vomiting, epigastric pain, belching.
- Position the adolescent/child left lateral or prone to provide comfort. Supine position is often uncomfortable.

CLIENT EDUCATION: Reinforce with the adolescent/child and family positioning to promote comfort.

Active Learning Scenario

A nurse is caring for a child in a hip spica cast. What should the nurse include in the care of this client? Use the ATI Active Learning Template: Therapeutic Procedure to complete this item.

NURSING INTERVENTIONS: List at least five actions the nurse should include in the child's care.

CLIENT EDUCATION: List at least six teaching points the nurse should include for the client and the client's parents.

Application Exercises

1. A nurse is assessing a child who has Legg-Calve-Perthes disease. Which of the following findings should the nurse expect? (Select all that apply.)
   - A. Longer affected leg
   - B. Hip stiffness
   - C. Back pain
   - D. Limited ROM
   - E. Limp with walking

2. A nurse is caring for a child who is suspected of having Legg-Calve-Perthes disease. The nurse should prepare the child for which of the following diagnostic procedures?
   - A. Bone biopsy
   - B. Genetic testing
   - C. CT scan
   - D. Radiographs

3. A nurse is caring for an infant and notices an audible click in their left hip. Which of the following diagnostic test should the nurse expect the provider to perform? (Select all that apply.)
   - A. Barlow test
   - B. Manipulation of foot and ankle
   - C. Babinski sign
   - D. Ortolani test
   - E. Ponseti method

4. A nurse is caring for a toddler who has been placed in hip spica cast. The toddler's parent asks the nurse why a Pavlik harness is not being used. Which of the following responses should the nurse make?
   - A. "The Pavlik harness is used for children with scoliosis, not hip dysplasia."
   - B. "The Pavlik harness is used for school-age children."
   - C. "The Pavlik harness cannot be used for your child because her condition is too severe."
   - D. "The Pavlik harness is used for infants less than 6 months of age."

5. A nurse providing perioperative teaching with an adolescent client and their parents who is scheduled for spinal instrumentation for scoliosis. Which of the following statements by the adolescent indicates understanding?
   - A. "I will go home the same day of surgery."
   - B. "I will have minimal pain."
   - C. "I may need a blood transfusion."
   - D. "I will not be able to eat until the day after surgery."

1. B, D, E. **CORRECT:** Legg-Calve-Perthes disease is a condition that is characterized by impaired circulation to the femoral head that results in aseptic necrosis. The nurse should expect the following findings: intermittent painless limp, hip stiffness, limited ROM, hip/thigh/knee pain, and shortening of the affected leg.
   A. A child who has Legg-Calve-Perthes exhibit shortening of the affected leg.
   C. A child who has Legg-Calve-Perthes exhibits a painless intermittent limp.

   Ⓝ NCLEX® Connection: Physiological Adaptation, Pathophysiology

2. A. A bone biopsy is used to diagnose conditions such a malignancies and infections.
   B. Legg-Calve-Perthes-disease is not a genetic disorder; therefore, genetic testing is not indicated.
   C. **CORRECT:** Legg-Calve-Perthes disease is a condition that is characterized by impaired circulation to the femoral head that results in aseptic necrosis. The nurse should anticipate a provider prescription for radiograph of hip and pelvis to determine diagnosis of this condition.
   D. An echocardiogram is used to diagnose cardiovascular conditions therefore this is not indicated for Legg-Calve-Perthes- disease, which is a musculoskeletal disorder.

   Ⓝ NCLEX® Connection: Reduction of Risk Potential, Therapeutic Procedures

3. A, D. **CORRECT:** The nurse should identify that an audible clicking sound in the left hip could be indicative of a developmental dysplasia hip disorder. Therefore, the nurse anticipate that the provider would check for this condition by performing the Barlow and Ortolani screening test by flexing the infant's hips and knees in a right-angle position.
   B. Manipulation of the foot and ankle is use check for clubfoot.
   C. Babinski reflex is used to check for neurological deficits by stroking the infant's lateral foot.
   E. Ponseti method is used to treat clubfoot.

   Ⓝ NCLEX® Connection: Reduction of Risk Potential, Illness Management

4. D. **CORRECT:** A Pavlik harness is used to manage developmental dysplasia of hip disorders. It is applied to an infant who is less than 6 months of age. After six months of age, the Pavlik harness is not indicated, and surgical correction is recommended in addition to spica casting. A Pavlik harness is too small for a toddler.

   Ⓝ NCLEX® Connection: Reduction of Risk Potential, Therapeutic Procedures

5. A. Spinal instrumentation surgery requires admission to pediatric intensive care unit (ICU), following surgery.
   B. The adolescent can experience mild to moderate pain following surgery. Therefore, their pain will be monitored frequently and managed by a self-controlled analgesic pump if prescribed.
   C. **CORRECT:** There is a chance for blood lost following surgery. Therefore, the adolescent will be given the opportunity for autologous donation prior to surgery. In the event of severe blood lost, the adolescent, may require a blood transfusion.
   D. The adolescent can eat following surgery as prescribed. The provider may start on clear liquid and advance as tolerated diet.

   Ⓝ NCLEX® Connection: Reduction of Risk Potential, Therapeutic Procedures

Active Learning Scenario Key

Using the ATI Active Learning Template: Therapeutic Procedure

NURSING INTERVENTIONS

- Assess and maintain the hip spica cast.
- Perform frequent neurovascular checks.
- Perform range of motion with the unaffected extremities.
- Perform frequent assessment of skin integrity, especially in the diaper area.
- Assess for pain control using an age-appropriate pain tool. Intervene as indicated.
- Evaluate hydration status frequently.
- Assess elimination status daily.

CLIENT EDUCATION

- Reinforce teaching regarding positioning, turning, neurovascular assessments, and care of the cast.
- Note color and temperature of toes on casted extremity.
- Give sponge baths to avoid wetting the cast.
- Use a waterproof barrier around the genital opening of spica cast to prevent soiling with urine or feces.
- Educate regarding care after discharge with emphasis on using appropriate equipment (stroller, wagon, car seat) for maintaining mobility.

Ⓝ NCLEX® Connection: Reduction of Risk Potential, Therapeutic Procedures

UNIT 2   SYSTEM DISORDERS
SECTION: MUSCULOSKELETAL DISORDERS

CHAPTER 29

Chronic Neuromusculoskeletal Disorders

Chronic problems associated with mobility can be reflective of a problem with the musculoskeletal system or the result of a disorder related to the neural pathway extending from the brain's cortex to the neuromuscular junction.

Cerebral palsy

- Cerebral palsy (CP) is a nonprogressive impairment of motor function, especially that of muscle control, coordination, and posture.
- CP can cause abnormal perception and sensation; visual, hearing, and speech impairments; seizures; and cognitive disabilities.
- CP manifests differently in each child. Developmental outcomes vary and are dependent on the severity of the injury.
- CP is classified as congenital (present at birth) or acquired (obtained after birth).
- CP is clinically classified as
  - Spastic (pyramidal): accounts for up to 80% of CP cases
  - Dyskinetic (non-specific, extrapyramidal): accounts for up to 15% of CP cases
  - Ataxic (non-spastic, extrapyramidal)

ASSESSMENT

RISK FACTORS

The exact cause of CP is not known. Prenatal, perinatal, and postnatal risk factors known to be associated with CP include the following.

Prenatal
- Malnutrition or drug use
- Genetic, chromosome abnormalities
- Infections
- Placenta insufficiency
- Bleeding
- Rh incompatibility

Perinatal
- Maternal chorioamnionitis
- Maternal infection, sepsis, seizures, preeclampsia
- Low birth weight

- PROM, long labor, premature birth
- Meconium aspiration
- Asphyxia

Postnatal
- Existing brain anomalies, anoxia to the brain
- Multiple births
- Stroke
- Brain injury
- Cerebral infections
- Head trauma (shaken baby syndrome)

EXPECTED FINDINGS

- Motor
  - Gagging or choking with feeding
  - Poor sucking
  - Consistent tongue thrusting
  - Asymmetric crawl
  - Early hand preference
  - Toe walking
- Reflex
  - Persistent primitive reflexes (Moro or tonic neck)
  - Hyperreflexia
- Posturing
  - Rigid posture and extremities,
  - Scissoring and extension of legs
- Muscle tone
  - Arching back
  - Difficulty diapering child
  - Stiff posture
- Associated problems and conditions
  - Vision, speech, or hearing impairments
  - Seizures
  - Cognitive/intellect impairment
  - Impaired social relationships
  - Parents report difficulty meeting developmental milestones

Spastic CP (pyramidal)
- Hypertonicity (muscle tightness or spasticity); increased deep tendon reflexes; clonus; and poor control of motion, balance, and posture
- Impairments of fine and gross motor skills
- Can present in all four extremities (tetraplegia); all extremities affected, lower more than upper (diplegia); three limbs (triplegia); one limb (monoplegia); or one side of the body (hemiplegia);
- Gait can appear crouched with a scissoring motion of the legs with feet plantar flexed.
- Babinski reflex

Dyskinetic CP (non-spastic, extrapyramidal)
- Athetoid: Findings include involuntary jerking movements that appear slow, writhing, and wormlike. These movements involve the extremities, trunk, neck, face, and tongue.
- Dystonic: Slow, twisting movements affect the trunk or extremities with abnormal posturing from muscle contractions. Drooling and speech impairment related to involvement of the muscles of pharynx, larynx, and oral regions.

Ataxic CP (non-spastic, extrapyramidal)
- Evidence of wide-based gait, lack of coordination with purposeful movements, such as reaching for an object
- Poor ability to do repetitive movements

DIAGNOSTIC PROCEDURES

Complete neurologic assessment

Metabolic and genetic testing

General movements assessment in children older than 2 years and younger than 5 years of age

MRI: Used to evaluate structures or abnormal areas

NURSING ACTIONS
- Assist the child to remain still during the procedure.
- Sedate the child if prescribed.

CLIENT EDUCATION: Provide emotional support.

EEG

Skull x-ray

Ultrasound

PATIENT-CENTERED CARE

NURSING CARE

- Individualize care to meet the needs of the child and family. Evaluate the need for hearing and speech evaluations.
- Promote independence with self-care activities as much as possible. Assist the client to maintain a positive self-image and a high level of self-esteem.
- Determine the extent of family coping and support.
- Assess the family's awareness of available resources.
- Assess the client's developmental level and monitor developmental milestones.
- Structure interventions and communications around the child's developmental level, rather than chronological age.
- Communicate with the child directly but include parents as needed. Qpcc
- Help the child to use augmented communication (electronic devices for speech and other types of communication tools [flash cards, picture boards, touch screen computers]).
- Include the family in physical care during hospitalization.
  - Ask the family about routine care and encourage them to provide it if appropriate.
  - Encourage the family to help verify the child's needs if communication is impaired.
- Maintain an open airway by elevating the head of the child's bed. (This is especially important if the child has increased oral secretions.) Qs
- Ensure suction equipment is available if required. Suction oral secretions as needed.
- Monitor for pain (especially with muscle spasms) using a developmentally appropriate pain tool.

- Administer medication for pain and/or spasms as prescribed.
- Ensure adequate nutrition.
  - Obtain and monitor daily weights.
  - Assess for the possibility of aspiration for children who are severely disabled.
  - Position upright after feeding.
  - Determine the child's ability to take oral nutrition.
  - Ascertain the correct positioning for feeding the child. Use head positioning and manual jaw control methods as needed.
  - Provide foods that are like foods eaten at home when possible. Administer nutritional supplements as prescribed.
  - Encourage foods high in fiber to prevent constipation.
  - Administer enteral feedings as prescribed if child has gastrostomy tube.
  - Maintain weight/height chart.
- Provide skin care.
  - Assess skin under splints and braces if applicable.
  - Maintain skin integrity by turning the child to keep pressure off bony prominences.
  - Keep skin clean and dry.
- Provide rest periods as needed.

THERAPEUTIC MANAGEMENT

MEDICATIONS

Baclofen

Prescribed intrathecal and administered via a surgically implanted pump for a child who has CP. Used as a centrally acting skeletal muscle relaxant that decreases muscle spasm and severe spasticity.

NURSING ACTIONS
- Monitor effectiveness of the medication.
- Monitor for adverse effects: nausea, vomiting, confusion, pruritis, drowsiness, dizziness, headaches, muscle weakness.

CLIENT EDUCATION
- Observe for expected responses of medications.
- Reinforce with the family the adverse effects of medications and when to call the provider.
- Instruct on how to use pump, site care and replacement of the pump medication every 4 to 6 weeks.

Diazepam

Skeletal muscle relaxant used to decrease muscle spasms and severe spasticity

NURSING ACTIONS
- Use in older children and adolescents.
- Monitor for drowsiness and fatigue.
- Monitor for hepatotoxicity.

CLIENT EDUCATION
- Observe for expected responses to medications.
- Monitor for adverse effects of the medication and call the provider.

Botulinum toxin A

- Administered IM
- Reduces spasticity in specific muscle groups (quadriceps)
- Used primarily for clients who have spasticity only in the lower extremities
- Decreases muscle movement by inhibiting the release of acetylcholine

NURSING ACTIONS: Monitor for temporary weakness and pain at the injection site.

CLIENT EDUCATION: Onset of the medication is 24 to 72 hr, with a peak of 2 weeks, lasting 3 to 6 months.

Antiepileptics

- Examples: Valproic acid, carbamazepine
- Inhibits seizure activity

Complementary and alternative therapies

- Herbal remedies Acupuncture
- Hyperbaric oxygen
- Aquatic exercise, assisted equine therapy, pet therapy
- Guided imagery, massage, music-color, and light therapy
- Mediation, hypnosis, prayer

INTERPROFESSIONAL CARE

Interprofessional team for a child who has CP can consist of the following members depending on the severity of the child's condition and the needs of the family: neurologist, pulmonologist, speech language pathologist, dietician, physical therapist, occupational therapist, orthopedics, pharmacist, social worker, genetic counselor, case manager, and/or psychiatrist.

- Coordinate care with interprofessional team).
- Initiate referral for technical aids that can assist with coordination, speaking, mobility, and an increased level of independence. Some children can benefit from the use of a voice-activated wheelchair.

Physical therapy (PT)

- Assist with providing ROM to strength muscles, promote endurance, prevent contractures/deformities, use of orthotic devices and adaptive equipment
- Orthotic devices: Braces, splints
- Adaptive equipment: Scooters, wheelchairs

Occupational therapy (OT)

- Provides training on how to perform ADPS independently and how to use adaptive equipment
- Feeding utensils, aids for ADLs

Speech therapy

- Special intervention programs
- Increase socialization

Surgical intervention

Orthopedic
- Correct contracture or other spastic deformities
- Tendon release

Neurological
- Dorsal rhizotomy

Gastrointestinal
- Gastrostomy: impaired swallowing, correct reflux, provide nutritional supplementation

CLIENT EDUCATION

- Adhere to therapeutic plan of care.
- Provide time for rest periods.
- Adhere to nutritional guidelines and feeding schedule, utilize feeding techniques if changes were made during hospitalization.
- Adhere to medication regimen.
- Ensure regular dental hygiene and examinations by provider.
- Provide developmental stimulation.
- Participate in developmentally appropriate recreational activities.
- Understand proper wound care if needed.
- Understand ankle-foot orthoses if prescribed.
- Utilize pulmonary hygiene techniques.
- Obtain recommended immunizations.
- Coordinate interprofessional team with cares.
- Identify resources needed (respite care).
- Consider participation in a support group for CP.

COMPLICATIONS

Aspiration

NURSING ACTIONS
- Keep the child's head elevated.
- Keep suction available if copious oral secretions are present or the child has difficulty with swallowing foods or fluids. Qs

CLIENT EDUCATION
- Perform appropriate feeding techniques to decrease the risk of aspiration.
- Take CPR classes.

Potential for injury

NURSING ACTIONS
- Make sure the child's bed rails are raised to prevent falls from the bed.
- Pad side rails and wheelchair arms to prevent injury.
- Secure the child in mobility devices (wheelchairs).
- Encourage the child to receive adequate rest to prevent injury at times of fatigue.
- Encourage the use of helmets, seat belts, and other safety equipment.

CLIENT EDUCATION: Perform appropriate safety precautions.

Spina bifida

Spinal bifida is a neural tube defect (NTD) present at birth and is characterized by failure of the osseous spine to close with CNS effects.

Spina bifida occulta: Mostly affects the lumbosacral area and is not visible externally. Surface of the vertebral bone is missing; no spinal cord involvement.

Spina bifida cystica: Protrusion of the sac is visible
- Meningocele: The sac contains spinal fluid and meninges. Increased risk for infection if ruptures. No neurologic deficits.
- Myelomeningocele (most common): The sac contains spinal fluid, meninges, and nerves. Failure of the neural tube to close causes decreased motor and sensory function.

ASSESSMENT

RISK FACTORS

- Medications/substances taken during pregnancy
- Maternal malnutrition
- Insufficient folic acid intake during pregnancy
- Exposure to radiation or chemicals during pregnancy
- Genetic predisposition

EXPECTED FINDINGS

SUBJECTIVE FINDINGS
- Presence of risk factors in prenatal history
- Family history of neural tube defects

PHYSICAL ASSESSMENT FINDINGS
Occulta
- Dimpling in the lumbosacral area (occulta)
- Port wine angioma nevi (flat area of pigmentation)
- Dark hair tufts
- Subcutaneous lipoma

Cystica (findings vary depending on the location of sac)
- Flaccid muscles flaccid paralysis, absent deep tendon reflex
- Lack of bowel control
- Constant dribbling of urine or urine overflow
- Foot contractures
- Spinal curvature abnormalities (scoliosis, kyphosis)
- Protruding sac midline of the osseous spine

LABORATORY TESTS

MATERNAL BLOOD TESTS: Blood alpha-fetoprotein during the second trimester of gestation indicate possible NTD.

INFANT BLOOD TESTS: Blood cultures to determine causative pathogen if appropriate.

DIAGNOSTIC PROCEDURES

PRENATAL
- **Ultrasound** can show visual defect.
- **Amniocentesis** is done following elevated alpha-fetoprotein levels to detect anencephaly or myelomeningocele.
- **Chorionic villus sampling.**

INFANT FOLLOWING BIRTH: MRI, ultrasonography, and CT to evaluate spinal cord and brain, myelography, spinal x-ray (Occulta).

PATIENT-CENTERED CARE

NURSING CARE

- Assess for infant-parent attachment.
- Assess the sac (cystica).
- Perform a routine newborn assessment.
- Assess the level of neurologic involvement.
- Obtain accurate output measurements.
- Assess head circumference and fontanels.
- Initiate measures to prevent infection.
- Perform neurologic assessments.
- Educate the parents about intermittent bladder catheterizations if needed.

INTERPROFESSIONAL CARE

Neurosurgeon, neurologist, urologist, orthopedics, pediatrician, physical therapy, occupational therapy, speech language pathologist, and social worker

THERAPEUTIC PROCEDURES

Closure of a myelomeningocele sac is done as soon as possible to prevent complications of injury and infection. Risk for the development of hydrocephalus.

PREOPERATIVE NURSING ACTIONS
- Prepare the infant/parents for surgery (within the first 24 to 72 hr after birth).
- Protect the sac from injury.
- Place infant in an incubator or radiant warmer if needed, without clothing.

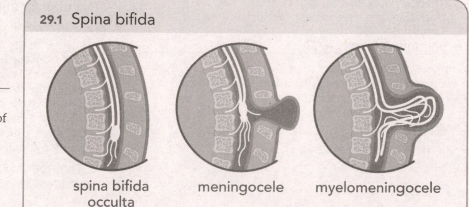

29.1 Spina bifida

spina bifida occulta   meningocele   myelomeningocele

- Apply a sterile, moist, non–adhering dressing with sterile 0.9% sodium chloride on the sac, changing it every 2 hr. Q EBP
- Do not remove dressing if becomes dry; add more sterile solution (sodium chloride).
- Inspect the sac closely for leaks, irritation, abrasions, and localized indications of infection.
- Assess for systemic indications of infection (fever, irritability, and lethargy).
- Place infant in the prone position.
- Administer IV antibiotic as prescribed.
- Avoid rectal temperatures.
- Avoid putting pressure on the sac.
- Measure head circumference to establish a baseline measurement.
- Report leakage of fluid.

PREOPERATIVE CLIENT EDUCATION: There will be decreased motor and sensory functions of lower extremities.

POSTOPERATIVE NURSING ACTIONS
- Monitor vital signs.
- Monitor I&O and weight.
- Assess for indications of infection.
- Check for pain using age-appropriate pain tool and provide management for pain as needed Provide incision care. Keep clean. Do not allow urine or feces to contaminate incision.
- Assess for manifestations of increased intracranial pressure.
- Use paper tape.
- Assess for CSF leakage.
- Maintain prone position until other positions are prescribed.
- Resume oral feedings.
- Provide range of motion (ROM) to extremities.

CLIENT EDUCATION

- Understand proper postoperative care at home.
- Understand ROM techniques depending on disability.

ONGOING CARE
- Assess and measure head circumference.
- Assess skin integrity.
- Assess for allergies (latex allergy).
- Assess cognitive development.
- Assess bladder and bowl functioning.
- Educate the parents about intermittent bladder catheterizations if needed.
- Assess motor development.
- Monitor for infections.
- Address body image concerns.
- Offer support to the family.
- Assist the child with independence through the lifespan.
- Assist the family with obtaining medical equipment/ services needed at home.

COMPLICATIONS

Skin ulceration

Caused by prolonged pressure in one area

NURSING ACTIONS
- Monitor skin for breakdown.
- Reposition frequently to prevent pressure on bony prominences.

CLIENT EDUCATION: Monitor skin integrity.

Latex allergy

The child is at an increased risk for a latex allergy. Allergy responses range from urticaria to wheezing, which can progress to anaphylaxis. A latex allergy is linked to allergies to certain foods (bananas, avocados, kiwi, and chestnuts).

NURSING ACTIONS
- Assist with testing for allergy.
- Reduce exposure.

CLIENT EDUCATION
- Avoid exposing the child to latex.
- Be aware of household items that can contain latex (water toys, pacifiers, plastic storage bags).
- Observe for indications of allergic reaction and report them to the provider.
- Understand proper use of epinephrine. Q S
- Wear allergy alert necklace or bracelet to identify latex allergy.

Increased intracranial pressure

- Caused by shunt malfunction or hydrocephalus.
- Prepare for surgery for shunt or shunt revision.

MANIFESTATIONS
- Infants: high-pitched cry, lethargy, vomiting, bulging fontanels, and/or widening cranial suture lines, increased head circumference
- CHILDREN: headache, lethargy, nausea, vomiting, double vision, decreased school performance of learned tasks, decreased level of consciousness, seizures

NURSING ACTIONS
- Use gentle movements when performing ROM exercises.
- Minimize environmental stressors (noise, frequent visitors).
- Assess and manage pain.

CLIENT EDUCATION: Observe for manifestations of shunt malfunction and hydrocephalus and notify the provider if necessary.

Bladder issues

The child who has myelomeningocele is at an increased risk for neurogenic bladder dysfunction (spasms, flaccidity).

NURSING ACTIONS
- Monitor for indications of bladder dysfunction.
- Monitor for indications of bladder infection.
- Monitor for blood in the urine.
- Administer antispasmodics or perform intermittent catheterizations as needed.
- Prepare the child and parents for surgery if needed.

CLIENT EDUCATION: Perform proper care of stoma (vesicostomy) if applicable.

Orthopedic issues

Corrections of associated potential problems (clubfoot, scoliosis, and other malformations of the feet and legs)

NURSING ACTIONS
- Monitor for indications of infection.
- Administer pain medications.
- Prepare the child and parents for surgery if needed.
- Provide cast care if cast is present.
- Monitor for neurologic deficits.
- Perform passive ROM exercises, position, and stretching exercises.

CLIENT EDUCATION
- Educate the family about indications of infection.
- Educate the family about cast and splint care if indicated.

Bowel control measures

- Increased risk for constipation
- Administer laxatives and fiber supplements as prescribed.
- Administer antegrade continence enemas (ACE) every 1 to 2 days as needed for older children. Instill solution directly into colon to empty out the bowels to obtain bowel continence.

Juvenile idiopathic arthritis

- Juvenile idiopathic arthritis (JIA) is a chronic autoimmune inflammatory disease affecting joints and other tissues.
- The chronic inflammation of the synovium of the joints leads to wearing down and damage to the articular cartilage.
- JIA is rarely life-threatening, and it can subside over time, but it can result in residual joint deformities and altered joint function.
- Classifications of JIA include systemic, oligoarthritis, psoriatic, enthesitis, polyarthritis (with and without rheumatoid factor), and undifferentiated.

ASSESSMENT

RISK FACTORS

- Immunogenic susceptibility
- Environmental triggers
- Genetic predisposition
- Female gender

EXPECTED FINDINGS

PHYSICAL ASSESSMENT FINDINGS
- Joint swelling, stiffness (tend to be worse in morning or after inactivity)
- Mobility limitations
- Fever
- Rash
- Gait with a limp
- Delayed growth

LABORATORY TESTS

- Elevated C-reactive protein can be present.
- Erythrocyte sedimentation rate (ESR) can be elevated.
- CBC with differential can show elevated WBCs, especially during exacerbations.
- Antinuclear antibodies (ANA) indicate an increased risk for uveitis.
- Rheumatoid factor is rarely detected in children.

DIAGNOSTIC PROCEDURES

- Radiographic studies can be used for baseline comparison. X-rays can demonstrate increased synovial fluid in the joint, which causes soft tissue swelling or widening of the joint. Later findings can include narrowed joint spaces.
- Slit lamp eye examination is used to diagnosis uveitis. It can be performed every 6 months for adolescents with pauciarticular arthritis.
- Arthrocentesis: analysis of synovial fluid

PATIENT-CENTERED CARE

NURSING CARE

- Care is primarily in an outpatient setting.
- Goal is to control pain, minimize damage from inflammation, preserve joint functioning and promote normal growth and development.
- Assist the child with an exercise program.
- Evaluate the child's pain and response to prescribed analgesics.
- Encourage a support group.
- Encourage the child to participate in a physical therapy program to increase mobility and prevent deformities.
- Encourage daily physical activity as tolerated.
- Encourage full ROM exercises.
- Apply heat or warm moist packs to the affected joints to promote comfort.
- Promote appropriate exercises (swimming).
- Encourage warm baths (paraffin [hands] or whirlpools).
- Identify alternate ways for the child to meet developmental needs, especially during periods of exacerbation.
- Encourage self-care by allowing adequate time for completion. Qpcc
- Encourage a well-balanced diet with adequate fluid intake.
- Encourage participation in school and contact with peers.
- Collaborate with the school nurse and teachers to arrange for care during the school day (medication administration, in-school physical therapy, extra sets of books, split days).

CLIENT EDUCATION

- Practice relaxation techniques and nonpharmacological pain management.
- Exacerbation worsens with illnesses.
- Schedule routine follow up with provider and regular eye exams.

THERAPEUTIC MANAGEMENT

MEDICATIONS

Nonsteroidal anti-inflammatory medications

Ibuprofen, naproxen, diclofenac, indomethacin, and tolmetin control pain and inflammation

CLIENT EDUCATION

- NSAIDs should be taken with food to minimize gastric irritation.
- Report changes in stool and GI discomfort or increase in bruising immediately.
- Take as directed. Often prescribed 4 times a day for 6 to 8 weeks (even if feeling better).

Disease-Modifying Antirheumatic Drugs (DMARDs)

Methotrexate slows joint degeneration and progression of rheumatoid arthritis when NSAIDs do not work alone. Administered weekly in a low dose.

NURSING ACTIONS

Monitor liver function tests and CBC regularly. Medication can cause bone marrow suppression, liver toxicity and is teratogenic and carcinogenic.

CLIENT EDUCATION

- Avoid alcohol.
- Utilize effective birth control to avoid birth defects while taking this medication.
- Take at bedtime to prevent nausea.

Glucocorticoids

Prednisone provides relief of inflammation and pain. They are reserved for life-threatening complications, severe arthritis, pericarditis, and uveitis.

NURSING ACTIONS

- Administer topical (ocular), orally, or IV (severe). An injection directly into the intra-articular space of the affected joint can provide effective pain relief.
- Administer at the lowest effective dose for short-term therapy and then discontinue by tapering the dose.

CLIENT EDUCATION

- Weight gain, especially in the face, is a common adverse effect.
- Monitor height and weight.
- An alteration in growth is a possible long-term complication of corticosteroids.
- Avoid exposure to potentially infectious agents.
- Practice healthy eating habits.

Biologic DMARDs

Etanercept is a tumor necrosis factor alpha-receptor inhibitor, that is used when methotrexate is not effective for immunosuppressive action by decreasing the inflammatory response.

NURSING ACTIONS

- Infliximab can be given IV in outpatient setting.
- Administer a tuberculin skin test prior to starting etanercept and yearly while taking the medication.
- Administer etanercept once or twice each week by subcutaneous injection.
- Monitor for lymphomas.

CLIENT EDUCATION

- Observe for allergic reactions.
- Report findings of infection.
- Avoid exposure to infectious agents.

THERAPEUTIC PROCEDURES

- Often delayed until child's growth is complete
- Synovectomy after all other interventions fail
- Joint replacement in older children

INTERPROFESSIONAL CARE

Physical therapist, occupational therapist, ophthalmologist, dentist, rheumatologist, dietitian, social worker, school nurse, counselors, and psychologists.
- Physical Therapy:
  - Assist with preventing deformities and improving muscle strength
  - Provide guidance on positioning, stretching, splinting, exercise, ROM

COMPLICATIONS

Joint deformity and functional disability

Risk for contractures, changes in growth plate, leg length changes

NURSING ACTIONS
- Reinforce the individualized therapeutic plan of care.
- Advocate for the child when treatments are not producing expected results.
- Encourage the child and family to adhere to the treatment regimen.
- Encourage self-care and active participation in an exercise program.

Systemic

Risk for pericarditis, endocarditis, myocarditis, anemia

NURSING ACTIONS
- Monitor for labs.
- Monitor EKG.

Psychosocial

Risk for mood disorders such as depression or anxiety

NURSING ACTIONS
- Monitor for changes in mood.
- Refer to psychologist as need.
- Inform parents to report changes in mood.

Muscular dystrophy

Muscular dystrophy (MD) is a group of inherited disorders with progressive degeneration of symmetric skeletal muscle groups causing progressive muscle weakness and wasting, which can lead to disability and deformity. Onset of disease, pace of progression, and muscle group affected depend on the type of MD.
- **Duchenne (pseudohypertrophic) muscular dystrophy** (DMD) is the most common form of MD. Inherited as an X-linked recessive trait, DMD has an onset between 3 and 5 years of age. age. Rapid progression with life expectancy of 15-30 years. Fat tissue replace muscles in lower limbs (gastrocnemius).
- **Facioscapulohumeral muscular dystrophy** is an autosomal dominant inherited disorder with the age of onset occurring during early adolescence. Progression is slow with normal life span. Characterized by facial weakness and inversion of the shoulders.
- **Limb-girdle muscular dystrophy** is an autosomal dominant and recessive, heterogeneous disorder. It appears later in childhood with a slow progression.

ASSESSMENT

RISK FACTORS

Family genetic history

EXPECTED FINDINGS (DUCHENNE)

PHYSICAL ASSESSMENT FINDINGS
- Fatigue
- Muscle weakness beginning in the lower extremities
- Unsteady gait, with a waddle
- Lordosis
- Delayed motor skill development
- Frequent falling
- Gowers' sign: Difficulty getting out of bed, rising from a seated position, or climbing stairs

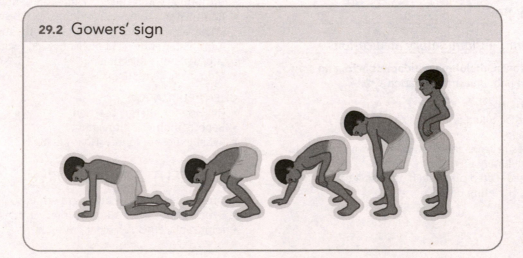

29.2 Gowers' sign

- Gowers' sign: Child walks hands up legs for support while going to a standing position
- Learning difficulties
- Mild cognitive delays that do not worsen with disease progression
- Progressive difficulty walking with possible loss of ability to walk
  - Often occurs by the age of 12 years (DMD)
- Progressive muscle atrophy of face, chest, and neck
- Respiratory and cardiac difficulties as the disease progresses

LABORATORY TESTS

- Blood polymerase chain reaction (PCR) to detect the dystrophin gene mutation
- Blood creatine kinase (CK): elevated and can be elevated prior to manifestations
- Genetic analysis

DIAGNOSTIC PROCEDURES

- Muscle biopsy
- EMG

PATIENT-CENTERED CARE

NURSING CARE

- Encourage and provide for genetic counseling.
- Assess and monitor the following.
  - Ability to perform ADLs
  - Respiratory function, including depth, rhythm, and rate of respirations during sleep and daytime hours
  - Cardiac function
  - The child and parents understanding of long-term effects
  - The child and parents' coping and support system
- Maintain optimal physical function for as long possible.
  - Encourage the child to be independent for as long as possible and to perform ADLs.
  - Perform ROM exercises and provide appropriate physical activity. Include stretching exercises, strength and muscle training, and breathing exercises. ○EBP
  - Maintain proper body alignment and encourage the child to reposition self frequently to avoid skin breakdown.
  - Assist with orthoses and braces as prescribed.
- Maintain respiratory functioning.
  - Monitor oxygen saturation levels.
  - Encourage the use of incentive spirometry.
  - Position the child to enhance expansion of lungs.
  - Provide supplemental oxygen as prescribed.
  - Provide noninvasive ventilation as prescribed.
  - Encourage the use of airway clearance devices (mechanical cough in-exsufflator [MIE]).

- Encourage adequate fluid intake.
- Monitor and encourage adequate nutritional intake.
  - Low calorie, high protein and fiber.
  - Administer stool softeners as prescribed
- Encourage routine physical exams and immunizations.
- Facilitate discussion of end-of-life decisions when appropriate.

CLIENT EDUCATION
- Understand proper use of a mechanical cough device.
- Encourage parents to consider assistance with care as disease progresses (respite care, long-term care, palliative care, and home-health care).
- Recommend a referral for the child and parents to support groups for MD.

THERAPEUTIC MANAGEMENT

MEDICATIONS

Corticosteroids

Prednisone increases muscle strength

NURSING ACTIONS
- Monitor for infection.
- Monitor for adverse effects.
- Teach child/parents to avoid infectious agents, take as prescribed, and monitor for adverse effects and report these findings to provider.

INTERPROFESSIONAL CARE

Neurologist; genetic counselor; physical therapist, occupational therapist, respiratory therapists, dietitian, case manager, social worker, nurses, school teacher, psychiatrist

THERAPEUTIC PROCEDURES

- Surgery can be indicated for release or repair of contractures
- Gastrostomy tube (maintain nutrition, swallowing impairment)
- Tracheostomy (maintain airway patency)

COMPLICATIONS

- Obesity
- Contractures
- Scoliosis
- Infections

RESPIRATORY COMPROMISE

Progressive weakening of respiratory muscles decreases the child's ability to maintain adequate respirations. There is a risk for the development of pneumonia.

NURSING ACTIONS

- Help the child turn hourly or more frequently.
- Have the child use deep breathing and coughing.
- Suction as needed.
- Administer oxygen as prescribed.
- Use intermittent positive pressure ventilation and mechanically- assisted cough devices if indicated.
- Administer antibiotics as prescribed.

CLIENT EDUCATION: Discuss mechanical ventilation options with the child and parents.

Active Learning Scenario

A nurse is caring for a child who has a new prescription for baclofen. Use the ATI Active Learning Template: Medication to complete this item.

THERAPEUTIC USES

MEDICATION ADMINISTRATION

COMPLICATIONS: List adverse effects of baclofen.

CLIENT EDUCATION: Include two teaching points.

Active Learning Scenario Key

Using the ATI Active Learning Template: Medication

THERAPEUTIC USES: Used as a centrally acting skeletal muscle relaxant that decreases muscle spasm and severe spasticity. Indicated for the treatment of cerebral palsy.

NURSING ADMINISTRATION

- Prescribed intrathecal and administered via a specialized, surgically implanted pump.
- Monitor effectiveness of the medication.

COMPLICATIONS

- Muscle weakness
- Drowsiness
- Nausea, vomiting
- Confusion
- Dizziness
- Headaches
- Pruritis

CLIENT EDUCATION

- Reinforce teaching with the child/parents about expected responses of medications.
- Reinforce adverse effects of medications with the child/parent and inform when to call the provider.
- Instruct on how to use pump, site care, and replacement of the pump medication every 4 to 6 weeks.

(N) *NCLEX® Connection: Pharmacological and Parenteral Therapies, Medication Administration*

Application Exercises

1. A nurse planning care for a toddler who has cerebral palsy. Which of the following interventions should the nurse include?

   A. Structure interventions according to the toddler's chronological age.

   B. Determine the toddler's need for an evaluation of hearing ability.

   C. Monitor the toddler's pain level routinely using a numeric rating scale.

   D. Provide total care for ADLs.

2. A nurse admitting a child who has cerebral palsy and is experiencing muscle spasms. Which of the following medications should the nurse expect the provider to prescribe? (Select all that apply.)

   A. Baclofen

   B. Diazepam

   C. Oxybutynin

   D. Methotrexate

   E. Prednisone

3. A nurse is caring of an infant who has a myelomeningocele. Which of the following actions should the nurse take?

   A. Encourage the guardian to cuddle the infant.

   B. Monitor the infant's temperature rectally.

   C. Maintain the infant in a supine position.

   D. Apply a sterile, moist dressing on the sac.

4. A nurse providing discharge teaching with the parents of a school-age child who has juvenile idiopathic arthritis. Which of the following instructions should the nurse include? (Select all that apply.)

   A. Provide extra time for their child to complete ADLs.

   B. Apply cold compresses to affected joints.

   C. Take ibuprofen on an empty stomach.

   D. Remain home from school during periods of exacerbation.

   E. Perform range-of-motion exercises.

5. A nurse is assessing a child who has muscular dystrophy. Which of the following findings should the nurse expect? (Select all that apply.)

   A. Purposeless, involuntary, abnormal movements

   B. Sac protruding from spinal column

   C. Muscular weakness in lower extremities

   D. Upward slant to the eyes

   E. Waddling and unsteady gait

1. A. The nurse should structure interventions according to the child's developmental level and not their chronological age.
   B. **CORRECT**: A child who has cerebral palsy is at risk for sensory impairments of their vision and hearing. Therefore, the nurse should implement interventions to evaluate the toddler's hearing.
   C. The nurse should monitor the toddler's pain by using a developmentally appropriate pain tool such as the FACES pain scale.
   D. The toddler will require total care for their ADLs but the nurse should encourage independence and active participation.

   Ⓝ *NCLEX® Connection: Physiological Adaptation, Alterations in Body Systems*

2. A. **CORRECT:** The nurse should anticipate prescriptions for baclofen and diazepam. Baclofen is a centrally acting skeletal muscle relaxant that decreases muscle spasm and severe spasticity.
   B. **CORRECT:** The nurse should anticipate prescriptions for baclofen and diazepam. Diazepam is a skeletal muscle relaxant that decreases muscle spasms and severe spasticity.
   C. Oxybutynin is an antispasmodic, anticholinergic medication that decreases bladder spasms.
   D. Methotrexate is a cytotoxic disease-modifying antirheumatic drug that slows joint degeneration and progression of rheumatoid arthritis. It is used for children who have juvenile idiopathic arthritis (JIA).
   E. Prednisone is a corticosteroid that increases muscle strength for children who have muscular dystrophy. It decreases inflammation in children who have JIA.

   Ⓝ *NCLEX® Connection: Pharmacological and Parenteral Therapies, Expected Actions/Outcomes*

3. A. Prior to surgery, the parents should not cuddle the infant because this can place pressure on the sac and can cause rupture.
   B. Rectal temperatures are not recommended because the infant is at risk for rectal prolapse because of relaxed bowel sphincter this can cause injury.
   C. The infant is positioned prone to prevent pressure on the sac.
   D. **CORRECT:** A myelomeningocele is neural tube defect in which a sac is protruding through the vertebral column. It can rupture which increase the infant's risk for developing infection. Therefore, the nurse should assist with protect the sac applying a sterile moist dressing that is moistened with sterile sodium chloride this will prevent drying and rupturing.

4. A, E. **CORRECT:** The nurse should inform the parents to provide extra time for their child to complete their ADLs to foster the child's independence because JIA can cause discomfort with joint movement. Perform range-of motion exercises should also be reinforce this will prevent contractures and deformities.
   B. The application of cold compress is not recommended because this can cause further discomfort. The application of warm moist heat to the affected joints will assist with alleviating discomfort.
   C. Ibuprofen should be taken with food to minimize GI adverse effects.
   D. During exacerbation, the child should continue their activities such as attending school and use measure to alleviate discomfort..

   Ⓝ *NCLEX® Connection: Physiological Adaptation, Pathophysiology*

5. C, E. **CORRECT:** A child who has muscular dystrophy can have the following findings: muscle weakness and waddling unsteady gait due to the degeneration of muscle fibers.
   A. Purposeless, involuntary movements is a finding for a child who has cerebral palsy.
   B. A sac protruding from the spinal column is a finding for a child who has myelomeningocele.
   D. Upward slant to eyes is a finding for a child who has trisomy disorder.

   Ⓝ *NCLEX® Connection: Physiological Adaptation, Alterations in Body Systems*

When reviewing the following chapters, keep in mind the relevant topics and tasks of the NCLEX outline, in particular:

Health Promotion and Maintenance

HEALTH PROMOTION/DISEASE PREVENTION: Educate the client on actions to promote/maintain health and prevent disease.

Pharmacological and Parenteral Therapies

PARENTERAL/INTRAVENOUS THERAPY: Apply knowledge and concepts of mathematics/nursing procedures/psychomotor skills when caring for a client receiving intravenous and parenteral therapy.

PHARMACOLOGICAL PAIN MANAGEMENT: Administer medications for pain management.

EXPECTED ACTIONS/OUTCOMES: Use clinical decision making/critical thinking when addressing expected effects/outcomes of medications.

Reduction of Risk Potential

LABORATORY VALUES: Compare client laboratory values to normal laboratory values.

POTENTIAL FOR COMPLICATIONS OF DIAGNOSTIC TESTS/TREATMENTS/PROCEDURES: Evaluate responses to procedures and treatments

Basic Care and Comfort

ELIMINATION: Provide skin care to clients who are incontinent.

NUTRITION AND ORAL HYDRATION: Provide/maintain special diets based on the client diagnosis/nutritional needs and cultural considerations.

Physiological Adaptation

ALTERATIONS IN BODY SYSTEMS
Provide care to a client with an infectious disease.

Educate client about managing health problems

FLUID AND ELECTROLYTE IMBALANCES: Apply
knowledge of pathophysiology when caring for the
client with fluid and electrolyte imbalances.

PATHOPHYSIOLOGY: Identify pathophysiology
related to an acute or chronic condition.

ILLNESS MANAGEMENT: Educate client
regarding an acute or chronic condition

HEMODYNAMICS: Manage the care of a client with alteration
in hemodynamics, tissue perfusion and/or hemostasis.

UNEXPECTED RESPONSE TO THERAPIES: Recognize signs
and symptoms of client complications and intervene.

CHAPTER 16

UNIT 2   SYSTEM DISORDERS

SECTION: INTEGUMENTARY DISORDERS

CHAPTER 30

Skin Infections and Infestations

Skin infections are bacterial, viral, or fungal. Arthropod bites and stings are caused by flies, mosquitoes, chiggers, bees, fire ants, mites, ticks, spiders, and scorpions. Skin infestations include scabies and lice.

Skin infections

- Bacterial infections include impetigo contagiosa, pyoderma, folliculitis, furuncle, carbuncle, cellulitis, and staphylococcal scalded skin syndrome.
- Viral infections include verruca, verruca plantaris, herpes simplex virus, varicella zoster virus, and molluscum contagiosum.
- Fungal infections include tinea capitis, tinea corporis, tinea cruris, tinea pedis/unguium, and candidiasis.

ASSESSMENT

RISK FACTORS

Bacterial

- Contact with infected person
- Congenital or acquired immunodeficiency disorders
- Immunosuppression

Viral

Contact with infected person

Fungal

- Contact with infected person
- Geographic area

EXPECTED FINDINGS

History of causative agent/exposure
- Bacterial **(30.1)**
- Viral **(30.2)**
- Fungal **(30.3)**

LABORATORY TESTS

Cultures (bacterial, viral, fungal)

30.1 Bacterial skin infections

	CAUSATIVE ORGANISM	MANIFESTATIONS	MANAGEMENT
Impetigo contagiosa	Staphylococcus	Reddish macule becomes vesicular	Topical bactericidal or triple antibiotic ointment
		Erupts easily leaving moist erosion on the skin, secretions dry forming honey-colored crusts	Oral or parenteral antibiotics for severe cases
		Spreads peripherally and by direct contact	*Methicillin-resistant Staphylococcus aureus (MRSA) is managed with vancomycin.*
		Pruritus common	
Pyoderma	Staphylococcus	Deeper infection into the dermis	Cleanse with soap and water
	Streptococcus	Possible systemic effects (fever, lymphangitis)	Bathe using antibacterial soap
			Launder washcloths and towels separately to prevent bacterial spread
			Apply mupirocin to lesions
			Systemic antibiotics
Folliculitis (pimple)	*Staphylococcus aureus* Methicillin-resistant *Staphylococcus aureus* (MRSA)	Infection of a hair follicle	Apply warm moist compresses
			Clean skin often
			Topical antibiotic medications
			Systemic antibiotics for severe cases
Furuncle (boil)	*Staphylococcus aureus* MRSA	Larger swollen, red lesion of a single hair follicle	Incision, draining, and irrigation of severe lesions
Carbuncle (multiple boils)	*Staphylococcus aureus* MRSA	More extensive swollen, red lesions involving multiple hair follicles Face, buttocks, neck	For MRSA infections, soak in diluted bleach solution
Cellulitis	Streptococcus Staphylococcus *Haemophilus influenzae*	Firm, swollen, red area of the skin and subcutaneous tissue Possible systemic effects (fever, malaise)	Oral or parenteral antibiotics Rest and immobilize affected area Acute care for systemic manifestations
Staphylococcal scalded skin syndrome	*Staphylococcus aureus*	Rough-textured skin with macular erythema Epidermis becomes wrinkled within 2 days with large bullae appearing	Systemic antibiotics Burow's solution or saline for gentle cleansing Compresses of 0.25% silver nitrate Acute hospitalization IV fluids, analgesics, bandaging

30.2 Viral skin infections

	CAUSATIVE ORGANISM	MANIFESTATIONS	MANAGEMENT
Verruca (warts)	Human papillomavirus	Elevated, rough, gray-brown firm papules Can occur anywhere on the skin Can be single or in groups	Individualized destructive therapy (surgical removal, electrocautery, cryotherapy, laser)
Verruca plantaris (plantar warts)		Flat warts on the plantar surface of the feet Possibly surrounded by hyperkeratosis	Caustic solution applied to wart Wear insoles with holes to decrease pressure for 2 to 3 days Soak affected area for 20 min Repeat treatment until wart falls off
Cold sore, fever blister	Herpes simplex virus type 1	Near a mucocutaneous area (lips, nose, buttock, genitalia) Group of vesicles that itch and burn	Apply Burrow solution during weeping stage Oral antiviral (acyclovir) to reduce duration
Genital herpes	Herpes simplex virus type 2	After drying, form a crusty area followed by exfoliation Healing occurs in 8 to 10 days Possible lymphadenopathy	Oral antiviral (valacyclovir) for genital herpes
Herpes zoster *Shingles*	Varicella zoster virus	Neurologic pain, hyperesthesias, or itching Rash, vesicular lesions appear near afferent nerve endings	Use oral or topical analgesics Apply moist compresses Zoster vaccine recomended for clients who are greater than 50 years of age
Molloscum contagiosum	Poxvirus	Flesh-colored papules on stalks (extremities, face, trunk)	Resolves spontaneously in 18 months Complicated cases: remove pox chemically or with curettage, cryotherapy or electrodessication

30.3 Fungal skin infections

	CAUSATIVE ORGANISM	MANIFESTATIONS	MANAGEMENT
Tinea capitis (ringworm of the scalp)	Trichophyton tonsurans Microsporum audouinii Microsporum canis	Scaly, circumscribed lesion with alopecia on the scalp Pruritic	Use of selenium sulfide shampoos Oral griseofulvin Kerion-griseofulvin and oral corticosteroids for 2 weeks Complicated cases: oral ketoconazole Treat infected pets (especially cats), if necessary
Tinea corporis (ringworm of the body)	Trichophyton rubrum Trichophyton mentagrophytes Microsporum canis	Round or oval erythematous scaling patch Spreads peripherally and unilaterally and clears centrally	Oral griseofulvin Topical antifungal (tolnaftate, clotrimazole) Treat infected pets
Tinea cruris (jock itch)	Epidermophyton floccosum Trichophyton rubrum Trichophyton mentagrophytes	Medial and proximal aspect of the thigh and crural folds May include the scrotum Pruritic Round erythematous scaling patch Spreads peripherally and clears centrally	Clotrimazole or ciclopirox twice a day for 2 to 4 weeks Ciclopirox or clotrimazole griseofulvin for severe infections Wear light-colored socks, well-ventilated shoes Burrow's solution or soaks
Tinea pedis (athlete's foot)	Trichophyton rubrum Trichophyton interdigitale Epidermophyton floccosum	Between toes or on the plantar surface of the feet Maceration and fissuring lesions between the toes and patches with tiny vesicles on the plantar surface of the foot	
Candidiasis (moniliasis)	Candida albicans	Found in moist areas of the skin surface White exudate, peeling inflamed areas that bleed easily Pruritic	Topical antifungal ointment (miconazole, nystatin) *Miconazole, clotramizole (vulvovaginal)*

30.4 Arthropod bites and stings

	MANIFESTATIONS	MANAGEMENT
Mosquitoes, fleas, flies	Variable, from no reaction to hypersensitivity reaction Papular urticaria Firm papules	Use antipruritic agent. Administer oral and topical antihistamines. Take soothing baths.
Bees, wasps, hornets, fire ants, yellow jackets	Local reaction: small red itchy wheal that is warm to the touch Systemic reaction (mild to severe): generalized edema, pain, nausea and vomiting, confusion, respiratory problems, and shock	Scrape or pull out stinger as quickly as possible. Cleanse with soap and water. Apply cool compresses. Apply home products (baking soda, lemon juice). Administer topical and oral antihistamines. Epinephrine and corticosteroids for severe cases.
Chiggers	Bites on warm parts of the body Variable, from no reaction to hypersensitivity reaction Papular urticaria Firm papules	Systemic steroids for severe cases
Ticks	Attaches to the skin with head embedded Firm, discrete, pruritic nodule at site Possible urticaria or persistent localized edema	Remove by pulling straight up with steady, even pressure with tweezers to remove the tick. Remove any remaining parts using a sterile needle. Cleanse site with soap and disinfectant.

	Lyme disease: tick infected with *Borrelia burgdorferi*
	Can appear in any of these stages:
	Stage 1: 3 to 30 days following bite
	• Erythema migrans at site
	• Chills, fever, itching, headache, fainting, stiff neck, muscle weakness, bull's eye rash at the site of the bite
	Stage 2: occurs 3 to 10 weeks following bite
	  ○ Systemic involvement begins (neurologic, cardiac, and musculoskeletal)
	  ○ Paralysis or weakness in the face, muscle pain, swelling in large joints (knees), fever, fatigue, splenomegaly
	Stage 3: 2 to 12 months following bite
	  ○ Systemic involvement is advanced (musculoskeletal pain that includes the muscles, tendons, bursae, and synovia); possible arthritis, deafness, cardiac complications, and encephalopathy.
	  ○ Abnormal muscle movement and weakness, numbness and tingling, speech problems
		Observe clients bitten by a tick for 30 days
		Antibiotic (single dose) for clients who meet criteria
		Antibiotic (2- to 3-week course) for clients who have confirmed disease
		Doxycycline for children older than 8 years and amoxicillin or cefuroxime for children under 8 years. Cefuroxime for children who have an allergy to penicillin

Brown recluse spider	Mild sting leads to transient erythema and blister Pain 2 to 8 hr following bite Star-shaped purple area in 3 to 4 days Necrotic ulceration in 7 to 14 days	Cool compresses Antibiotic, corticosteroids Analgesic for pain Possible skin graft
Black widow spiders	Mild sting leads to swollen, painful, and erythematous site Dizziness, weakness, and abdominal pain Possible delirium, paralysis, seizures, and death	Cleanse bite with antiseptic. Apply cool compresses. Administer antivenin. Administer muscle relaxant. Administer analgesics.
Scorpions	Intense pain Erythema, burning, numbness Restlessness and vomiting Ascending paralysis: seizures, weakness, increase in pulse, thirst, salivation, dysuria, pulmonary edema leading to coma and death	Position site in dependent position. Keep child calm. Administer antivenin. Analgesic for pain. Admit to intensive care unit for close monitoring.

PATIENT-CENTERED CARE

NURSING CARE

- Assess the general condition of the affected area.
- Assess for evidence of associated infection.
- Assist in preventing the child to itch or touch the affected areas.
- Teach the importance of proper hand hygiene.

CLIENT EDUCATION

Perform methods to avoid the spread of infections.
- Use appropriate hand hygiene.
- Avoid sharing clothing, hats, combs, brushes, or towels. (fungal infections).
- Keep the child from touching the affected area by using distraction.
- Do not squeeze vesicles.
- Apply topical medications as prescribed.
- Teach how to administer medications as prescribed and monitor for adverse effects.

Arthropod Bites and Stings

Scorpions, black widow, and brown recluse spiders inject venom that requires immediate attention.

ASSESSMENT

RISK FACTORS

Geographic area

EXPECTED FINDINGS

History of causative agent/exposure (30.4)

PATIENT-CENTERED CARE

NURSING CARE (30.4)

CLIENT EDUCATION

- Prevent secondary infections.
- Children at risk for or who have a history of severe reactions should wear a medical alert identification bracelet. Qs
- Parents should keep a home emergency kit of epinephrine if child has history of severe reaction.
- Inspect skin after possible exposure.
- Prevent bites.
  - Avoid areas of tall grass.
  - Use insect repellent.
  - Avoid contact with insects.
  - Avoid wood piles.
  - Inspect and treat pets, carpets, and furniture.
  - Avoid flowery prints and bright clothing.
  - Avoid perfumes and colognes.

Skin Infestations

- Scabies mite, Sarcoptes scabiei, is spread by direct contact with an infected person. The mite burrows into the skin and lays eggs.
- (Pediculus humanus capitis) Pediculosis capitis (head lice), is spread by direct contact with an infected person, bedding, and objects (hair brush, clothing). The life span of the adult louse life is 1 month and they can live up to 48 hr without a human host. The female lays eggs at night, close to the skin surface and at the junction of the hair shaft. The nits hatch in 7 to 10 days.

ASSESSMENT

RISK FACTORS

Anyone is at risk for developing both conditions

Scabies: continuous close personal contact

EXPECTED FINDINGS

Itching (30.5)

DIAGNOSTIC TESTS

Scabies: examination under a microscope

PATIENT-CENTERED CARE

NURSING CARE (30.5)

- Teach the child and parents about the medications. Qpcc
- Assess for infestation.
- **Scabies**: Pencil-like marks on skin.
- **Head lice**: Adult lice are hard to see: small, grayish-tan, and no wings. Nits look like dandruff on the hair shaft and are firmly attached.
- Assess for secondary skin infection.

CLIENT EDUCATION

- Avoid home remedies, as it can worsen infection.
- Understand correct laundering of potentially infected clothing, bedding.
- Bag items that cannot be laundered into tightly sealed bag for 14 days.
- Boil combs, brushes and hair accessories for 10 min or soak in lice-killing products for 1 hr.
- Avoid sharing of personal items.

30.5 Skin infestations

	MANIFESTATIONS	NURSING INTERVENTIONS
Scabies mite: Sarcoptes scabiei	Intensely itchy, especially at night Rash, especially between fingers, popliteal folds, and inguinal regions Thin, pencil-like marks on the skin. Mites look like black dot on end of a grayish-brown burrow **INFANTS** Widespread on the body Pimples on the trunk Blisters on the palms of the hands and soles of the feet **YOUNG CHILDREN:** Most common on head, neck, shoulders, palms, and soles **OLDER CHILDREN:** Most common on hands, wrists, genitals, and abdomen	Apply a scabicide (5% permethrin cream) over the entire body to remain on the skin for 8 to 14 hr; repeat in 1 to 2 weeks. Treat entire family and persons that have been in contact with infected person during and 60 days after infection. Wash underwear, towels, clothing, and sleepwear in hot water. Vacuum carpets and furniture. Apply calamine lotion or cool compresses until itching subsides following treatment. Difficult cases: May use oral ivermectin.
Pediculosis capitis (head lice): Pediculus humanus capitis	Intense itching Small, red bumps on the scalp Nits (white specks) on the hair shaft	1% permethrin shampoo Spinosad 0.9% topical suspension for children 4 years and older. Benzyl alcohol 5% in infants 6 months and older. Remove nits with a nit comb, repeat in 7 days after shampoo treatment Wash clothing, bedding in hot water with detergent. Place items unable to be laundered in a sealed plastic bag for 14 days. Difficult cases: use malathion 0.5%

Application Exercises

1. A nurse is caring for a child who has cellulitis on the hand. Which of the following actions should the nurse take?

   A. Administer oral antibiotics.

   B. Cleanse area using Burrow solution.

   C. Prepare for cryotherapy.

   D. Apply a topical antifungal medication.

2. A nurse is planning care for a child who has tinea capitis. Which of the following actions should the nurse include in the plan of care? (Select all that apply.)

   A. Treat infected house pets.

   B. Use selenium sulfide shampoo.

   C. Cleanse area with Burrow solution.

   D. Administer antiviral medication.

   E. Use moist, warm compresses.

3. A nurse is assessing an infant who has scabies. Which of the following findings should the nurse expect? (Select all that apply.)

   A. Presence of nits on the hair shaft

   B. Pencil-like marks on hands

   C. Blisters on the soles of the feet

   D. Small, red bumps on the scalp

   E. Pimples on the trunk

4. A nurse is teaching a parent of a child who has pediculosis capitis. Which of the following instructions should the nurse include in the teaching?

   A. Apply mayonnaise to the affected area at night.

   B. Treat all household pets.

   C. Use an over-the-counter medication containing 1% permethrin.

   D. Discard the child's stuffed animals.

5. A nurse is teaching a group of parents about preventing insect bites. Which of the following information should the nurse include in the teaching? (Select all that apply.)

   A. Wear perfumes when outside.

   B. Avoid areas of tall grass.

   C. Wear bright-colored clothing.

   D. Wear insect repellent.

   E. Check house pets frequently.

Active Learning Scenario

A nurse is teaching a group of caregivers about preventing skin infections. Use the ATI Active Learning Template: System Disorder to complete this item.

CLIENT EDUCATION: Describe five teaching points.

Active Learning Scenario Key

Using the ATI Active Learning Template: System Disorder
CLIENT EDUCATION
- Use good hand hygiene.
- Avoid sharing clothing, hats, combs, brushes, and towels.
- Keep the child from touching the affected area by using distraction.
- Do not squeeze vesicles.
- Apply topical medications as prescribed.
- Teach how to administer medications as prescribed and monitor for adverse effects.

Ⓝ *NCLEX® Connection: Health Promotion and Maintenance, Health Promotion/Disease Prevention*

Application Exercises Key

1. A. **CORRECT:** Oral antibiotics are often prescribed for the treatment of cellulitis.
   B. Cleansing with Burow's solution is recommended for staphylococcal scalded skin syndrome or herpes simplex virus.
   C. Cryotherapy is recommended for human papillomavirus.
   D. Topical antifungal medications are indicated for the treatment of candidiasis or tinea corporis.

Ⓝ *NCLEX® Connection: Physiological Adaptation, Alterations in Body Systems*

2. A. **CORRECT:** Tinea capitis can be transmitted from household pets, especially cats, to persons. Pets should be treated, if infected.
   B. **CORRECT:** Selenium sulfide shampoo is recommended for use for children who have tinea capitis.
   C. A topical antifungal medication is recommended for children who have tinea capitis.
   D. Tinea capitis is a fungal infection. Antifungal medications are administered.
   E. Moist, warm compresses are applied for bacterial skin infections and not recommended for children who have tinea capitis.

Ⓝ *NCLEX® Connection: Physiological Adaptation, Alterations in Body Systems*

3. A. Presence of nits on the hair shaft is a manifestation of pediculosis capitis.
   B. **CORRECT:** Pencil-like marks on hands is a manifestation of scabies.
   C. **CORRECT:** Blisters on the soles of the feet is a manifestation of scabies.
   D. Small, red bumps on the scalp are a manifestation of pediculosis capitis.
   E. **CORRECT:** Pimples on the trunk is a manifestation of scabies.

Ⓝ *NCLEX® Connection: Physiological Adaptation, Pathophysiology*

4. A. Home remedies (mayonnaise) increase the risk of infection and should be avoided.
   B. Pediculosis capitis is transmitted person-to-person; household pets are not hosts.
   C. **CORRECT:** Pediculosis capitis is treated with 1% permethrin, which can be purchased over the counter.
   D. Items that cannot be placed in the laundry can be placed in a sealed bag for 14 days to kill the lice.

Ⓝ *NCLEX® Connection: Physiological Adaptation, Alterations in Body Systems*

5. A. Perfumes attract insects and should be avoided.
   B. **CORRECT:** Insects live in tall grasses; these areas should be avoided.
   C. Bright-colored clothing attracts insects and should be avoided.
   D. **CORRECT:** Insect repellent should be applied to prevent insect bites.
   E. **CORRECT:** House pets should be inspected and treated for insects to prevent exposing family members.

Ⓝ *NCLEX® Connection: Health Promotion and Maintenance, Health Promotion/Disease Prevention*

CHAPTER 31 # Dermatitis and Acne

Common skin conditions of the pediatric population include contact dermatitis, atopic dermatitis, and acne.

Contact dermatitis

Contact dermatitis is an inflammatory, hypersensitive reaction of the skin. It is caused when the skin comes into contact with chemicals or other irritants (feces, urine, soaps, poison ivy, animals, metals, dyes, medications).

Diaper dermatitis can be caused by exposure to an irritant: (urine (increased pH), stool, skin friction, chemicals, soaps, or detergents) that come in prolonged or excessive contact with the diaper/perineal area. It can also be a result of Candida albicans.

Seborrheic dermatitis (cradle cap, blepharitis, otitis externa) has an unknown etiology but is most common in infancy and puberty.

ASSESSMENT

RISK FACTORS

- Diaper dermatitis: Use of diapers, infrequent diaper changing, excessive stooling
- Contact dermatitis: Exposure to an irritant

EXPECTED FINDINGS

Pruritus

PHYSICAL ASSESSMENT FINDINGS
Depends on the cause of the irritant and the client
- **Contact dermatitis**
  - Red bumps that can form moist, weeping blisters
  - Skin warm and tender to the touch
  - Presence of oozing, drainage, or crusts
  - Skin becomes scaly, raw, or thickened
- **Diaper dermatitis**
  - Mild: scattered erythematous papules, minor irritation
  - Moderate: erosions and macerations, extensive erythema, pain
  - Severe: extensive glistening erythema, skin erosions, papules, pustules, nodules, pain
- **Seborrheic dermatitis**
  - Thick, adherent lesions
  - Patches that are yellow and scaly

PATIENT-CENTERED CARE

NURSING CARE

Diaper dermatitis
- Change diapers frequently.
- Promptly remove soiled diapers.
- Cleanse diaper/perineal area with a nonirritating cleanser or plain warm water.
- Use soft cloths and commercial wipes (free of alcohol and fragrances) to cleanse the diaper/perineal area.
- Expose the affected area to air.
- Apply a skin barrier, such as zinc oxide. Do not wash it off with each diaper change.

Contact dermatitis: Remove irritant, and limit further exposure.

Poisonous plant exposure
- Cleanse exposed area as soon as possible by flushing it with cold running water.
- Clothes, shoes should be cleansed in hot water with detergent.
- Apply calamine lotion, Burrow's solution compresses, or natural colloidal oatmeal baths.
- Use topical corticosteroid gel.
- Oral corticosteroids for severe reactions or for irritation on the face, neck, or genitalia.

Seborrheic dermatitis
- Encourage parents to perform daily scalp/hair hygiene.
- Treat by gently scrubbing the scalp to remove scaly lesions and crusted patches. May apply petrolatum or mineral oil to scalp to soften lesions overnight.
- Use a fine-tooth comb to remove the loosened crusts from the scalp/hair.
- Use an antiseborrheic (contains sulfur and salicylic acid) shampoo daily.

MEDICATIONS

Antihistamines

Hydroxyzine or diphenhydramine
Administer in cases of allergic/medication reactions.

CLIENT EDUCATION
- Educate the child's family on the importance of the medication and administering on schedule.
- Reinforce the sedating effect of some antihistamines and the need for parents to monitor the child and provide for safety during use Qs

Antibiotics

Used to treat secondary infections.

CLIENT EDUCATION: Educate the family about the importance of continuing the medication as prescribed.

Antifungal ointments

Clotrimazole
Used to treat Candida albicans associated with diaper dermatitis.

CLIENT EDUCATION: Educate the family on the importance of the medication and administering schedule.

CLIENT EDUCATION

- Change diapers frequently.
- Avoid bubble baths and harsh soaps.
- Wear long sleeves and pants when there is risk of possible exposure to irritants.
- Remove an offending agent as soon as exposure takes place.
- Practice proper hand hygiene.

COMPLICATIONS

Bacterial infections

Caused by breaks in the skin from scratching.

NURSING ACTIONS
- Monitor the area for manifestations of infection.
- Keep fingernails trimmed short.
- Cleanse the area with mild soap and water.
Administer antipruritics and antibiotics.

CLIENT EDUCATION: Educate the family and child about avoiding offending agents. Qpcc

Atopic dermatitis

- Atopic dermatitis (AD) is a type of eczema (eczema describes a category of integumentary disorders, not a specific disorder with a determined etiology) that is characterized by pruritus and associated with a history of allergies that are of an inherited tendency (atopy).
- Classifications of atopic dermatitis are based on the child's age, how the lesions are distributed, and the appearance of the lesions.
- AD cannot be cured but can be well-controlled.

ASSESSMENT

RISK FACTORS

- Presence of allergic condition and family history of atopy
- Previous skin disorder and exacerbation of present skin disorder
- Exposure to irritating and/or causative agents
- Genetic predisposition
- Geographic location

EXPECTED FINDINGS

- Recent exposure to any irritant (medication, food, soap, contact with animals)
- Intense pruritus

PHYSICAL ASSESSMENT FINDINGS
- Unaffected skin can appear dry and rough.
- Hypopigmentation of skin can occur in small, diffuse areas.
- Pallor surrounds the nose, mouth, and ears.
- A bluish discoloration is present underneath the eyes.
- Lymphadenopathy occurs, especially around affected areas.

INFANTS

Onset at 2 to 6 months of age with spontaneous remission by 3 years of age

DISTRIBUTION: Generalized distribution of lesions on cheeks, scalp, neck, and feet, as well as extensor surfaces of extremities

LESIONS
- Erythema
- Vesicles, papules
- Weeping, oozing, crusting, scaling

CHILDREN

Onset at 2 to 3 years of age with 90% of children having manifestations by 5 years of age; can follow infantile eczema

DISTRIBUTION: Lesions in the flexural areas (antecubital and popliteal fossae, neck), wrists, ankles, and feet with symmetric involvement

LESIONS
- Clusters
- Erythematous or flesh-colored papules
- Dry
- Lichenification
- Keratosis pilaris

ADOLESCENTS

Onset at age 12 and can continue into adulthood

DISTRIBUTION: Similar distribution to children

LESIONS
- Same as for children
- Dry, thick
- Confluent papules

PATIENT-CENTERED CARE

NURSING CARE

- Assess and monitor the skin frequently.
- Keep skin hydrated with tepid baths. Two or three baths may be given daily with one prior to bedtime.
- Use a mild skin cleanser if needed during baths. After bathing, pat, do not rub, skin. Apply an emollient or moisturizer immediately after bathing and drying while skin is still moist.
- Dress the child in cotton clothing. Avoid wool and synthetic fabrics.
- Avoid excessive heat and perspiration, which increases itching.
- Avoid irritants (bubble baths, soaps, perfumes, fabric softeners).
- Provide support to the child and family.
- Wash skin folds and genital area frequently with water.
- Assist in identifying causative agent.
- Keep child's nail short and filed smooth to eliminate sharp edges.

THERAPEUTIC MANAGEMENT

MEDICATIONS

Antihistamines

Hydroxyzine or diphenhydramine
Used to manage severe pruritis

CLIENT EDUCATION
- Reinforce the sedating effect of some antihistamines and the need for parents to monitor the child during use.
- Reinforce safety of the child when using sedating antihistamines. Qs

Loratadine or fexofenadine
Oral antihistamine for antipruritic effect

NURSING ACTIONS: Administer as prescribed.

CLIENT EDUCATION: It is preferred for use during the daytime.

Antibiotics

Antibiotics are used to treat secondary infections.

Topical corticosteroids

Topical corticosteroids may be used intermittently to reduce or control flare-ups. They can be low-, moderate-, or high-potency and are prescribed based on the degree of skin involvement (extremity versus eyelids), age of the child, and consequences from adverse effects.

Topical immunomodulators (nonsteroidal)

Tacrolimus or pimecrolimus
- Used to decrease inflammation during flare-ups
- Safe to apply to face

NURSING ACTIONS
- Use for children older than 2 years of age.
- Use at the start of an exacerbation of AD when skin turns red and starts to itch.

CLIENT EDUCATION
- Observe for manifestations of infection.
- Change diapers when wet or soiled.
- Keep nails short and trimmed.
- Place gloves or cotton socks over hands for sleeping.
- Dress young children in soft, cotton, one-piece, long-sleeve, long-pant outfits.
- Remove items that can promote itching (woolen blankets, scratchy fabrics). Use cotton items whenever possible.
- Use mild detergents to wash clothing and linens. The wash cycle can be repeated without soap.
- Avoid latex products, second-hand smoke, furry pets, dust, and molds.
- Encourage tepid baths (can use a mild skin cleanser if needed) at least daily. Avoid scrubbing the skin and using bubble bath.
- Soaking in bathtub is recommended for less than 10 minutes. Apply prescribed medications and moisturizers immediately after bathing when skin is still moist.
- Apply wet wraps overnight as prescribed for severe pruritis (Apply gauze that is moisten water to affected area, wrap a dry gauze over the moistened gauze.
- Follow specific directions regarding topical medications, soaks, and baths. Emphasize the importance of understanding the sequence of treatments to maximize the benefit of therapy and prevent complications.
- Use a room humidifier or vaporizer.
- Maintain treatment to prevent flare-up.
- Follow up with the provider as directed.
- Participate in support groups.

Therapeutic Procedures

- Phototherapy: affected areas exposed to UV light for at least 2-3 times per week

Complementary and alternative therapies

- Topicals: coconut/sunflower oil, vitamin B12
- Vitamins and supplements: Vitamin D, fish oil, melatonin, turmeric
- Other: acupuncture, meditation, yoga, massage

COMPLICATIONS

Infection

Caused by breaks in the skin from scratching

NURSING ACTIONS
- Keep nails trimmed.
- Administer antipruritics.
- Monitor the area for manifestations of infection.
- Cleanse the area with mild cleanser and water.

CLIENT EDUCATION: Educate the family and child to avoid offending agents. Qpcc

Acne

- Acne also known as acne vulgaris, is the most common skin condition during adolescence.
- Acne is self-limiting and not life-threatening. However, it poses a threat to self-image and self-esteem for adolescents.
- Acne involves the pilosebaceous follicles (hair follicle and sebaceous gland complex) of the face, neck, chest, and upper back.
- Propionibacterium acnes is the bacteria associated with inflammation in acne.

ASSESSMENT

RISK FACTORS

- Acne has a genetic link.
- More common in males.
- Age: common during adolescence
- Hormonal fluctuations can result in acne flares.
- The use of cosmetic products containing ingredients (petrolatum and lanolin) can increase acne outbreaks.
- Adolescents working at fast-food restaurants can have an increased incidence of acne due to exposure to cooking grease.
- There is a possible dietary link with acne and the intake of high glycemic index foods and dairy products.

EXPECTED FINDINGS

Report of exacerbations and remissions

PHYSICAL ASSESSMENT FINDINGS

- Lesions (comedones) are either open (blackheads) or closed (whiteheads). Both are most often found on the face, neck, back, and chest.
- P. acnes can lead to inflammation manifesting as papules, pustules, nodules, or cysts.

PATIENT-CENTERED CARE

NURSING CARE

- Discuss the process of acne with the adolescent and family.
- Discuss the importance of adherence with the prescribed plan of care.

CLIENT EDUCATION
- Gently wash the face and other affected areas, avoiding scrubbing and abrasive cleaners.
- Observe for adverse effects of prescribed medications.

MEDICATIONS

Tretinoin

Interrupts abnormal keratinization that causes microcomedones

CLIENT EDUCATION
- Tretinoin can irritate the skin. Wait 20 to 30 min after washing the face before applying to decrease skin irritation.
- Use a pea-size amount of medication and apply at night.
- Avoid sun exposure.
- Use sunscreen (SPF 15 or greater).

Benzoyl peroxide

Antibacterial agent

NURSING ACTIONS
- Inhibits growth of P. acnes.
- Benzoyl peroxide can bleach bed linens, towels, and clothing, but not skin.

Topical and oral antibacterial agents

Inhibits growth of P. acnes

NURSING ACTIONS
- Various topical antibacterial agents (clindamycin, azelaic acid, dapsone) may be used. Assess and monitor for allergic reactions.
- Every-other-day application decreases adverse effects (drying of the skin, burning sensations, and erythema).
- Oral antibacterial medications (tetracycline, doxycycline, erythromycin, minocycline) are indicated for severe acne that is unresponsive to topical agents.
- Avoid sun exposure due to photosensitivity.
- Use sunscreen with an SPF of 15 or greater when exposure to sun is unavoidable.

Isotretinoin

Affects factors involved in the development of acne

NURSING ACTIONS

- Isotretinoin is only prescribed by dermatologists for severe acne that is unresponsive to other therapies.
- Adverse effects include dry skin and mucous membranes, dry eyes, decreased night vision, headaches, photosensitivity, elevated cholesterol and triglycerides, depression, suicidal ideation, and/or violent behaviors.
- Monitor for mood or behavioral changes.
- Isotretinoin is teratogenic. Therefore, it is contraindicated in women of childbearing age who are not taking oral contraceptives. If sexually active, the client must agree to use two forms of effective contraception for 1 month before and during treatment, and at least 1 month following treatment.

CLIENT EDUCATION: Adverse effects include dry skin and mucous membranes, dry eyes, decreased night vision, headaches, photosensitivity, elevated cholesterol and triglycerides, depression, suicidal ideation, and violent behaviors.

Oral contraceptive pills

Decreases endogenous androgen production and bioavailability, resulting in decreased acne development

NURSING ACTIONS

- Indicated only for adolescent females.
- Therapy is combined with a topical acne treatment.

CLIENT EDUCATION

- Reinforce that adherence to the therapeutic plan is essential to preventing acne flares.
- Encourage the child to eat a balanced, healthy diet.
- Encourage sleep, rest, and daily exercise.
- Wash the affected area gently with a mild cleanser once or twice daily, and not to pick or squeeze comedones.
- Encourage frequent shampooing of hair.

- Encourage support of the adolescent and family members to assist the adolescent in coping with body-image changes. Qpcc
- Wear protective clothing and sunscreen when outside.
- Use sunscreen with an SPF of 15 or greater when exposure to sun is unavoidable.
- Reinforce the need for follow-up and monitoring of cholesterol and triglycerides for adolescents who are taking isotretinoin.
- Reinforce the importance of using effective contraception while taking isotretinoin.

COMPLICATIONS

Psychosocial impairment

Causes: stress, decreased self-esteem, depression (related to cosmetic appearance)

NURSING ACTIONS

- Monitor for mood or behavioral changes
- Encourage verbalization of feelings

CLIENT EDUCATION

- Encourage adherence to treatment plan
- Report changes in mood

Skin scarring

- Caused by lesions skin from scratching or delay in treatment of acne, that causes permanent scaring
- Scars can be atrophic (loss of tissue damage) or hypertrophic (increased tissue formation such as keloids).
- Therapeutic management: topical medications, injectable steroids, silicone dressings, punch excision, cryosurgery, dermabrasion, microdermabrasion.
- Explain to adolescent and family that therapy will improve the appearance of skin.

Active Learning Scenario

A nurse is teaching a guardian of a child who has eczema. Use the ATI Active Learning Template: System Disorder to complete this item.

ALTERATION IN HEALTH (DIAGNOSIS)

CLIENT EDUCATION: Include at least five teaching points.

Active Learning Scenario Key

Using the ATI Active Learning Template: System Disorder

ALTERATION IN HEALTH (DIAGNOSIS): Eczema describes a category of integumentary disorders, not a specific disorder with a determined etiology, that is characterized by pruritus and associated with a history of allergies that are of an inherited tendency (atopy).

CLIENT EDUCATION
- Observe for manifestations of infection.
- Change diapers when wet or soiled.
- Keep nails short and trimmed.
- Place gloves or cotton socks over hands for sleeping.
- Dress young children in soft, cotton, one-piece, long-sleeve, long-pant outfits.
- Remove items that can promote itching (woolen blankets, scratchy fabrics). Use cotton items whenever possible.
- Use mild detergent to wash clothing and linens. The wash cycle can be repeated without soap.
- Avoid latex products, second-hand smoke, furry pets, dust, and molds.
- Encourage tepid baths without the use of soap. Avoid oils and powders.
- Follow specific directions regarding topical medications, soaks, and baths.
- Emphasize the importance of understanding the sequence of treatments to maximize the benefit of therapy and prevent complications.
- Avoid overheating the bedroom during winter months. Use a room humidifier.
- Maintain treatment to prevent flare-ups.
- Follow up with the provider as directed.
- Participate in support groups.

Ⓝ *NCLEX® Connection: Physiological Adaptation, Illness Management*

Application Exercises

1. A nurse is teaching the guardian of an infant who has seborrheic dermatitis of the scalp. Which of the following instructions should the nurse include in the teaching?

   A. Use petrolatum to help soften and remove patches from the scalp.

   B. Keep infant away from others when patches are present.

   C. Avoid washing patches from infant's hair.

   D. Apply a compress with Burrow's solution to patches.

2. A nurse is planning care for an infant who has diaper dermatitis. Which of the following actions should the nurse include in the plan of care? (Select all that apply.)

   A. Apply talcum powder with every diaper change.

   B. Allow the buttocks to air dry.

   C. Use commercial baby wipes to cleanse the area.

   D. Change diapers frequently.

   E. Apply zinc oxide ointment to the affected area.

3. A nurse is caring for a child who has contact dermatitis due to poison ivy. Which of the following actions should the nurse take? (Select all that apply.)

   A. Remove the clothing over the rash.

   B. Initiate contact isolation precautions while the rash is present.

   C. Expose the rash to a heat lamp for 15 min.

   D. Cleanse the affected skin with hydrogen peroxide solution.

   E. Apply calamine lotion to the skin.

4. A nurse is assessing an infant who has eczema. Which of the following findings should the nurse expect? (Select all that apply.)

   A. Generalized distribution of lesions

   B. Papules

   C. Ecchymosis in flexural areas

   D. Crusting lesions

   E. Keratosis pilaris

5. A nurse is caring for an adolescent who has acne and is receiving prescribed isotretinoin. Which of the following laboratory findings should the nurse plan to monitor?

   A. Cholesterol and triglycerides

   B. BUN and creatinine

   C. Blood potassium

   D. Blood sodium

Application Exercises Key

1. A. **CORRECT:** Recommend that the guardian use petrolatum, vegetable oil, or mineral oil to help soften and remove scales and crusted areas.
   B. Seborrheic dermatitis is not contagious, so it is not necessary to keep the infant away from others.
   C. Washing the infant's hair daily with an antiseborrheic shampoo can help remove scales and crusted areas and can help prevent recurrence.
   D. Burrow's solution compresses are not recommended because this can cause further complications

   Ⓝ *NCLEX® Connection: Physiological Adaptation, Alterations in Body Systems*

2. A. Talcum powder can cake and cause inhalation injury. It should not be used for infants who have diaper dermatitis.
   B. **CORRECT:** Allowing the buttocks to air dry facilitates thorough drying of the skin and should be included in the plan of care.
   C. Commercial baby wipes contain chemicals that can irritate the skin. They should not be used for infants who have diaper dermatitis.
   D. **CORRECT:** Diapers should be changed frequently, and soiled diapers should be removed promptly.
   E. **CORRECT:** Zinc oxide ointment protects the skin from moisture and irritation and should be included in the plan of care.

   Ⓝ *NCLEX® Connection: Basic Care and Comfort, Elimination*

3. A. **CORRECT:** Removing the irritant from the skin will decrease the child's exposure. Remove the clothing over the affected area.
   B. Poison ivy is not spread by contact with the rash. Once the plant oils are removed, it cannot be transmitted to others.
   C. Avoid using a heat lamp, which can cause skin burns.
   D. Cleanse the affected area with cold running water, followed by soap and water as soon as possible following exposure.
   E. **CORRECT:** Apply calamine lotion to assist in relieving discomfort.

   Ⓝ *NCLEX® Connection: Physiological Adaptation, Alterations in Body Systems*

4. A. **CORRECT:** Generalized distribution of lesions is an expected finding in infants who have eczema.
   B. **CORRECT:** Papules are an expected finding in infants who have eczema.
   C. Lesions, rather than ecchymosis, in the flexural areas are an expected finding in children 2 years of age and older.
   D. **CORRECT:** Crusting lesions are an expected finding in infants who have eczema.
   E. Keratosis pilaris is an expected finding in children 2 years of age and older.

   Ⓝ *NCLEX® Connection: Physiological Adaptation, Pathophysiology*

5. A. **CORRECT:** Adverse effects of isotretinoin include elevated cholesterol and triglycerides. Plan to monitor these laboratory values during treatment.
   B. Medications (cephalosporins and furosemide) can alter blood BUN and creatinine levels. However, they do not to be monitored in clients taking isotretinoin.
   C. Medications (diuretics and corticosteroids) can alter blood potassium levels. However, it does not need to be monitored in clients taking isotretinoin.
   D. Medications (IV fluids and corticosteroids) can alter the blood sodium level. However, it does not need to be monitored in clients taking isotretinoin.

   Ⓝ *NCLEX® Connection: Pharmacological and Parenteral Therapies, Expected Actions/Outcomes*

NCLEX® Connections

When reviewing the following chapters, keep in mind the relevant topics and tasks of the NCLEX outline, in particular:

Client Needs: Pharmacological and Parenteral Therapies

ADVERSE EFFECTS/CONTRAINDICATIONS/SIDE EFFECTS/ INTERACTIONS: Provide information to the client on common side effects/adverse effects/potential interactions of medications and inform the client when to notify the primary health care provider.

MEDICATION ADMINISTRATION
Review pertinent data prior to medication administration.

Educate client on medication self–administration procedures.

Client Needs: Reduction of Risk Potential

DIAGNOSTIC TESTS: Monitor the results of diagnostic testing and intervene as needed.

POTENTIAL FOR COMPLICATIONS FROM SURGICAL PROCEDURES AND HEALTH ALTERATIONS: Apply knowledge of pathophysiology to monitoring for complications.

SYSTEM-SPECIFIC ASSESSMENTS: Recognize trends and changes in client condition and intervene as needed.

Client Needs: Physiological Adaptation

ALTERATIONS IN BODY SYSTEMS: Educate client about managing health problems.

ILLNESS MANAGEMENT: Apply knowledge of client pathophysiology to illness management.

MEDICAL EMERGENCIES: Apply knowledge of pathophysiology when caring for a client experiencing a medical emergency.

PATHOPHYSIOLOGY: Identify pathophysiology related to an acute or chronic condition.

UNIT 2   SYSTEM DISORDERS
SECTION: ENDOCRINE DISORDERS

CHAPTER 32   *Diabetes Mellitus*

Diabetes mellitus is characterized by a partial or complete metabolic deficiency of insulin. Type 1 is characterized by destruction of pancreatic beta cells. Type 2 arises when the body fails to use insulin properly combined with insulin insufficiency.

Diabetes mellitus is a contributing factor for the development of cardiovascular disease, hypertension, renal failure, blindness, and stroke as individuals age.

ASSESSMENT

RISK FACTORS

- Genetics can predispose a person to the occurrence of type 1 and type 2 diabetes mellitus.
- Toxins and viruses can predispose an individual to diabetes by destroying the beta cells, leading to type 1 diabetes mellitus.
- Obesity, physical inactivity, high triglycerides (greater than 250 mg/dL), and hypertension can lead to insulin resistance and type 2 diabetes mellitus. Ⓠᴱᴮᴾ

EXPECTED FINDINGS

BLOOD GLUCOSE ALTERATIONS
- **Hypoglycemia**: blood glucose less than 60 mg/dL
  - Hunger, lightheadedness, and shakiness
  - Anxiety and irritability
  - Pallor, cool skin
  - Diaphoresis
  - Irritability
  - Normal or shallow respirations
  - Tachycardia and palpitations
  - Strange or unusual feelings
  - Decreasing level of consciousness
  - Difficulty in thinking and inability to concentrate
  - Change in emotional behavior
  - Slurred speech
  - Headache and blurred vision
  - Seizures leading to coma
- **Hyperglycemia**: blood glucose usually greater than 250 mg/dL
  - Thirst
  - Polyuria (early), oliguria (late)
  - Nausea, vomiting, abdominal pain
  - Skin that is warm, dry, and flushed with poor turgor
  - Dry mucous membranes

- Confusion
- Weakness
- Lethargy
- Weak pulse
- Diminished reflexes
- Rapid, deep respirations with acetone/fruity odor due to ketones (Kussmaul respirations)
- Recurrent vaginal yeast (early indication of type 2)

LABORATORY TESTS

DIAGNOSTIC CRITERIA FOR DIABETES
- An 8-hr fasting blood glucose level of 126 mg/dL or more
- A random (casual) blood glucose of 200 mg/dL or more with manifestations of diabetes
- An oral glucose tolerance test of 200 mg/dL or more in the 2-hr sample
- Hba1c greater than 6.5%

Fasting blood glucose

CLIENT EDUCATION: Ensure that the child has fasted (no food or drink other than water) for 8 hr prior to the blood draw. Antidiabetic medications should be postponed until after the level is drawn.

ORAL GLUCOSE TOLERANCE TEST

CLIENT EDUCATION
- Instruct the child to consume a balanced diet for the 3 days prior to the test, then, to fast for 8 hr prior to the test. A fasting blood glucose level is drawn at the start of the test.
- The child is then instructed to consume a specified amount of glucose. Blood glucose levels are drawn every 30 min for 2 hr.
- The child must be assessed for hypoglycemia throughout the procedure.

Glycosylated hemoglobin (HbA1c)

Used to evaluate diabetes management by providing an average of the child's blood glucose level over a period of about 3 months. The expected reference range is 4% to 6%, but an acceptable target for children who have diabetes can be 6.5% to 8% depending on the child's age and ability to tolerate lower blood glucose levels.

DIAGNOSTIC PROCEDURES

Self-monitored blood glucose (SMBG) Ⓠᴾᶜᶜ

- Blood glucose monitoring is essential to management of diabetes. Measurements should be assessed at a minimum before meals and at bedtime.
- Follow or ensure that the child follows the proper procedure for blood sample collection and use of a glucose meter.

CLIENT EDUCATION

- Instruct the child to check the accuracy of the strips with the control solution provided.
- Advise the child to keep a record of the SMBG that includes time, date, blood glucose level, insulin dose, food intake, and other events that can alter glucose metabolism (activity level or illness).

PATIENT-CENTERED CARE

NURSING CARE Qᴛᴄ

- Monitor the following.
  - Vital signs
  - Blood glucose levels and factors affecting levels (other medications, diet, and/or activity)
  - I&O and weight
  - Skin integrity and healing status of any wounds, paying close attention to the feet and folds of the skin
  - Findings of poor glucose control (paresthesias, visual changes, recurrent infections)
  - Dietary practices
  - Exercise patterns
  - The child's proficiency at self-monitoring blood glucose
  - The child's proficiency at self-administering medication
- Follow agency policy for nail care. Some protocols allow for trimming toenails straight across with clippers and filing edges with a nail file. If clippers or scissors are contraindicated, the child should file the nails straight across.
- Teach personal hygiene.
- Caution the child against wearing sandals, walking barefoot, or wearing shoes without socks.
- Teach the child to cleanse cuts with warm water and mild soap, gently dry, and apply a dry dressing. Instruct the child and parents to monitor healing and seek intervention promptly.
- Teach the child the importance of having medical identification.
- Examine the child's eyes yearly.
- Emphasize the importance of regular dental and health care visits.
- Provide nutritional guidelines.
  - Read labels for nutritional value.
  - Meal planning is based on the requirements of growth and development of the child.
  - Plan meals to match the timing of food to activity, and the onset, peak and duration of antidiabetic medications. Calories and food composition should be similar each day.
  - Eat at regular intervals and do not skip meals.
  - Count grams of carbohydrates consumed.
  - Recognize that 15 g of carbohydrates are equal to 1 carbohydrate exchange.
  - Avoid high-fat and high-sugar/high-carbohydrate food items.
  - Use artificial sweeteners in moderation.

- Teach appropriate techniques for SMBG, including obtaining blood samples, recording and responding to results, and correctly handling supplies and equipment.
- Assist with an exercise plan.
  - Children active with team sports will require a snack 30 min prior to activity.
  - Prolonged activities will require food intake every 45 to 60 min.
  - Adjustment in diet and medications can be required with changes in activities.
- Teach the child illness management guidelines.
  - Monitor blood glucose and urinary ketone levels every 3 hr.
  - Continue to take antidiabetic agents. However, dosages can differ.
  - Encourage sugar-free, noncaffeinated liquids to prevent dehydration.
  - Meet carbohydrate needs by eating soft foods if possible. If not, consume liquids that are equal to the usual carbohydrate content.
  - Rest.
  - Call the provider for the following.
    - Blood glucose greater than 240 mg/dL
    - Positive ketones in the urine
    - Disorientation or confusion
    - Rapid breathing
    - Vomiting occurs more than once
    - Liquids cannot be tolerated
- Teach manifestations of hypoglycemia (tremors, diaphoresis, anxiety, nervousness, chills, headache, confusion, labile, difficulty focusing, hunger, dizziness, pallor, palpations).
  - Check blood glucose levels.
  - Follow guidelines outlined by the provider or diabetes educator. Guidelines can include the following. Qꜱ
    - Treat with 10 to 15 g simple carbohydrate (1 tbsp sugar). Examples are 4 oz orange juice, 8 oz milk, 2 to 3 glucose tablets, or 4 oz regular soft drink.
    - For mild reactions, use milk or fruit juice.
    - Monitor blood glucose frequently.
    - Recheck blood glucose after 15 min to determine if additional carbohydrates are required.
    - Follow with complex carbohydrate.
    - If the child is unconscious or unable to swallow, administer glucagon SC or IM and notify the provider. Administer simple carbohydrate as soon as tolerated. Watch for vomiting, and take precautions against aspiration.
- Teach manifestations of hyperglycemia (lethargy, confusion, thirst, nausea, vomiting, abdominal pain, manifestations of dehydration, rapid respirations, fruity breath).
  - Encourage oral fluid intake.
  - Administer insulin as prescribed.
  - Test urine for ketones, and report if findings they remain high.
  - Consult the provider if manifestations persist or progress.

33.1 Rate of onset, peak, and duration of action by insulin type

	TYPE	ONSET	PEAK	DURATION
Rapid-acting	Insulin lispro	15 to 30 min	30 min to 3 hr	3 to 5 hr
Short-acting	Regular insulin	30 min to 1 hr	1 to 5 hr	6 to 10 hr
Intermediate-acting	NPH insulin	1 to 2 hr	4 to 14 hr	14 to 24 hr
Long-acting	Insulin glargine U-100	1 to 4 hr	None	24 hr

MEDICATIONS

- Insulin is used to manage type 1 diabetes.
- The rate of onset, peak, and duration of action varies for each different type of insulin.

Insulin pumps
- Delivers a programmed amount of insulin on a consistent basis.
- Boluses can be administered before meals.

Insulin injections
- Self-administered injections two or more times per day.
- Mixing insulin: usually rapid-and intermediate-acting

NURSING ACTIONS
- Do not mix insulin glargine with other insulin due to incompatibility.
- Observe the child and/or parent drawing up and administering the insulin injection, and offer additional instruction as indicated.
- Observe the child and/or parent using the insulin pump and offer additional instruction as indicated.

CLIENT EDUCATION
Perform self-administration of insulin.
- Rotate injection sites (prevents lipohypertrophy) within one anatomic site four or six injections before switching to another anatomic site (prevents day-to-day changes in absorption rates).
- Inject at a 90° angle. (Use pinch technique if skin is thin.) Aspiration for blood is not necessary.
- When mixing a rapid- or short-acting insulin with a longer-acting insulin, draw up the shorter-acting insulin into the syringe first and then the longer-acting insulin (this reduces the risk of introducing the longer-acting insulin into the vial of the shorter-acting insulin).

INTERPROFESSIONAL CARE

- Refer the child and family to a diabetes nurse educator for comprehensive education in diabetes management.
- Referrals often include pediatric endocrinologist, nutritionist, and exercise physiologist.
- School teachers, school nurses, guidance counselors, and coaches should also be involved.

COMPLICATIONS

Diabetic ketoacidosis (DKA)

- DKA is an acute, life-threatening condition characterized by hyperglycemia (greater than 330 mg/dL), glycosuria, and acidosis (pH 7.30 and bicarbonate 15 mmol/L), resulting in the breakdown of body fat for energy and an accumulation of ketones from the blood, urine, and lungs. The onset is rapid, and the mortality rate is high.
- Causes of DKA include insufficient insulin, acute stress, and poor management of acute illness.

NURSING ACTIONS
- Admit the child to an intensive care unit.
  - Place the child on a cardiac monitor.
  - Obtain venous access for administration of fluids, electrolytes, and insulin.
- Assess subjective and objective data for DKA.
  - Ketone levels in the blood and urine
  - Blood glucose levels
  - Labs: glucose, electrolytes, BUN, ABG, CBC
  - Fruity scent to the breath
  - Mental confusion
  - Dyspnea
  - Nausea and vomiting
  - Dehydration
  - Weight loss
  - Electrolyte imbalances
  - Untreated: Coma, which can progress to death
- Provide rapid isotonic fluid (0.9% sodium chloride) replacement to maintain perfusion to vital organs. Large quantities are often required to replace losses. Monitor for evidence of fluid volume excess and cerebral edema.
- When blood glucose levels approach 250 mg/dL, add glucose to IV fluids in order to maintain 120 to 240 mg/dL blood glucose levels. Administer regular insulin continuously through an IV infusion at 0.1 unit/kg/hr.
- Monitor glucose levels hourly, or more frequently if required.

- Monitor blood potassium levels. Potassium levels will initially be elevated. With insulin therapy, potassium will shift into cells and the child will need to be monitored for hypokalemia. Provide potassium replacement therapy in IV fluids as indicated by laboratory values. Make sure urinary output is adequate before administering potassium.
- Administer sodium bicarbonate by slow IV infusion for severe acidosis (pH less than 7.0). Monitor potassium levels because a correction of acidosis that occurs too quickly can lead to hypokalemia. Monitor closely for changes in level of consciousness.
- Administer oxygen to children who are cyanotic and whose arterial oxygen level is less than 80%.

CLIENT EDUCATION: Reinforce instructions to manage diabetes. Qᴘᴄᴄ

Long-term complications

- Kidney disease
- Eye disease
- Neurologic complications

Active Learning Scenario

A nurse is teaching the parents of a school-age child who has type 1 diabetes mellitus. Use the ATI Active Learning Template: System Disorder to complete this item.

ALTERATION IN HEALTH (DIAGNOSIS)

MEDICATIONS: List the types of insulin used for children who have type 1 diabetes mellitus.

NURSING CARE: Describe eight interventions.

CLIENT EDUCATION: Describe three client outcomes.

Application Exercises

1. Sort the following clinical manifestation into the correct category: Hypoglycemia or Hyperglycemia
   A. Diaphoresis
   B. Diminished reflexes
   C. Fruity breath odor
   D. Irritability
   E. Pallor
   F. Polyuria
   G. Tachycardia
   H. Thirst
   I. Tremors
   J. Warm, dry skin

2. A nurse is reviewing sick-day management with a parent of a child who has type 1 diabetes mellitus. Which of the following should the nurse include in the teaching?(Select all that apply.)
   A. Monitor blood glucose levels every 3 hr.
   B. Discontinue taking insulin until feeling better.
   C. Drink 8 oz of fruit juice every hour.
   D. Test urine for ketones.
   E. Call the provider if blood glucose is greater than 240 mg/dL.

3. A nurse is teaching a child who has type 1 diabetes mellitus about self-care. Which of the following statements by the child indicates understanding of the teaching?
   A. "I should skip breakfast when I am not hungry."
   B. "I should increase my insulin with exercise."
   C. "I should drink a glass of milk when I am feeling irritable."
   D. "I should draw up the NPH insulin into the syringe before the regular insulin."

4. A nurse is teaching a school-age child who has diabetes mellitus about insulin administration. Which of the following should the nurse include in the teaching?
   A. "You should inject the needle at a 30-degree angle."
   B. "You should combine your glargine and regular insulin in the same syringe."
   C. "You should aspirate for blood before injecting the insulin."
   D. "You should give four to six injections in one area before switching sites."

5. A nurse is caring for a child who has type 1 diabetes mellitus. The nurse should recognize that which of the following are manifestations of diabetic ketoacidosis? (Select all that apply.)
   A. Blood glucose 58 mg/dL
   B. Weight gain
   C. Dehydration
   D. Mental confusion
   E. Fruity breath

Application Exercises Key

1. **HYPOGLYCEMIA:** A, D, E, G, I;
   HYPERGLYCEMIA: B, C, F, H, J

   Manifestation of hypoglycemia include pallor, irritability, tremors, diaphoresis, and tachycardia. Manifestations of hyperglycemia include thirst, warm, dry skin, polyuria, fruity breath odor, and diminished reflexes.

   (N) *NCLEX® Connection: Reduction of Risk Potential, System–Specific Assessments*

2. A, D, E. **CORRECT:** When taking action while reviewing sick day management with the parent of a child who has type 1 diabetes mellitus, the nurse should instruct the parent to monitor the blood glucose every three hours to help identify hyperglycemic or hypoglycemic episodes. The nurse should also instruct the parent to test the urine for ketones to assist in early detection of ketoacidosis. Additionally, the parent should be instructed to notify the provider of blood glucose levels greater than 240 mg/dL to obtain further instructions in caring for the hyperglycemia.
   B. A child who is experiencing illness should continue taking insulin during to prevent hyperglycemic episodes.
   C. A child who is experiencing illness should drink fluids without sugars.

   (N) *NCLEX® Connection: Physiological Adaptation, Alterations in Body Systems*

3. A. A child who has diabetes should eat three meals per day with snacks and avoid skipping meals to prevent hypoglycemic episodes.
   B. The insulin requirements of a child who has type 1 diabetes will decrease with exercise. Increasing the amount of insulin with exercise could precipitate a hypoglycemic episode.
   C. **CORRECT:** When evaluating the outcomes of teaching during the care of a child who has type 1 diabetes mellitus, the nurse should identify that the statement, "I should drink a glass of milk when I am feeling irritable" indicates understanding of the teaching. Irritability is an early manifestation of hypoglycemia. A glass of milk contains approximately 15 g of carbohydrates and will help prevent worsening of the hypoglycemia.
   D. Regular insulin should be drawn up into the syringe prior to drawing up NPH to avoid altering the regular insulin.

   (N) *NCLEX® Connection: Physiological Adaptation, Alterations in Body Systems*

4. A. Instruct the child to inject the needle at a 90° angle.
   B. Instruct the child to not mix glargine with any other insulin due to incompatibility.
   C. Instruct the child that it is not necessary to aspirate for blood prior to administering insulin.
   D. **CORRECT:** When taking action during the care of a school-aged child who has diabetes mellitus, the nurse should instruct the child to administer four to six injections in one area, about 2.5 cm (1 in) apart before switching to another site.

   (N) *NCLEX® Connection: Pharmacological and Parenteral Therapies, Medication Administration*

5. C, D, E. **CORRECT:** When analyzing cues during the care of a child who has type 1 diabetes mellitus, the nurse should recognize that dehydration, mental confusion, and a fruity odor to the breath are manifestations of diabetic ketoacidosis.
   A. Diabetic ketoacidosis is classified as a blood glucose level greater than 300 mg/dL.
   B. Children who have diabetic ketoacidosis display weight loss.

   (N) *NCLEX® Connection: Physiological Adaptation, Medical Emergencies*

Active Learning Scenario Key

Using the ATI Active Learning Template: System Disorder

ALTERATION IN HEALTH (DIAGNOSIS): Diabetes mellitus is characterized by a partial or complete metabolic deficiency of insulin.

MEDICATIONS
- Insulin lispro: Rapid-acting
- Regular insulin: Short-acting
- NPH insulin: Intermediate-acting
- Insulin glargine U-100: Long-acting

NURSING CARE
- Monitor for manifestations of hyperglycemia and hypoglycemia.
- Provide nail care according to policy.
- Teach wound care.
- Provide nutritional guidelines.
- Encourage yearly eye exams.
- Encourage dental and medical follow-up.
- Teach self-monitoring of blood glucose.
- Teach guidelines to follow when sick.
- Teach about medications.

CLIENT EDUCATION
- The child will have blood glucose levels within the prescribed range.
- The child will maintain a glycosylated hemoglobin within the target range.
- The child and/or family will be able to administer insulin.
- The child and/or family will be able to monitor for complications and intervene as necessary.
- The child and/or family will maintain adequate dietary intake to support growth and development.

(N) *NCLEX® Connection: Physiological Adaptation, Alterations in Body Systems*

CHAPTER 33 Growth Hormone Deficiency

Human growth hormone (GH), somatotropin, is a naturally occurring substance that is secreted by the pituitary gland. GH is important for normal growth, development, and cellular metabolism. A deficiency in GH prevents somatic growth throughout the body.

Other hormones that work with GH to control metabolic processes include adrenocorticotropic hormone (ACTH), thyroid stimulating hormone (TSH), and the gonadotropins: follicle-stimulating hormone (FSH) and luteinizing hormone (LH).

Hypopituitarism is the diminished or deficient secretion of pituitary hormones (primarily GH). Consequences of the condition depend on the degree of the deficiency.

ASSESSMENT

RISK FACTORS

- Structural factors (tumors, trauma, structural defects, surgery)
- Heredity disorders
- Other pituitary hormone deficiencies (deficiencies of TSH or ACTH)
- Most often, GH deficiencies are idiopathic

EXPECTED FINDINGS

PHYSICAL ASSESSMENT FINDINGS
- Short stature but proportional height and weight
- Delayed epiphyseal closure
- Increased insulin sensitivity
- Delayed or altered dentition
- Underdeveloped jaw
- Delayed sexual development
- Linear growth velocity consistently less than −1 standard deviation (SD) for age, or an absolute height of less than −2 SD

LABORATORY TESTS

Plasma insulin–like growth factor–1 (IGF–1) and IGF binding protein–3 (IGFBP–3) levels

Further evaluation is indicated if the values are one standard deviation below the mean for age.

NURSING ACTIONS
- Collect the appropriate amount of blood for the test.
- Explain the laboratory procedure to the family and child.

CLIENT EDUCATION: The child should fast the night before the test. Qpcc

DIAGNOSTIC PROCEDURES

GH stimulation

GH stimulation testing is generally done for children who have a low level of IGF–1 and IGFBP–3, and short stature.

NURSING ACTIONS
- Draw baseline blood sample between 0600 and 0800.
- Administer medication that triggers the release of GH (arginine or GH–releasing hormone).
- Obtain blood sample every 15–30 min for a 3-hr period following medication administration.

CLIENT EDUCATION
- Nothing to eat or drink 10 to 12 hr before the test.
- Limit activity 10 to 12 hr before the test.

Radiologic assessments

- Assess skeletal maturity by comparing epiphyseal centers to age–appropriate published standards.
- A general skeletal survey is done in children under 3 years of age; older children should have radiographs of the hands and wrists. This will provide information about growth as well as epiphyseal function.
- A series of skull films can detect structural abnormalities (small sella turcica).

NURSING ACTIONS: Assist in positioning the child.

Computed tomographic scanning, magnetic resonance imaging

Used to identify tumors or other brain lesions

NURSING ACTIONS: Monitor the child during the procedure.

CLIENT EDUCATION: Provide emotional support. Qpcc

Evaluation of the growth curve

NURSING ACTIONS
- Accurately obtain and plot height and weight measurements on an appropriate growth chart.
- Assess height velocity or height over time.
- Determine height-to-weight relationship.
- Project target height in context of genetic potential.

PATIENT-CENTERED CARE

NURSING CARE

- The child's height and weight are measured and marked on a growth chart as part of every visit to the provider.
  - The height of a child is more affected than weight. Bone age usually matches height age.
- Assess and monitor effectiveness of GH replacement. GH is supplied by recombinant DNA technology.
- Administer other hormone replacements (thyroid hormone) if prescribed.
- Provide support to the child and family regarding psychosocial concerns (altered body image, depression). Reassure the child and family that there are no cognitive delays or deficits.
- Stress the importance of maintaining realistic expectations based on the child's age and abilities.

MEDICATIONS

Somatropin

Used as human growth hormone replacement therapy when growth hormone deficiency is present. Stimulates growth of bone and skeletal muscle.

NURSING ACTIONS

- Administer the medication via subcutaneous injections into the abdomen, thigh, buttock, or back of upper arm.
- Use cautiously in children who are receiving insulin.
- Rotate injection sites to prevent tissue atrophy.
- Administer at bedtime to promote the effectiveness of the medication. (GH generally peaks during sleep.)

INTERPROFESSIONAL CARE

- Consult with an endocrinologist.
- Psychological counseling can be indicated to help the child and family cope during this period of time.

CLIENT EDUCATION

- There should not be any significant adverse effects when GH replacement therapy is used in appropriate doses for GH deficiency.
- GH will assist with muscle growth and help improve self-esteem.
- Understand how to administer medication by subcutaneous injection for home use. Qᴘᴄᴄ
- Instruct the child and parents that GH should be administered 6 to 7 days a week.
- Educate the parents on the need for compliance with injections.
- Encourage the child and family to seek evaluation during early adulthood to determine the need for continued replacement therapy.
- Child, family, and health care team make the decision to stop treatment together. If growth is not equal to or greater than 2.5 cm (1 inch)/year, treatment is discontinued.

COMPLICATIONS

GH deficiency without hormone replacement can result in disruption of vertical growth, delayed epiphyseal closure, delayed bone age, delayed sexual development, and premature aging later in life.

Application Exercises

1. A nurse is assessing a child who has short stature. Which of the following findings should the nurse identify as a manifestation of a growth hormone deficiency?

   A. Delayed or altered dentition

   B. Height proportionally greater than weight

   C. Oversized jaw

   D. Early-onset puberty

2. A nurse is caring for a child who has short stature and is being evaluated for growth hormone deficiency. Which of the following diagnostic tests should the nurse anticipate including in the plan of care? (Select all that apply.)

   A. CT scan of the head

   B. Skeletal x-rays

   C. GH stimulation test

   D. Serum IGF-1

   E. DNA

3. A nurse is caring for a school-age child who has GH deficiency. The child's asks the nurse how long the child will need to take growth hormone injections. Which of the following responses should the nurse make?

   A. "Injections are usually continued until age 10 for girls and age 12 for boys."

   B. "Injections continue until your child reaches the fifth percentile on the growth chart."

   C. "Injections might be stopped once your child grows less than 1 inch per year."

   D. "The injections will need to be administered throughout your child's entire life."

4. A nurse is providing education to the parents of a child who has a growth hormone deficiency. Which of the following should the nurse include in the teaching as complications of untreated growth hormone deficiency? (Select all that apply.)

   A. Delayed sexual development

   B. Premature aging

   C. Advanced bone age

   D. Short nature

   E. Increased epiphyseal closure

Active Learning Scenario

A nurse is planning care for a child who is to undergo a growth hormone (GH) stimulation test. What interventions should the nurse include in the plan of care? Use the ATI Active Learning Template: Nursing Skill to complete this item.

NURSING INTERVENTIONS: Include two preprocedure nursing actions and three intraprocedure actions.

Active Learning Scenario Key

Using the ATI Active Learning Template: Nursing Skill
NURSING INTERVENTIONS

Preprocedure
- Ensure child has nothing to eat or drink 10 to 12 hr prior to procedure.
- Limit child's activity 10 to 12 hr prior to procedure.

Intraprocedure
- Draw baseline blood sample between 0600 and 0800.
- Administer medication that triggers the release of GH (arginine or GH-releasing hormone).
- Obtain blood sample every 30 min during a 3-hr period following medication administration.

Ⓝ *NCLEX® Connection: Reduction of Risk Potential, Diagnostic Tests*

Application Exercises Key

1. A. **CORRECT:** When analyzing cues during the assessment of a child who has a short stature, the nurse should identify delayed or altered dentition as a manifestation of growth hormone deficiency. component to the short stature.
   B. Height greater than weight is unexpected.
   C. An underdeveloped jaw is an expected finding.
   D. Delayed sexual development is an expected finding.

Ⓝ *NCLEX® Connection: Reduction of Risk Potential, Diagnostic Tests*

2. A, B, C, D. **CORRECT:** When generating solutions for the care of a child who has short stature and is being evaluated for growth hormone deficiency, the nurse should anticipate including a CT of the head, skeletal x-rays, a GH stimulation test, and a serum IGF-1 test into the plan of care. A CT scan of the head is conducted to determine whether there is a structural component to the short stature. Skeletal x-rays are conducted to determine the development of the bones. A GH stimulation test is conducted to confirm diagnosis of GH deficiency. A serum IGF-1 is obtained as a preliminary test to determine GH deficiency. DNA testing is not a diagnostic test to determine GH deficiency.

Ⓝ *NCLEX® Connection: Physiological Adaptation, Pathophysiology*

3. A. Standards for stopping therapy include a bone age of more than 14 years for females or more than 16 years for males.
   B. While the child's growth is tracked on growth charts, stopping treatment is not based on percentile markings.
   C. **CORRECT:** When taking action during the care of a child who has GH deficiency, the nurse should instruct the parent that the child will need to continue growth hormone injections until the child growth slows to less than 2.5 cm (1 in) per year.
   D. Injections are stopped once sufficient growth is obtained, which will be variable among clients.

Ⓝ *NCLEX® Connection: Pharmacological and Parenteral Therapies, Medication Administration*

4. A, B, D. **CORRECT:** When taking action and providing education to the parents of a child who has a growth hormone deficiency, the nurse should include in the teaching that complications of untreated growth hormone deficiency include delayed sexual development, premature aging, and short stature. A complication of untreated growth hormone deficiency includes delayed bone age. A complication of untreated growth hormone deficiency includes delayed epiphyseal closure.

Ⓝ *NCLEX® Connection: Physiological Adaptation, Pathophysiology*

NCLEX® Connections

When reviewing the following chapters, keep in mind the relevant topics and tasks of the NCLEX outline, in particular:

Basic Care and Comfort

NONPHARMACOLOGICAL COMFORT INTERVENTIONS: Provide nonpharmacological comfort measures.

Safety and Infection Control

STANDARD PRECAUTIONS/TRANSMISSION-BASED PRECAUTIONS/SURGICAL ASEPSIS
Understand communicable diseases and the modes of organism transmission.

Apply principles of infection control.

Health Promotion and Maintenance

HEALTH PROMOTION/DISEASE PREVENTION
Inform the client of appropriate immunization schedules.

Educate client about health promotion and maintenance recommendations.

Assist the client in maintaining an optimum level of health.

Physiological Adaptation

ALTERATIONS IN BODY SYSTEMS
Identify signs, symptoms, and incubation periods of infectious diseases.

Apply knowledge of nursing procedures, pathophysiology, and psychomotor skills when caring for a client who has an alteration in body systems.

ILLNESS MANAGEMENT: Implement interventions to manage the client's recovery from an illness.

Pharmacological and Parenteral Therapies

ADVERSE EFFECTS/CONTRAINDICATIONS/ SIDE EFFECTS/INTERACTIONS
Identify a contraindication to the administration of a medication to the client.

Provide information to the client on common side effects/ adverse effects/potential interactions of medications and inform the client when to notify the primary health care provider.

Reduction of Risk Potential

POTENTIAL FOR ALTERATIONS IN BODY SYSTEMS:
Compare current client data to baseline client data.

POTENTIAL FOR COMPLICATIONS FROM SURGICAL PROCEDURES AND HEALTH ALTERATIONS: Apply knowledge
of pathophysiology to monitoring for complications.

CHAPTER 34

CHAPTER 34 *Immunizations*

Administration of a vaccine stimulates the immune system to produce antibodies against a specific disease. Vaccines contain the infectious organism, but it is either killed or weakened to prevent causing the disease. Antibodies disappear after they destroy the infection/antigen, but memory cells are formed to protect from future exposures to that same infection. This builds immunity against that antigen to protect against future exposure.

The Advisory Committee on Immunization Practices (ACIP) makes recommendations and creates guidelines regarding immunizations. Children who are born preterm should receive the dose of each vaccine according to the immunization schedule. The most up-to-date information can be found at the Centers for Disease Control and Prevention website.

CHILDHOOD IMMUNIZATIONS

For children who have missed scheduled immunizations, use the "catch-up" schedule located on the CDC website. (34.1)

PURPOSE

- Decrease or eliminate certain infectious diseases in society.
- Prevent infectious diseases and their complications.

34.1 Childhood immunizations

	MINIMUM AGE	NUMBER OF DOSES	SCHEDULE	CONSIDERATIONS
HEPATITIS B (HEPB)	Birth	Three	Birth 1 to 2 months 6 to 18 months	Minimum of 4 weeks between doses one and two. Minimum of 8 weeks between doses two and three. Final dose no earlier than age of 24 weeks of age and at least 16 weeks after first dose. Should be withheld for infants born prematurely and weighing less than 2,000 g if the mother is negative for hepatitis B.
ROTAVIRUS (RV)	6 weeks	Two (RV1) or Three (RV5)	2 and 4 months (Rotarix [RV1]) or 2, 4, and 6 months (RotaTeq [RV5])	Maximum age for the first dose is 24 weeks, 6 days. Maximum age for the last dose is 8 months, 0 days. Series should not be initiated for children 15 weeks, 0 days or older.
DIPHTHERIA, TETANUS, AND ACELLULAR PERTUSSIS (DTAP)	6 weeks	Five	2 months 4 months 6 months 15 to 18 months 4 to 6 years	Minimum of 6 months between doses three and four. Dose four can be given as early as 12 months of age Dose five dose is not needed if dose four was given at 4 years of age or older.
TETANUS, DIPHTHERIA, AND ACELLULAR PERTUSSIS (TDAP); TETANUS AND DIPHTHERIA (TD)	11 years	One (Tdap) Every 10 years (Td)	11 to 12 years then Booster every 10 years (Td)	Administer one dose to adolescents who are pregnant (with each pregnancy) regardless of timing of previous Td or Tdap vaccine (between 27 and 36 weeks of gestation). Booster with Td every 10 years after administration of Tdap. Administer Tdap or Td according to recommendations for wounds. If wound is minor and clean and more than 10 years have elapsed since last tetanus dose, administer Tdap or Td. For all other wounds, Tdap or Td should be administered if greater than 5 years have elapsed.

	MINIMUM AGE	NUMBER OF DOSES	SCHEDULE	CONSIDERATIONS
HAEMOPHILUS INFLUENZAE TYPE B (HIB)	6 weeks	Four 4: Hib (PRP-T) or Three 3: Hib (PRP-OMP)	2 months 4 months 6 months (only if four-dose series) 12 to 15 months (booster dose with any Hib-containing vaccine)	Administer Hiberix as a booster dose at 12 months to 4 years of age only if a prior dose of Hib was received. Only 1 dose is recommended for children who are 15 months of age or older, and not immunized.
PNEUMOCOCCAL CONJUGATE (PCV13)	6 weeks	Four	2 months 4 months 6 months 12 to 15 months	Follow current recommendations for dual vaccination series with PCV13 and PPSV23 for children who have high-risk conditions.
INACTIVATED POLIOVIRUS (IPV)	6 weeks	Four	2 months 4 months 6 to 18 months 4 to 6 years	Final dose should be administered on or after the age of 4 years and at least 6 months from the previous dose.
INACTIVATED INFLUENZA VACCINE (IIV)	6 months	Yearly	Yearly	Must be 2 years or older to receive live, attenuated influenza vaccine (LAIV). Children who have medical conditions that predispose them to influenza should not receive LAIV. Administer starting with availability, usually in early fall. Administration recommendations can change yearly because the vaccine is created with different influenza strains each year.
MEASLES, MUMPS, RUBELLA (MMR)	12 months	Two	12 to 15 months 4 to 6 years	Administer one dose to infants age 6 to 11 months if traveling internationally. However, a two-dose series is still recommended starting at 12 to 15 months. Dose two of the series can be given prior to the age of 4 years if it has been at least 4 weeks since the first dose.
VARICELLA (VAR)	12 months	Two	12 to 15 months 4 to 6 years	Dose two of the series can be given prior to the age of 4 years if it has been at least 3 months since the first dose.
HEPATITIS A (HEPA)	12 months	Two	12 to 23 months 6 to 18 months following	Administer the final dose 6 to 18 months after the first. Two-dose series is recommended for anyone over the age of 2 years who needs immunity to hepatitis A virus.
MENINGOCOCCAL CONJUGATE (MENACWY)	2 months (MenACWY-CRM) 9 months (MenACWY-D)	One	11 to 12 years 16 years (booster)	Follow recommendations for earlier administration to children who have high-risk conditions or who travel to areas with hyperendemic or epidemic rates of meningococcal disease.
MENINGOCOCCAL (MENB)	10 years	Two or three dose series	16 to 18 years	Maximum age 23 years. Administer 2 doses of Bexsero at least 1 month apart. Trumenba is given in 2 doses at least 6 months apart; clients who have certain risk factors should receive 3 doses of Trumenba at 0, 1 to 2 months, and 6 months time spacing.
HUMAN PAPILLOMAVIRUS (HPV)	9 years	Two or three dose series	11 to 12 years 6 to 12 months following	If first dose is administered prior to 15 years of age, administer 2 doses. The 2nd dose should be administered at 6-12 months, after the first dose. If first dose administered after 15 years of age, administer a total of 3 doses. The 2nd dose should be administered 1-2 months after the first dose. The 3rd dose should be administered within 6 months of the 2nd dose.

34.2 Immunization considerations

	ADVERSE EFFECTS	CONTRAINDICATIONS	PRECAUTIONS
DTAP	**Mild** • Redness, swelling, and tenderness at the injection site • Poor appetite • Vomiting • Low fever • Behavioral changes (drowsiness, irritability, anorexia) **Moderate** • Inconsolable crying for 3 hr or more • Fever 40.6° C (105° F) or higher • Seizures (with or without fever) • Shock-like state **Severe:** Acute encephalopathy (rare)	Occurrence of encephalopathy within 7 days following prior doses of the vaccine	Occurrence of Guillain-Barré syndrome within 6 weeks of prior dose of tetanus toxoid Progressive neurologic disorders; uncontrolled seizures Acute illness that is moderate/severe with or without fever
HIB	Redness, swelling, warmth, and tenderness at the injection site Fever greater than 37.8° C (101° F), vomiting, diarrhea, and crying	Age younger than 6 weeks	
RV	Irritability Mild, temporary diarrhea or vomiting Intussusception	History of intussusception Severe combined immunodeficiency (SCID), which is a rare disorder that is inherited	Chronic gastrointestinal disease Spina bifida Bladder exstrophy Immunocompromised (other than SCID)
MMR	Mild: Local reactions (rash; fever; swollen glands in cheeks and/or neck) **Moderate** • Pain at the site of the injection • Joint pain and stiffness lasting for days to weeks • Febrile seizure • Low platelet count **Severe** • Transient thrombocytopenia	Pregnancy Immunodeficiency	History of thrombocytopenia or thrombocytopenic purpura Anaphylactic reaction to eggs, gelatin, or neomycin Transfusion with blood product containing antibodies within the prior 3 months Simultaneous tuberculin skin testing
VAR	**Mild** • Tenderness and swelling at injection site • Fever • Rash (mild) possible for up to 1 month after vaccination **Moderate:** Seizures **Severe** • Pneumonia • Low blood count (extremely rare) • Severe brain reactions (extremely rare)	Pregnancy Anaphylactic reaction to gelatin or neomycin Immunodeficiency	Transfusion with blood product containing antibodies within the prior 3 to 11 months Treatment with antiviral medication within 24 hr prior to immunization (avoid taking antivirals for 14 days following immunization) Treatment with immunosuppressants (corticosteroids) for 2 weeks or longer Cancer Aspirin or products containing aspirin
PCV13	Swelling, redness and tenderness at site of injection Fever Irritability Drowsiness Anorexia Headache Chills	Anaphylactic reaction to any vaccine containing diphtheria toxoid	

		ADVERSE EFFECTS	CONTRAINDICATIONS	PRECAUTIONS
HEPA		Tenderness at the injection site Headache Anorexia Malaise Low grade fever	Severe allergy to latex	
HEPB		Tenderness at the injection site Temperature of 37.7° C (99.9° F) or higher	Anaphylactic allergy to yeast	Infant weight less than 2 kg (4 lb, 6.4 oz)
IIV		• Swelling, redness and tenderness at the injection site • Hoarseness • Fever • Malaise • Headache • Cough • Aches Severe: • Increased risk for Guillain-Barré syndrome • Increased risk of seizures in young children receiving PCV13 and/or DTaP simultaneously		Occurrence of Guillain-Barré syndrome within 6 weeks of prior influenza vaccine The CDC currently recommends that a client who has a history of egg allergy can receive any recommended and age-appropriate influenza vaccine, regardless of the severity of the allergy. The vaccine should be administered in a medical setting by a provider who can recognize and respond to severe allergic reactions. Moderate or severe acute illness The CDC and ACIP currently recommend that children who have a history of an egg allergy may receive any approved, age-appropriate influenza vaccine. Those who have a history of severe egg allergy should receive their immunization in a medical setting in which manifestations of severe allergic reaction can be recognized and managed in a timely manner.
LAIV		Vomiting, diarrhea Cough Fever Headache Myalgia Nasal congestion, runny nose Wheezing	2-4 years of age with history of asthma or wheezing Pregnancy	Occurrence of Guillain-Barré syndrome within 6 weeks of prior influenza vaccine History of asthma for greater than 5 years Treatment with antiviral medication within 48 hr prior to immunization (avoid taking antivirals for 14 day following immunization) Certain chronic conditions The CDC and ACIP currently recommend that children who have a history of an egg allergy may receive any approved, age-appropriate influenza vaccine. Those who have a history of severe egg allergy should receive their immunization in a medical setting in which manifestations of severe allergic reaction can be recognized and managed in a timely manner.
MENACWY		Redness and tenderness at the injection site Fever		
MENB		Injection site pain Headache Fatigue Muscle pain	Prior hypersensitivity Bexsero: latex allergy (prefilled syringes contain latex)	Use Bexsero in pregnancy only if clearly indicated; add client to pregnancy registry. Trumenba safety is not established for children under 10 years of age.
HPV9		Redness, swelling and tenderness at the injection site Mild to moderate fever Headache Fainting (shortly after receiving the vaccine)	Severe allergy to yeast	Pregnancy
IPV		Tenderness at the injection site	Anaphylactic reaction to neomycin, streptomycin or polymyxin B	Pregnancy

CONTRAINDICATIONS, AND PRECAUTIONS

- A severe allergic reaction (anaphylaxis) can occur in response to any vaccine and is a contraindication for receiving further doses of that vaccine or other vaccines containing that substance. Qᴇʙᴘ
- Moderate or severe illnesses with or without fever are precautions to receiving immunizations.
- The common cold and other minor illnesses are not contraindications to immunizations.
- Severe febrile illness is a contraindication to all immunizations.
- Do not administer live virus vaccines (varicella or MMR) to a child who is severely immunocompromised, pregnant, or has received treatment that provides acquired passive immunity (blood products) within 11 months.
- Precautions to immunizations require providers to analyze data and weigh the risks that come with immunizing or not immunizing. (34.2)

NURSING ADMINISTRATION

- Ensure consent has been obtained from the child's guardian prior to administration.
- Prior to administration, provide vaccine information sheets (VIS) and review the content with guardians and older children. Include the publication date of each VIS given in documentation.
- Reassure guardians that there is no association of autism with the MMR vaccine.
- Give IM immunizations in the vastus lateralis or ventrogluteal muscle in infants and young children, and into the deltoid muscle for older children and adolescents.
- Give subcutaneous injections in the outer aspect of the upper arm or anterolateral thigh.
- Select needle size based on the route, site, age, and amount of medication. Adequate needle length reduces the incidence of swelling and tenderness at the injection site. Qᴘᴄᴄ
- Use strategies to minimize discomfort.
  - Provide distraction.
  - Apply a topical anesthetic prior to injection.
  - Give infants a concentrated oral sucrose solution 2 min prior to, during, and 3 min after immunization administration.
  - Use non-nutritive sucking (pacifiers) during procedure.
- Have emergency medications and equipment on standby in case the child experiences an allergic response (anaphylaxis [rare]).
- Encourage caregivers to use comforting measures during and after the procedure (applying cool compresses to injection site, gentle movement of involved extremity).
- Provide praise afterward.
- Apply a colorful bandage, if appropriate.

- Document the administration of the vaccine.
  - Date, route, and site of immunization
  - Type, manufacturer, lot number, and expiration date of the vaccine
  - Evidence of informed consent from the guardian
  - Name, address and title of administering nurse
- Encourage guardian to maintain up-to-date immunizations for the child.
- Instruct guardians to avoid administering aspirin to the child to treat fever or local reaction following administration of a live virus vaccine due to the risk of developing Reye syndrome.
- Instruct the family to observe for complications and notify the provider if adverse effects occur.
- Report any adverse reactions to the Vaccine Adverse Event Reporting System (VAERS).

NURSING EVALUATION OF MEDICATION EFFECTIVENESS

Depending on therapeutic intent, effectiveness can be evidenced by the following.

- Improvement of local reaction to immunization with absence of pain, fever, and swelling at the site of injection
- Development of immunity

Active Learning Scenario

A nurse is preparing to administer LAIV, 9v-HPV, and MenACWY to a 12 year-old client. Use the ATI Active Learning Template: Medication to complete this item.

COMPLICATIONS: Include adverse effects for each vaccine.

Active Learning Scenario Key

Using the ATI Active Learning Template: Medication
COMPLICATIONS

LAIV
- Allergic reaction
- Vomiting and/or diarrhea
- Cough
- Fever
- Headache
- Myalgia
- Nasal congestion/runny nose

9v-HPV
- Redness, swelling and tenderness at the injection site
- Mild to moderate fever
- Headache
- Fatigue
- Fainting (shortly after receiving the vaccine)

MᴇɴACWY
- Allergic reaction
- Redness and tenderness at the injection site
- Fever

Ⓝ *NCLEX® Connection: Health Promotion and Maintenance, Health Promotion/Disease Prevention*

Application Exercises

1. A nurse is planning to administer recommended immunizations to a 2-month-old infant. Which of the following vaccines should the nurse plan to give? (Select all that apply.)

   A. Rotavirus (RV)

   B. Diphtheria, tetanus, and acellular pertussis (DTaP)

   C. *Haemophilus influenzae* type b (Hib)

   D. Hepatitis A (HepA)

   E. Pneumococcal conjugate (PCV13)

   F. Inactivated poliovirus (IPV)

2. A nurse is planning to administer recommended immunizations to a 4-year-old child. Which of the following vaccines should the nurse plan to give? (Select all that apply.)

   A. Inactivated poliovirus (IPV)

   B. *Haemophilus influenzae* type b (Hib)

   C. Measles, mumps, rubella (MMR)

   D. Varicella (VAR)

   E. Hepatitis B (HepB)

   F. Diphtheria, tetanus, and acellular pertussis (DTaP)

3. A nurse is preparing to administer the varicella vaccine to an adolescent. Which of the following questions should the nurse ask to determine whether there is a contraindication to administering the vaccine?

   A. "Do you have an allergy to eggs?"

   B. "Have you ever had encephalopathy following immunizations?"

   C. "Are you currently taking corticosteroid medication?"

   D. "Have you ever had an anaphylactic reaction to yeast?"

4. A nurse is caring for a 15-month-old child in a clinic. Based on the chart below, which of the following actions should the nurse take?

IMMUNIZATION RECORD

HepB: 1 month, 2 months, 12 months

Rotavirus: 2 months, 4 months, 6 months

DTaP: 2 months, 4 months, 6 months

Hib: 2 months, 4 months, 12 months

IPV: 2 months, 4 months, 6 months

MMR: 12 months

Varicella: 12 months

HepA: 12 months

NURSES NOTES

Temperature: 37.8° C (100.1° F)

Sore throat

Family history of seizures

   A. Administer DTaP vaccine.

   B. Administer rotavirus vaccine.

   C. Hold immunizations until fever subsides.

   D. Administer hepatitis A vaccine.

5. A nurse is preparing to administer immunizations to a 4-month-old infant. Which of the following actions should the nurse take to provide atraumatic care?

   A. Administer 81 mg of aspirin.

   B. Use the Z-track method when injecting.

   C. Ask the parents to leave the room during the injection.

   D. Provide sucrose solution on the pacifier.

Application Exercises Key

1. A. **CORRECT:** RV is given as a two-or three-dose series starting at 2 months of age.
   B. **CORRECT:** DTaP is given as a five-dose series starting at 2 months of age.
   C. **CORRECT:** Hib is given as a three-or four-dose series starting at 2 months of age.
   D. HepA is given as a two-dose series starting at 12 months of age.
   E. **CORRECT:** PCV13 is given as a four-dose series starting at 2 months of age.
   F. **CORRECT:** IPV is given as a four-dose series starting at 2 months of age.

   Ⓝ *NCLEX® Connection: Health Promotion and Maintenance, Health Promotion/Disease Prevention*

2. A. **CORRECT:** Four doses of IPV are given during childhood with a dose given at 4 years of age.
   B. The series of Hib vaccines is complete by the age of 15 months.
   C. **CORRECT:** Two doses of MMR are given during childhood with a dose given at 4 years of age.
   D. **CORRECT:** Two doses of VAR are given during childhood with a dose given at 4 years of age.
   E. The series of HepB vaccines is complete by the age of 18 months.
   F. **CORRECT:** Five doses of DTaP are given during childhood with a dose given at 4 years of age.

   Ⓝ *NCLEX® Connection: Health Promotion and Maintenance, Health Promotion/Disease Prevention*

3. A. The varicella vaccine is contraindicated for clients who have an allergy to gelatin or neomycin.
   B. DTaP vaccine is contraindicated for clients who have a history of encephalopathy within 7 days following prior doses of the vaccine.
   C. **CORRECT:** Varicella vaccine is contraindicated for clients who have been taking corticosteroids or other medications that affect the immune system for 2 weeks or longer.
   D. HepB vaccine is contraindicated for clients who have had an anaphylactic reaction to yeast.

   Ⓝ *NCLEX® Connection: Pharmacological and Parenteral Therapies, Adverse Effects/Contraindications/Interactions*

4. A. **CORRECT:** Five diphtheria, tetanus, and acellular pertussis immunizations are given during childhood, with one at 15 months of age.
   B. This child completed the three-dose rotavirus vaccine series at age 6 months.
   C. Temperature of 37.8° C (100.1° F) is not a contraindication to administering immunizations.
   D. Two hepatitis A immunizations are given during childhood, with the second one 6 to 18 months after the first.

5. A. Administering aspirin to the infant can increase the risk for developing Reye syndrome.
   B. Using the Z-track method is not recommended with immunizations.
   C. Separating the caregivers from the infant can produce anxiety in the infant.
   D. **CORRECT:** Allowing an infant to suck on a pacifier with sucrose solution can decrease pain with immunizations and is an appropriate action for the nurse to take in providing atraumatic care.

   Ⓝ *NCLEX® Connection: Basic Care and Comfort, Non–Pharmacological Comfort Interventions*

UNIT 2   SYSTEM DISORDERS

SECTION: IMMUNE AND INFECTIOUS DISORDERS

CHAPTER 35

Communicable Diseases

Communicable diseases are spread through airborne, droplet, or direct contact transmission. Most communicable diseases can be prevented with immunizations.

Antibiotics and antitoxins reduce serious complications. Primary prevention refers to immunizations. Secondary prevention controls the spread of the disease to others.

See immunization recommendations at the CDC website.

HEALTH PROMOTION AND DISEASE PREVENTION

Conjunctivitis

SPREAD: Direct contact (viral and bacterial)

INCUBATION: Depends on the infection

COMMUNICABILITY
- Viral: Appears secondary to a viral infection; starts in one eye, spreads to the other; clears on its own in 7 to 14 days.
- Bacterial: Clears with topical antibiotics.
- Allergic: Occurs in people who have other allergic conditions; clears with allergy medications.

ISOLATION PRECAUTIONS
- Viral conjunctivitis: Contact
- Bacterial conjunctivitis: Standard

Infectious mononucleosis/Epstein Barr virus

SPREAD: Oral secretions

INCUBATION: 30 to 50 days

COMMUNICABILITY
- Healthy people can carry EBV in saliva, transmitting the virus for a lifetime.
- People who have mononucleosis can transmit for weeks.

ISOLATION PRECAUTIONS: Standard

Erythema infectiosum (fifth disease)/parvovirus B19

SPREAD
- Respiratory secretions
- Transfusion of blood or blood products

INCUBATION: 4 to 14 days, sometimes up to 21 days

COMMUNICABILITY: Onset of manifestations before rash appears

ISOLATION PRECAUTIONS: Droplet

Mumps/paramyxovirus

SPREAD: Direct contact with respiratory droplets

INCUBATION: 14 to 21 days

COMMUNICABILITY: Immediately before and after swelling begins

ISOLATION PRECAUTIONS: Droplet

Pertussis (whooping cough)/Bordetella pertussis

SPREAD
- Direct or indirect contact with respiratory secretions
- Droplet
- Indirect contact with freshly contaminated articles

INCUBATION: 6 to 20 days, usually 7 to 10 days

COMMUNICABILITY: Greatest during catarrhal stage before onset of paroxysmal stage

ISOLATION PRECAUTIONS: Droplet

Rubella (German measles)/rubella virus

SPREAD: Direct or indirect contact with respiratory secretions

INCUBATION: 14 to 21 days

COMMUNICABILITY: 7 days before to 5 days after the rash appears

ISOLATION PRECAUTIONS: Droplet

Rubeola (measles)/rubeola virus

SPREAD: Direct or indirect contact with respiratory secretions

INCUBATION: 10 to 20 days

COMMUNICABILITY: 4 days before to 5 days after the rash appears

ISOLATION PRECAUTIONS: Airborne

Varicella (chickenpox)/varicella-zoster virus

SPREAD
- Direct or indirect contact with respiratory secretions
- Contact with contaminated objects

INCUBATION: 2 to 3 weeks, usually 14 to 16 days

COMMUNICABILITY: 1 to 2 days before lesions appear until all lesions have formed crusts

ISOLATION PRECAUTIONS
- Airborne
- Contact

ASSESSMENT

RISK FACTORS

- History of communicable disease
- Immunocompromised status
- Crowded living conditions
- Poor sanitation
- Poor nutrition
- Poor oxygenation and impaired circulation
- Chronic illness
- Recent exposure to a known case of a communicable disease
- Not immunized or up-to-date on immunizations
- Prodromal manifestations

EXPECTED FINDINGS

Conjunctivitis

- Pink or red color in the sclera of the eyes
- Swelling of the conjunctiva
- Excessive tearing
- Yellow-green, purulent discharge from the eyes (bacterial)
- Crusting of the eyelids in the morning (bacterial)
- Watery eye discharge (viral)

Fifth disease (Erythema infectiosum)

BEFORE RASH (SEVERAL DAYS): Fever, runny nose, headache

RASH (7 DAYS TO SEVERAL WEEKS)
- Red rash on face (slapped cheek) which appears from day 1 to 4
- Maculopapular red spots symmetrically distributed on upper and lower extremities progressing proximal to distal surfaces through 1 week
- Secondary itchy rash that can appear on rest of body, especially on the soles of the feet

Measles (rubeola)

3 TO 4 DAYS PRIOR TO RASH
- Mild to moderate fever
- Conjunctivitis
- Fatigue
- Cough, runny nose, red eyes, sore throat

RASH
- Koplik spots (tiny white spots) appear in mouth 2 days before rash
- Red or reddish-brown rash beginning on the face spreading downward
- Spike in fever with rash

Infectious mononucleosis/Epstein Barr virus

- Fever
- Lethargy
- Sore throat
- Swollen lymph glands
- Loss of appetite
- Headache
- Increased WBC
- Atypical lymphocytes
- Splenomegaly
- Hepatic involvement

Mumps

- Painful, swollen parotid glands
- Fever and muscle aches
- Headache
- Earache made worse by chewing
- Fatigue and loss of appetite

Pertussis (whooping cough)

- Common cold manifestations: runny nose, congestion, sneezing, mild fever, mild cough (catarrhal stage)
- Severe coughing starts in 1 to 2 weeks (paroxysmal stage)
  - Coughing fits
  - Violent and rapid coughing
  - Loud "whooping" sound upon inspiration

Rubella (German measles)

- Low-grade fever and sore throat
- Headache
- Malaise
- Cough
- Lymphadenopathy
- Red rash that starts on the face and spreads to the rest of the body, lasting 2 to 3 days

Varicella (chickenpox)

MANIFESTATIONS 1 TO 2 DAYS PRIOR TO RASH
- Fever
- Fatigue
- Loss of appetite
- Headache

RASH
- Macules start in center of trunk, spreading to the face and proximal extremities.
- Progresses from macules, to papules, to vesicles, and crust formation follows.
- Scabs appear in approximately 1 week.

LABORATORY TESTS

- CBC
- Electrolyte panels
- Mono spot blood test for infectious mononucleosis

PATIENT-CENTERED CARE

NURSING CARE Q_TC

SYMPTOMATIC TREATMENT

- Administer an antipyretic for fever. Do not administer aspirin, due to the risk of Reye syndrome.
- Administer an antipruritic for severe itching.
- Administer analgesics for pain.
- Provide fluids and nutritious foods of the child's preference. Q_PCC
- Provide quiet diversional activities.
- Promote adequate rest with naps if necessary.
- Keep lights dim if the child develops photophobia.
- Keep the child out of the sun.
- Notify the child's school or day care center of the child's infection. Obtain a plan from the school so that the child can continue working on schoolwork at home.
- Notify the health department of communicable diseases.

SKIN CARE

- Provide calamine lotion for topical relief.
- Keep the skin clean and dry to prevent secondary infection.
- Keep the child cool, but prevent chilling.
- Dress the child in lightweight, loose clothing.
- Give baths in tepid water.
- Keep the child's fingernails clean and short.
- Apply mittens if the child scratches.
- Teach good oral hygiene. A sore throat can be managed with analgesics, lozenges, and saline rinses.
- Change linens daily.

MEDICATIONS

Antihistamine

Diphenhydramine hydrochloride and hydroxyzine used to control pruritus

NURSING ACTIONS

- Monitor the reaction to the medication, because some children can become hyperalert with the administration of a medication from this group.
- Monitor for drowsiness.
- Educate the family about safety precautions. Q_S

Antibiotic or antiviral therapy

- Acyclovir for high-risk clients who have varicella
- Antibiotics for pertussis
- Antibiotic eye drops for bacterial conjunctivitis

NSAIDs or acetaminophen

Decreases fever

NURSING ACTIONS

- Be alert for allergies.
- Teach parents the proper dosing for acetaminophen. Q_PCC

35.1 Activity Case Study

Scenario Introduction

Parker is a registered nurse in a pediatric clinic who is caring for Jasmine, an 8-year-old who was sent home from school the previous day for fever and malaise. Jasmine is brought to the office by her grandmother, Diann.

Scene 1

Parker: Good morning, Jasmine and Diann. My name is Parker. I will be the nurse taking care of you. What brought you guys in this morning?

Diann: Jasmine was sent home from school yesterday afternoon with a fever. She said she was just feeling "yucky." This morning she woke up with a rash on her chest that she said itches. She is still running a little fever and has not has much of an appetite for a few days.

Parker: Ok. Jasmine, I'm going to go and get Dr. Mallare so we can both look at your rash at the same time. Is that ok?

Jasmine: I guess so.

Scene 2

Dr. Mallare: Hi, Jasmine. I'm Dr. Mallare. I hear that you aren't feeling well today. Can you tell me about that?

Jasmine: I just don't feel very good, and I have an itchy rash on my chest.

Dr. Mallare: Do you mind if I take a look at the rash? That will help me to know what it is so I can help you feel better.

Jasmine: I guess that is ok. My grandma gets to stay while you look, right?

Dr. Mallare: Of course!

Scene 3

Dr. Mallare finds a generalized rash on Jasmine's chest and back with macular, popular, and vesicular lesions.

Dr. Mallare: Well, Jasmine and Diann, it looks like Jasmine has chickenpox. Has she been around anyone in the last couple of weeks who had them?

Diann: Yes, as a matter of fact she has! Her cousin had them a couple of weeks ago. Jasmine spent the night with her before we knew she had them.

Dr. Mallare: That makes perfect sense, and it's good to know where and when she was exposed. I am going to discuss her treatment plan with Parker. He will be back in shortly to talk to you and Jasmine about what you need to watch for and how we can help her feel a little better. Do you have any questions for me right now?

Diann. No, not at the moment.

Scene Conclusion

Dr. Mallare has provided Parker with discharge instructions to give to Diann and Jasmine.

CLIENT EDUCATION Q PCC

- Good hand hygiene prevents the spread of infection.
- Adhere to the antibiotic or antiviral therapy.
- Cover the nose and mouth when coughing or sneezing.
- Wash bed linens daily in mild detergent.
- If immunocompromised, seek prompt medical care if manifestations develop.
- Adolescents can participate in decision making.

COMPLICATIONS

Fifth disease: Self-limited arthritis and arthralgia (more common in adult females)

Mononucleosis: Ruptured spleen

Myocarditis: Fetal death if mother is infected during the second trimester of pregnancy

Mumps: Orchitis, encephalitis, meningitis, oophoritis, mastitis, deafness, myocarditis, arthritis, hepatitis

Pertussis
- Infants and children: pneumonia, seizures, apnea, encephalopathy, death, ear infections, hemorrhage, weight loss, hernias
- Teens and adults: weight loss, loss of bladder control, syncope, rib fractures, pneumonia

Rubella
- Complications generally rare with this communicable disease
- Birth defects (deafness; heart defects; cognitive deficits, liver, and spleen damage) in fetus of women infected during pregnancy

Rubeola: Ear infections, pneumonia, encephalitis, death, laryngitis

Varicella: Pneumonia, bleeding problems, bacterial infection of the skin, encephalitis

Active Learning Scenario

A nurse is planning care for a group of clients who have communicable diseases. Use the ATI Active Learning Template: Basic Concept to complete this item.

RELATED CONTENT: List the communicable diseases that require more than standard isolation precautions during hospitalization.

NURSING INTERVENTIONS: Identify the type of isolation precaution to be implemented with the communicable disease identified above.

Active Learning Scenario Key

Using the ATI Active Learning Template: Basic Concept
RELATED CONTENT
- Varicella
- Rubella
- Fifth disease
- Pertussis
- Mumps

NURSING INTERVENTIONS
- Airborne/contact: Varicella
- Droplet: Rubella, fifth disease, pertussis, mumps

Ⓝ *NCLEX® Connection: Safety and Infection Control, Standard Precautions/Transmission–Based Precautions/ Surgical Asepsis*

Application Exercises

1. A nurse is teaching a group of family members about communicable diseases. The nurse should include that which of the following is the best method to prevent a communicable disease?

   A. Hand washing

   B. Avoiding persons who have active disease

   C. Covering your cough

   D. Obtaining immunizations

2. A nurse in a pediatric clinic is providing discharge instructions to the caregiver of a child who has chickenpox (varicella). Which of the following instructions should the nurse include in the teaching? (Select all that apply.)

   A. The child is contagious until all vesicles have crusted.

   B. Calamine lotion may be applied to decrease itching.

   C. Fingernails should be kept short while lesions are present.

   D. Bed linens should be changed every other day.

   E. Bathe the child in tepid water.

3. A nurse is assessing a child who has chickenpox (varicella). Which of the following rashes should the nurse expect to depict chickenpox (varicella) lesions?

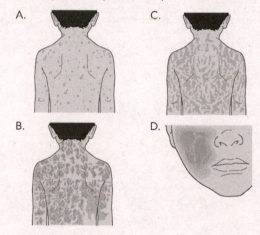

4. A nurse is assessing a client who has pertussis. Which of the following findings should the nurse expect? (Select all that apply.)

   A. Runny nose

   B. Mild fever

   C. Cough with whooping sound

   D. Swollen salivary glands

   E. Red rash

5. A nurse is caring for a child who has rubeola. The nurse should monitor for which of the following complications? (Select all that apply.)

   A. Otitis media

   B. Constipation

   C. Laryngitis

   D. Arthralgia

   E. Syncope

6. A nurse is teaching a group of family members about complications of communicable diseases. Which of the following communicable diseases can lead to pneumonia? (Select all that apply.)

   A. Rubella (German measles)

   B. Rubeola (measles)

   C. Pertussis (whooping cough)

   D. Varicella (chickenpox)

   E. Mumps

Application Exercises Key

1. A. Hand washing will decrease the spread of infection. However, this is not the best method to prevent communicable disease.
   B. Avoiding people who have active disease will decrease the spread of infection. However, this is not the best method to prevent communicable disease.
   C. Covering coughs will decrease the spread of infection. However, this is not the best method to prevent communicable disease.
   D. **CORRECT:** When providing teaching to a group of family members about prevention of communicable diseases, the nurse should include in the teaching that obtaining immunizations is the best prevention method for communicable diseases.

   Ⓝ *NCLEX® Connection: Safety and Infection Control, Standard Precautions/Transmission-Based Precautions/Surgical Asepsis*

2. A. **CORRECT:** When taking action and providing discharge instructions to the caregiver of a child who has chickenpox (varicella), the nurse should include in the teaching that the child is contagious until all vesicles have formed a crust.
   B. **CORRECT:** The nurse should also inform the caregiver that calamine lotion may be applied to decrease itching, fingernails should be kept short to help prevent scratching and secondary skin infections, and the child should be bathed in tepid, or lukewarm water, to decrease itching.
   C. **CORRECT:** The nurse should also inform the caregiver that calamine lotion may be applied to decrease itching, fingernails should be kept short to help prevent scratching and secondary skin infections, and the child should be bathed in tepid, or lukewarm water, to decrease itching.
   D. Bed linens should be changed every day.
   E. **CORRECT:** The nurse should also inform the caregiver that calamine lotion may be applied to decrease itching, fingernails should be kept short to help prevent scratching and secondary skin infections, and the child should be bathed in tepid, or lukewarm water, to decrease itching.

   Ⓝ *NCLEX® Connection: Physiological Adaptation; Alterations in Body Systems*

3. A. **CORRECT:** The nurse should identify that the generalized rash with macules, papules, and vesicles is the rash that is consistent with chickenpox (varicella).

4. A, B, C. **CORRECT:** When assessing a child who has pertussis the nurse should expect the child to have a runny nose, mild fever, and a cough with a whooping sound on inspiration.
   D. A child who has mumps will have enlarged lymph nodes.
   E. A child who has measles will have a red rash.

   Ⓝ *NCLEX® Connection: Physiological Adaptation, Alterations in Body Systems*

5. A, C. **CORRECT:** When analyzing cues during the care of a child who has rubeola, the nurse recognize that otitis media and laryngitis are complications of rubeola.
   B. Constipation is not a complication of rubeola.
   D. Arthralgia is a complication of fifth disease and mumps.
   E. Syncope is a complication of pertussis.

   Ⓝ *NCLEX® Connection: Physiological Adaptation, Alterations in Body Systems*

6. B, C, D. **CORRECT:** The nurse should include that rubeola, pertussis, and varicella are communicable diseases that can lead to pneumonia.
   A. Complications of rubella include birth defects (deafness; heart defects; mental, liver, and spleen damage) in the fetus of a woman infected during pregnancy.
   E. Complications of mumps include orchitis, encephalitis, meningitis, oophoritis, mastitis, and deafness.

   Ⓝ *NCLEX® Connection: Safety and Infection Control, Standard Precautions/Transmission-Based Precautions/Surgical Asepsis*

UNIT 2 SYSTEM DISORDERS
SECTION: IMMUNE AND INFECTIOUS DISORDERS

CHAPTER 36 *Acute Otitis Media*

Acute otitis media (AOM) is an infection of the structures of the middle ear. AOM is one of the most common acute illnesses in childhood. Otitis media with effusion (OME) is a collection of fluid in the middle ear but no infection.

Repeated infections can cause impaired hearing and speech. Many infections clear spontaneously in a few days. The majority of incidences are related to Eustachian tube malfunction.

ASSESSMENT

RISK FACTORS

- Eustachian tubes in children are shorter and more horizontal than those of adults. Otitis media is most common in the first 24 months of life and again when children enter school (ages 5 to 6). Otitis media occurs infrequently after age 7.
- Otitis media is usually triggered by a bacterial infection (Streptococcus pneumoniae, Haemophilus influenzae, Moraxella catarrhalis), a viral infection (respiratory syncytial virus or influenza), allergies, or enlarged adenoids.
- There is a lower incidence of otitis media in infants who are breastfed possibly due to the presence of immunoglobulin A (IgA) in breastmilk, and the semi-vertical feeding position of breastfed babies. Q EBP
- Incidence is higher in the winter and spring months.
- Exposure to large numbers of children (day care).
- Exposure to secondhand smoke.
- Cleft lip and/or cleft palate.
- Nonadherence with childhood immunizations.
- Down syndrome.

EXPECTED FINDINGS

- Recent history of upper respiratory infection
- Acute onset of changes in behavior
- Frequent crying, irritability, and fussiness
- Inconsolability
- Tugging at ear
- Turning head from side to side
- Reports of ear pain, loss of appetite, nausea, and vomiting
- Fever

PHYSICAL ASSESSMENT FINDINGS

- **AOM**
  - Rubbing or pulling on ear
  - Crying
  - Lethargy
  - Bulging yellow or red tympanic membrane
  - Purulent material in middle ear or drainage from external canal
  - Decreased or no tympanic movement with pneumatic otoscopy
  - Lymphadenopathy of the neck and head
  - Temperature: can be as high as 40° C (104° F)
  - Hearing difficulties and speech delays if otitis media becomes a chronic condition
- **OME**
  - Feeling of fullness in the ear
  - Orange discoloration of the tympanic membrane with decreased movement
  - Vague findings including rhinitis, cough, and diarrhea
  - Transient hearing loss and balance disturbances

DIAGNOSTIC PROCEDURES

Pneumatic otoscope

A pneumatic otoscope is used by a provider to visualize the tympanic membrane and middle ear structures and assess tympanic membrane movement.

NURSING ACTIONS: Gently pull the pinna down and back to visualize the tympanic membrane of a child younger than 3 years old. For a child older than 3 years, gently pull the pinna up and back.

PATIENT-CENTERED CARE

NURSING CARE

- Provide comfort measures.
  - Administer pain medication as needed.
  - Provide diversional activities.
- Place child in an upright position.
- Management of fevers.

THERAPEUTIC MANAGEMENT

- Management by a provider depends on the child's physical findings, age, and history.
- The American Academy of Pediatrics (AAP) recommend that providers wait and monitor a child who is 2 to 12 years of age, who has uncomplicated, nonrecurrent AOM for at least 2 to 3 days, prior to prescribing antibiotics.

MEDICATIONS

Acetaminophen or ibuprofen

Used to provide analgesia and reduce fever

Antibiotics

- Amoxicillin, amoxicillin-clavulanate, or azithromycin PO (5 to 10 days)
- Ceftriaxone IM (once)

NURSING ACTIONS
- Antibiotics are recommended for children over 6 months of age who have severe manifestations (increased pain or temperature above 39° C [102.2° F]) for more than 2 days, or for children 6 to 23 months with bilateral AOM and no manifestations.
- In other cases, antibiotic therapy can be withheld. If the child does not improve or worsens within 48 to 72 hours, antibiotics are started at that time.
- Administer in high doses orally, usually 80 to 90 mg/kg/day in two divided doses.
- The usual course of oral treatment is 10 days in children younger than 6 years of age. The course can be shorter for older children.
- IM is used for resistant organisms or for client-specific reasons (difficulty taking oral medications, inability to complete the oral course).

CLIENT EDUCATION
- The child should complete the total course of antibiotic treatment.
- Observe for manifestations of allergy to the antibiotic (rash or difficulty breathing). Qs

Topical anesthetics

Benzocaine or lidocaine ear drops can help relieve pain.

THERAPEUTIC PROCEDURES

Myringotomy and placement of tympanoplasty tubes can be indicated for a child who has multiple episodes of otitis media. This procedure can be performed by laser treatment.
- This procedure is performed in an outpatient setting with the administration of general anesthesia. It is usually completed in 15 min.
- A small incision is made in the tympanic membrane, and tiny plastic or metal tubes are placed into the eardrum to equalize pressure and minimize effusion.
- Recovery takes place in a PACU, and discharge usually occurs within 1 hr.
- Postoperative pain is not common and, if present, will be mild.
- The tubes usually come out spontaneously (in 8 to 18 months).

CLIENT EDUCATION
- Limit the child's activities for a few days following surgery.
- Notify the provider when tubes come out. This usually does not require replacement of tubes.
- Avoid getting water into the child's ears while the tubes are in place. The effectiveness of earplugs is not conclusive. Advise the guardians to follow the health care provider's instructions.

CLIENT EDUCATION

- Use comfort measures.
- Feed the child in an upright position when bottle- or breastfeeding.
- If drainage is present, clean the external ear with sterile cotton swabs. Apply antibiotic ointment.
- Avoid exposure of child to risk factors if possible (secondhand smoke, individuals with viral/bacterial respiratory infections).
- Seek medical care at initial manifestations of infections (change in behavior, tugging on ear).
- Maintain up-to-date immunizations.

COMPLICATIONS

Hearing loss and/or speech delays

NURSING ACTIONS
- Assess and monitor for deficits.
- Refer the child for audiology testing if needed.

CLIENT EDUCATION
Speech therapy may be necessary.

Application Exercises

1. A nurse is assessing an infant who has manifestations of acute otitis media (AOM). Which of the following assessment data should the nurse identify as risk factors for otitis media? (Select all that apply.)

   A. Breastfeeds without formula supplementation.

   B. Attends day care 4 days per week.

   C. Immunizations are up to date.

   D. History of a cleft palate repair.

   E. Parents smoke cigarettes outside.

2. A nurse is assessing an infant. Which of the following findings are clinical manifestations of acute otitis media? (Select all that apply.)

   A. Decreased pain in the supine position

   B. Rolling head side to side

   C. Loss of appetite

   D. Increased sensitivity to sound

   E. Crying

3. A nurse is caring for a toddler who has had rhinitis, cough, and diarrhea for 2 days. Upon assessment, it is noted that the tympanic membrane has an orange discoloration and decreased movement. Which of the following statements should the nurse make to the caregiver?

   A. "Your child has an ear infection that requires antibiotics."

   B. "Your child may have transient hearing loss."

   C. "Your child will need a decongestant until this condition clears."

   D. "Your child will need to have a myringotomy."

4. A nurse is caring for a toddler who has acute otitis media. Which of the following is the priority action for the nurse to take?

   A. Provide emotional support to the family.

   B. Educate the family on care of the child.

   C. Provide a diversional activity.

   D. Administer analgesics.

5. A nurse is caring for a toddler who has had three ear infections in the past 5 months. The nurse should identify that the toddler is at risk for developing which of the following long-term complications?

   A. Balance difficulties

   B. Rash

   C. Speech delays

   D. Mastoiditis

Active Learning Scenario

A nurse is caring for an infant who has acute otitis media for the first time. Use the ATI Active Learning Template: System Disorder to complete this item:

ALTERATION IN HEALTH (DIAGNOSIS)

NURSING CARE: Describe two interventions.

MEDICATIONS: List two.

CLIENT EDUCATION: Describe two teaching points.

COMPLICATIONS: Identify one.

Active Learning Scenario Key

Using the ATI Active Learning Template: System Disorder

ALTERATION IN HEALTH (DIAGNOSIS): Acute otitis media is an infection of the structures of the middle ear with rapid manifestations of infection.

NURSING CARE
- Comfort care with pain medications and distraction.
- Management of fevers
- Place child in an upright position

MEDICATIONS
- Amoxicillin, amoxicillin-clavulanate or azithromycin PO or ceftriaxone IM
- Acetaminophen or ibuprofen for pain and fever
- Benzocaine

CLIENT EDUCATION
- Inform the parents about comfort measures.
- Encourage the parents to feed the child in an upright position when bottle or breastfeeding.
- If drainage is present, clean the external ear with sterile cotton swabs. Apply antibiotic ointment.
- Teach parents to avoid risk factors (secondhand smoke, exposure to individuals with viral/bacterial respiratory infections).
- Stress the importance of seeking medical care at the onset of findings of infections (change in child's behavior, tugging on ear).
- Encourage the parents to keep the child's immunizations up to date.

POTENTIAL COMPLICATION: Hearing loss and/or speech delays

Ⓝ *NCLEX® Connection: Physiological Adaptation, Pathophysiology*

Application Exercises Key

1. B, D, E. **CORRECT:** When recognizing cues during the care of an infant who has manifestation of acute otitis media, the nurse should identify that attending daycare, having a history of cleft palate repair, and living with parents who smoke are risk factors for acute otitis media. Attending daycare increases the risk due to exposure to multiple children. Children who have had a cleft palate repair are more prone to AOM because micro-organisms can easily enter the Eustachian tubes. Children who live with parents who smoke cigarettes, even outside, are at a greater risk due to exposure to secondhand smoke.
   A. Breastfeeding helps to protect against AOM because breast milk contains secretory immunoglobulin A.
   C. The pneumococcal conjugate vaccine decreases the incidence of OM.

   Ⓝ *NCLEX® Connection: Health Promotion and Maintenance, Health Promotion/Disease Prevention*

2. B, C, E. **CORRECT:** When recognizing cues during the assessment of an infant, the nurse should recognize that rolling the head side to side, loss of appetite, and crying are manifestations of acute otitis media.
   A. Infants who have acute otitis media will have an increase in pain in the supine position from the fluid and pressure in the ear.
   D. Infants who have acute otitis media have a decreased sensitivity to sound from the fluid and pressure in the ear.

   Ⓝ *NCLEX® Connection: Physiological Adaptation, Pathophysiology*

3. A. Antibiotics are not recommended for OME.
   B. **CORRECT:** When analyzing cues during the care of a toddler who has had rhinitis, cough, and diarrhea for 2 days that is accompanied by a tympanic membrane with an orange discoloration and decreased movement, the nurse should identify that the toddler has manifestations of otitis media effusion (OME). Transient hearing loss is a complication of OME; therefore, the nurse should inform the guardians that the child may have transient hearing loss.
   C. Decongestants are not recommended for OME.
   D. Myringotomy is recommended for clients who have chronic OME.

   Ⓝ *NCLEX® Connection: Physiological Adaptation, Unexpected Response to Therapies*

4. A. Providing emotional support to the family will promote psychological well-being. However, it is not the priority action.
   B. Educating the family on the care of the child will promote recovery from illness. However, it is not the priority action.
   C. Providing a diversional activity for the toddler will help provide normalcy during care. However, it is not the priority action.
   D. **CORRECT:** When using Maslow's hierarchy of needs to prioritize hypothesis during the care of a toddler who has acute otitis media, the nurse should identify that the administration of analgesics can meet the toddlers physiologic need for pain relief. Therefore, this is the priority action to take.

   Ⓝ *NCLEX® Connection: Physiological Adaptation, Illness Management*

5. A. Balance difficulties can be present with otitis media. However, it is not a long-term complication.
   B. Although rash can indicate antibiotic sensitivity, it is not a long-term complication of otitis media.
   C. **CORRECT:** When analyzing cues during the care of a toddler who has had three ear infections in the past five months, the nurse should identify that the toddler is at risk for speech delays as a complication of recurrent otitis media.
   D. Mastoiditis can be a result of otitis media. However, it is not a long-term complication.

   Ⓝ *NCLEX® Connection: Physiological Adaptation, Pathophysiology*

UNIT 2　SYSTEM DISORDERS

SECTION: IMMUNE AND INFECTIOUS DISORDERS

CHAPTER 37　# HIV/AIDS

HIV infection is a viral infection in which the virus primarily infects a specific subset of T-lymphocytes, the CD4 T cells causing immune dysfunction. The virus impairs or destroys cells of the immune system and progressively destroys the body's ability to fight off infections. This leads to organ dysfunction and a variety of opportunistic illnesses in a weakened host. It is estimated that at least 20% of new HIV infections occur in adolescents and young adults. A goal of Healthy People 2030 is to decrease the number of new HIV infections by 90%.

ASSESSMENT

RISK FACTORS

- Infants can become infected perinatally or by ingesting breast milk from an HIV infected client
- Exposure to blood products or body fluids that contain the HIV virus
- Sexual assault survivor
- Risky behaviors (unprotected sexual activity and IV substance use)
- Sexually transmitted infections
- Lack of awareness of risk factors and modes of transmission

EXPECTED FINDINGS

37.1　HIV infection stages

	LESS THAN 12 MONTHS (CELLS/μL*)	1 TO 5 YEARS (CELLS/μL)	6 YEARS AND OLDER (CELLS/μL)
STAGE 1	1,500 or more	1,000 or more	500 or more
STAGE 2	750 to 1,499	500 to 999	200 to 499
STAGE 3	Less than 750	Less than 500	Less than 200

*CD4+ T-lymphocyte count
Source: CDC.gov

HIV clinical classification

To read more about HIV, go to the website of the Centers for Disease Control and Prevention.

Category N: Not symptomatic
No manifestations considered to be the result of HIV infection are present, or the child has only one of the conditions listed in the mildly symptomatic category.

Category A: Mildly symptomatic
Children have two or more of the following mildly symptomatic manifestations, but none of the conditions listed in the moderately or severely symptomatic categories.
- Lymphadenopathy
- Hepatomegaly
- Splenomegaly
- Recurrent upper respiratory infections, sinusitis, or otitis media

Category B: Moderately symptomatic
Children have more serious manifestations, including:
- Anemia
- Bacterial meningitis, pneumonia, or sepsis (single episode)
- Oropharyngeal candidiasis
- Cytomegalovirus infection
- Cardiomyopathy
- Herpes zoster
- Herpes simplex virus (HSV), HSV stomatitis, bronchitis, pneumonitis, or esophagitis
- Hepatitis
- Lymphoid interstitial pneumonia (LIP) or pulmonary lymphoid hyperplasia complex
- Leiomyosarcoma
- Toxoplasmosis

Category C: Severely symptomatic
Children who have the following conditions are considered severely symptomatic.
- Multiple serious bacterial infections (meningitis, bone or joint infection, abscesses of internal organ or body cavity, septicemia, mycobacterial pneumonia)
- Esophageal or pulmonary candidiasis, (bronchi, trachea, lungs)
- Cytomegalovirus disease (greater than 1 month of age with site other than liver, spleen, or lymph nodes)
- Bronchitis, pneumonitis, or esophagitis lasting longer than 1 month
- Kaposi's sarcoma
- Tuberculosis
- Encephalopathy with developmental delays
- Extrapulmonary cryptococcosis
- Cryptosporidiosis
- Disseminated histoplasmosis
- Pneumocystis carinii pneumonia
- Encephalopathy
- Septicemia
- Wasting syndrome
- Lymphoma

HIV infection: 13 to 20 years

Refer to **ADULT MEDICAL SURGICAL REVIEW MODULE, CHAPTER 87: HIV/AIDS.** Qᴘᴄᴄ

DIAGNOSTIC PROCEDURES

LABORATORY CRITERIA FOR DIAGNOSIS

- 18 months or older: Positive result from HIV antigen/antibody combination immunoassay followed by HIV-1/HIV-2 antibody differentiation immunoassay.
- Infants less than 18 months of age and were born to infected mothers: Positive result from polymerase chain reaction and virus culture.

PATIENT-CENTERED CARE

NURSING CARE

- Encourage a balanced diet that is high in calories and protein. Obtain the child's preferred food and beverages. Give nutritional supplements.
- Administer total parental nutrition if prescribed.
- Provide good oral care, and report abnormalities for treatment.
- Keep the child's skin clean and dry.
- Provide nonpharmacological methods of pain relief.
- Assess for pain, and provide adequate pain management. Use of medications can include nonsteroidal anti-inflammatory drugs (NSAIDs), acetaminophen, opioids, muscle relaxants, and/or a eutectic mixture of local anesthetics (lidocaine and prilocaine topical ointment) for numerous diagnostic procedures.
- Prevent infection. Qs
- Use standard precautions.
- Encourage deep breathing and coughing.
- Maintain good hand hygiene.
- Teach the child and parents to avoid individuals who have colds/infections/viruses.
- Encourage immunizations (pneumococcal vaccine and yearly seasonal influenza vaccine).
- Monitor for indications of opportunistic infections.
- Administer medications as prescribed for opportunistic infections.
- Provide psychosocial support to client and family and assist them in disclosing the diagnosis.
- Educate the child and caregivers about transmission of the virus (high-risk behaviors).
- Identify stressors affecting the family, and make appropriate referrals (school/community response to child, finances, access to health care).
- Discuss with adolescents the various routes of HIV transmission (sexual transmission, IV substance use).

MEDICATIONS

Antiretroviral medications

Antiretroviral medications are given at various stages of the HIV cycle to inhibit reproduction of the virus, therefore slowing progression of the HIV disease process.

- Combinations of antiretroviral medications are prescribed to decrease the client's development of medication resistance.
- Antiretroviral medication therapy is lifelong.

Nucleoside reverse transcriptase inhibitors: Zidovudine, didanosine, stavudine, lamivudine, and abacavir suppress the synthesis of viral DNA.

Non-nucleoside reverse transcriptase inhibitors: Delavirdine, efavirenz, nevirapine, doravirine, etravirine, and rilpivirine bind to the viral DNA, causing direct inhibition.

Protease inhibitors: Indinavir, ritonavir, nelfinavir, saquinavir, atazanavir, darunavir, fosamprenavir, tipranavir, and lopinavir inhibit an enzyme needed for the virus to mature.

NURSING ACTIONS

Monitor laboratory results (CBC, WBC, liver function tests). Antiretroviral medications can increase alanine aminotransferase, aspartate aminotransferase, bilirubin, mean corpuscular volume, high-density lipoproteins, total cholesterol, triglycerides, and blood glucose levels.

CLIENT EDUCATION

- Observe for adverse effects of the medications and perform ways to decrease the severity of the adverse effects.
- Take the medication on a regular schedule and do not miss doses.

Antibiotics

Trimethoprim–sulfamethoxazole

Administer to all infants who are born to infected mothers until HIV infection is excluded. QEBP

IV gamma globulin

To prevent recurrent or serious bacterial infections

INTERPROFESSIONAL CARE QTC

- Social services can help with access to health care and medication acquisition.
- Dietitian can assist with nutritional support and promote good nutrition.

CLIENT EDUCATION

- This illness is chronic and there is a need for lifelong medication administration.
- Notify the provider for manifestations requiring medical care, including headache, fever, lethargy, warmth, tenderness, redness at joints, and neck stiffness.
- Perform safe practice when using needles/syringes and administering medications.
- Discuss with adolescents the various routes of HIV transmission, including sexual transmission and IV substance use. Ensure the adolescent understands safe sex practices.

COMPLICATIONS

Failure to thrive

NURSING ACTIONS

- Obtain a baseline height and weight, and continue to monitor.
- Promote optimal nutrition. This can require the administration of total parenteral nutrition.
- Assess growth and development. Monitor for delays.
- Provide opportunities for normal development (age-appropriate toys, playing with children of the same age).

CLIENT EDUCATION: Consume appropriate nutrition to meet nutritional needs.

Pneumocystis carinii pneumonia

NURSING ACTIONS

- Assess and monitor respiratory status, which includes respiratory rate and effort, oxygen saturation, and breath sounds.
- Administer appropriate antibiotics.
- Administer an antipyretic and/or analgesics.
- Provide adequate hydration and maintain fluid and electrolyte balance.
- Use postural drainage and chest physiotherapy to mobilize and remove fluid from the lungs.
- Promote adequate rest.
- Educate the child and caregivers about the infectious process and how to prevent infection.
- Educate the child and caregivers about the importance of medication and the need to maintain the medication regimen.

Active Learning Scenario

A nurse is teaching a guardian of a child who has AIDS. Use the ATI Active Learning Template: System Disorder to complete this item.

COMPLICATIONS: List two complications of AIDS and include four nursing actions for each.

Application Exercises

1. A nurse is admitting a child who has HIV. The nurse should identify which of the following findings as an indication that the child is in the mildly symptomatic category of HIV? (Select all that apply.)

   A. Herpes zoster

   B. Anemia

   C. Oral candidiasis

   D. Hepatomegaly

   E. Lymphadenopathy

2. A nurse is admitting a child who has manifestations of severely symptomatic HIV. Which of the following findings should the nurse expect? (Select all that apply.)

   A. Kaposi's sarcoma

   B. Hepatitis

   C. Wasting syndrome

   D. Pulmonary candidiasis

   E. Cardiomyopathy

3. A nurse is teaching a parent of a child who has HIV. Which of the following information should the nurse include? (Select all that apply.)

   A. Obtain yearly influenza vaccination.

   B. Monitor a fever for 24 hr before seeking medical care.

   C. Avoid individuals who have colds.

   D. Provide nutritional supplements.

   E. Administer aspirin for pain.

4. A nurse is caring for a child who has HIV. Which of the following isolation precautions should the nurse implement?

   A. Contact

   B. Airborne

   C. Droplet

   D. Standard

5. A nurse is teaching a group of adolescents about HIV/AIDS. Which of the following statements should the nurse include in the teaching?

   A. "You can contract HIV through casual kissing."

   B. "HIV is transmitted through IV substance use."

   C. "HIV is now curable if caught in the early stages."

   D. "Antiretroviral therapy inhibits transmission of the HIV virus."

Active Learning Scenario Key

Using the ATI Active Learning Template: System Disorder

COMPLICATIONS

Failure to thrive
- Obtain a baseline height and weight, and continue to monitor.
- Promote optimal nutrition. This can require the administration of total parenteral nutrition.
- Assess growth and development. Monitor for delays.
- Provide opportunities for normal development (age-appropriate toys, playing with children of the same age).
- Educate the child and parents about appropriate nutrition and how to meet nutritional needs.

Pneumocystis carinii pneumonia (PCP)
- Assess and monitor respiratory status, which includes respiratory rate and effort, oxygen saturation, and breath sounds.
- Administer appropriate antibiotics.
- Administer an antipyretic and/or analgesics.
- Provide adequate hydration, and maintain fluid and electrolyte balance.
- Use postural drainage and chest physiotherapy to mobilize and remove fluid from the lungs.
- Promote adequate rest.
- Educate the child and parents about the infectious process and how to prevent infection.
- Educate the child and parents about the importance of medication and the need to maintain the medication regimen.

Ⓝ *NCLEX® Connection: Physiological Adaptation, Unexpected Response to Therapies*

Application Exercises Key

1. C, D, E. **CORRECT:** When recognizing cues during the admission of a child who has HIV, the nurse should identify hepatomegaly, lymphadenopathy, and reports of recurrent sinusitis as manifestations of the mildly symptomatic category of HIV.
   A. Herpes zoster is a manifestation of a child who is moderately symptomatic.
   B. Anemia is a manifestation of a child who is moderately symptomatic.

Ⓝ *NCLEX® Connection: Physiological Adaptation, Alterations in Body Systems*

2. A, C, D. **CORRECT:** When recognizing cues during the admission of a child who has HIV, the nurse should identify Kaposi's sarcoma, wasting syndrome, and pulmonary candidiasis as manifestations of the severely symptomatic category of HIV.
   B. Hepatitis is a manifestation of a child who is moderately symptomatic.
   E. Cardiomyopathy is a manifestation of a child who is moderately symptomatic.

Ⓝ *NCLEX® Connection: Physiological Adaptation, Alterations in Body Systems*

3. A, C, D. **CORRECT:** When taking action and teaching a parent of a child who has HIV, the nurse should include in the teaching that the child should receive a yearly influenza vaccine, avoid individuals who have colds, and be given nutritional supplements. The influenza vaccine and avoiding individuals who have colds help to prevent opportunistic infections. Nutritional supplements are recommended to promote improved nutrition in children who have HIV.
   B. The child who has HIV should receive prompt medical care for a fever, as this is an indication of an infection.
   E. Acetaminophen, NSAIDs, or opioids should be administered to a child who has pain.

Ⓝ *NCLEX® Connection: Physiological Adaptation, Illness Management*

4. A. Contact isolation precautions are used to protect transmission of disease that is skin-to-skin or direct contact.
   B. Airborne isolation precautions are used to protect transmission of disease that is small-particle droplets.
   C. Droplet isolation precautions are used to protect transmission of disease that is large-particle droplets.
   D. **CORRECT:** When caring for the child who has HIV, the nurse should implement standard isolation precautions.

Ⓝ *NCLEX® Connection: Safety and Infection Control, Standard Precautions/Transmission–Based Precautions/ Surgical Asepsis*

5. A. There is no evidence that casual contact (kissing) spreads the virus.
   B. **CORRECT:** When taking action and teaching a group of adolescents about HIV/AIDS, the nurse should include in the teaching that HIV is transmitted through IV substance use as well as through blood, semen, vaginal secretions, and breast milk." HIV is transmitted via blood, semen, vaginal secretions, and breast milk.
   C. Antiretroviral therapy slows the progression of HIV but does not cure the disease.
   D. Antiretroviral therapy suppresses the reproduction of the virus but do not prevent transmission from one individual to another.

Ⓝ *NCLEX® Connection: Safety and Infection Control, Standard Precautions/Transmission–Based Precautions/ Surgical Asepsis*

When reviewing the following chapters, keep in mind the relevant topics and tasks of the NCLEX outline, in particular:

Basic Care and Comfort

NUTRITION AND ORAL HYDRATION: Evaluate the impact of disease/illness on nutritional status of a client.

Pharmacological and Parenteral Therapies

EXPECTED ACTIONS/OUTCOMES: Evaluate client response to medication.

PHARMACOLOGICAL PAIN MANAGEMENT: Administer and document pharmacological pain management appropriate for client age and diagnoses.

Reduction of Risk Potential

DIAGNOSTIC TESTS
Monitor the results of diagnostic testing and intervene as needed.

Apply knowledge of related nursing procedures and psychomotor skills when caring for clients undergoing diagnostic testing.

POTENTIAL FOR COMPLICATIONS OF DIAGNOSTIC TESTS/ TREATMENTS/PROCEDURES: Use precautions to prevent injury and/or complications associated with a procedure or diagnosis.

THERAPEUTIC PROCEDURES
Provide preoperative care.

Educate client about treatments and procedures.

Physiological Adaptation

ILLNESS MANAGEMENT
Educate client regarding an acute or chronic condition.

Apply knowledge of client pathophysiology to illness management.

ALTERATIONS IN BODY SYSTEMS: Provide postoperative care.

PATHOPHYSIOLOGY: Identify pathophysiology
related to an acute or chronic condition.

Psychosocial Integrity

THERAPEUTIC COMMUNICATION: Encourage
client to verbalize feelings.

CHAPTER 38

CHAPTER 38 *Organ Neoplasms*

Caring for a child who has cancer requires compassion and competency. The nurse should provide individualized care and support to the child and the child's family. Pediatric cancers have a low rate of incidence compared to cancer in adults. However, some neoplasms occur predominantly in children.

For more information about neoplasms, refer to: Adult Medical Surgical Review Module Chapter 90: General Principles of Cancer, Adult Medical Surgical Review Module, Chapter 93: Cancer Disorders.

Wilms' tumor (nephroblastoma) is a malignancy that occurs in the kidneys or abdomen. The tumor is usually unilateral, with 10% of cases affecting both kidneys. Diagnosis typically occurs before age 5, with most cases diagnosed between 2 and 3 years of age. Metastasis is rare.

Neuroblastoma is a malignancy that occurs in the adrenal gland, sympathetic chain of the retroperitoneal area, head, neck, pelvis, or chest. It is usually manifested during the toddler years, with 95% of cases prior to age 10. Median age at diagnosis is 19 months. It is more common in males than females. Half of all cases have metastasized before diagnosis.

Treatment varies by child and can be any combination of surgery, chemotherapy, and radiation.

ASSESSMENT

RISK FACTORS

There are no known risk factors for Wilms' tumor or neuroblastoma. Q EBP

EXPECTED FINDINGS

Wilms' tumor

- Mass is usually found by caregivers during routine bathing or dressing of their child
- Painless, firm, nontender abdominal swelling or mass
- Fatigue, malaise, weight loss
- Fever
- Hematuria
- Hypertension
- Manifestations of metastasis include dyspnea, cough, shortness of breath, and chest pain

Neuroblastoma

- Manifestations depend upon the location and stage of the condition
- Palpable abdominal mass
- Weight loss, constipation, anorexia
- Diaphoresis, hypertension
- Manifestations of metastasis include jaundice, and dark pigmented nodules on the extremities, dyspnea, edema of face and neck

LABORATORY TESTS

Wilms' tumor

- BUN, creatinine
- CBC
- Urinalysis

Neuroblastoma

- CBC and coagulation studies
- Urine catecholamines (vanillylmandelic acid, homovanillic acid, dopamine, and norepinephrine)

DIAGNOSTIC PROCEDURES

NURSING ACTIONS
- Assess the child for allergies to dye or shellfish.
- Educate the parent and child prior to procedure on expectations.
- Assist the child to remain still during the procedure.
- Instruct the child to drink oral contrast if prescribed.
- Sedate the child if prescribed.
- Provide emotional support. Q PCC

Wilms' tumor

- Abdominal ultrasonography
- Abdominal and chest computed tomography (CT) scan
- Inferior venacavogram (rule out involvement with the vena cava)
- Bone marrow aspiration (rule out metastasis)

Neuroblastoma

- Skeletal survey
- Skull, neck, chest, abdominal, and bone CT scans
- Bone marrow aspiration (rule out metastasis)
- Metaiodobenzylguanidine scan (determine bone, bone marrow, and soft tissue involvement)
- Biopsy of tumor

PATIENT-CENTERED CARE

NURSING CARE

- If an abdominal tumor is suspected, do not palpate the abdomen.
- Use extreme caution when handling or bathing the client to prevent trauma to the tumor site. Qs
- Assess the child's and family's coping and support.
- Assess for developmental delays related to illness.
- Assess physical growth (height and weight).
- Provide education and support to the child and family regarding diagnostic testing, treatment plan, ongoing therapy, and prognosis.
- Monitor for findings of infection.
- Administer antibiotics as prescribed for infection.
- Keep the child's skin clean and dry.
- Provide oral hygiene.
- Provide age-appropriate diversional activities.
- Provide support to the child and family.
  - Avoid false reassurance.
  - Listen to the child's concerns.
  - Allow time for the child and family to discuss feelings regarding grief and loss.

THERAPEUTIC MANAGEMENT

Treatment for Wilms' tumor

- Varies according to the stage and histology of the tumor
- Surgical removal of the tumor and kidney soon after diagnosis
- Preoperative chemotherapy or radiation if both kidneys are involved to decrease the size of the tumors and potentially preserve one kidney
- Postoperative radiation and/or chemotherapy for children who have large tumors, metastasis, recurrence, and residual disease

Treatment for neuroblastoma

- Varies according to the tumor stage
- Surgical removal of the tumor
- Chemotherapy and/or radiation for metastasis and residual disease

Radiation

- Radiation is dose-calculated and usually delivered in divided treatments over several weeks.
- Radiation affects rapidly growing cells in the body. Therefore, cells that normally have a fast turnover can be affected in addition to cancer cells.

NURSING ACTIONS
- Take care when radiation is in use. Wear lead aprons.
- Educate the child and family about the procedure and provide support.

CLIENT EDUCATION Qpcc
- Do not wash off marks on skin that outline the targeted areas.
- Wash the marked areas with lukewarm water, use hands instead of a washcloth, pat dry, and take care not to remove the markings. Avoid using hot or cold water.
- Avoid use of soaps, creams, lotions, and powders unless they are prescribed.
- Wear loose cotton clothing.
- Keep the areas protected from the sun by wearing a hat and long-sleeved shirts.
- Seek medical care for blisters, weeping, and red/tender skin.

Chemotherapy

The child can have a long-term central venous access device or peripherally inserted central catheter in place.

Wilms' tumor
- Actinomycin D and vincristine.
- For tumors at more advanced stages, with unfavorable histology, or that recur after treatment, other medications (doxorubicin and cyclophosphamide) can be used.

Neuroblastoma: Various combination of agents are used: cyclophosphamide, doxorubicin, cisplatin, etoposide, vincristine, and carboplatin

NURSING ACTIONS
- Provide an antiemetic prior to administration of chemotherapy.
- Allow the child several food choices, including their favorite foods.
- Assess the mouth for mucosal ulcerations.
- Offer cool fluids to prevent dehydration and soothe sore mucous membranes.

CLIENT EDUCATION Qpcc
- Monitor for adverse effects of chemotherapy
- Receive immunizations and follow-up appointments.
- Perform good infection control practices.

ADVERSE EFFECTS OF CHEMOTHERAPY/RADIATION

Assess for adverse effects of chemotherapy and provide interventions to prevent and minimize manifestations.

- **Skin breakdown**
  - Inspect skin daily.
  - Examine rectal mucosa for fissures.
  - Avoid rectal temperatures.
  - Provide sitz baths as needed.
  - Reposition frequently.
  - Use a pressure reduction system.
- **Constipation**
  - Encourage a diet high in fiber.
  - Administer stool softeners and laxatives as needed.
  - Encourage fluids.
- **Foot drop**
  - Use a footboard in bed.
  - Wear high-top shoes.
  - Causes weakness and numbness of extremities.
  - Assist with ambulation.
- **Pain**
  - Collect data for pain.
  - Administer analgesics as prescribed.
  - Assist with determining the effectiveness of pain interventions.
  - For jaw pain, provide a soft or liquid diet.
- **Loss of appetite**
  - Monitor fluid intake and hydration status.
  - Weigh the child daily.
  - Monitor electrolyte values.
  - Provide small, frequent, well-balanced meals.
  - Encourage high protein and caloric foods and supplements.
  - Involve the child in meal planning.
  - Administer enteral nutrition if needed.
  - Ensure that chemotherapy is administered early in the day.
  - If nausea or vomiting is present, administer antiemetics prior to or after therapy (ondansetron).
- **Hemorrhage cystitis**
  - Encourage fluids.
  - Encourage frequent voiding.
  - Ensure that chemotherapy is administered early in the morning to promote adequate fluid intake and voiding.
  - Administer mesna to provide protection to the bladder.

Bone marrow suppression:
Resulting in anemia, neutropenia, and/or thrombocytopenia

- NURSING ACTIONS
  - Monitor vital signs and report them to the health care provider. Report a temperature greater than 37.8° C (100° F).
  - Monitor for findings of infection (lung congestion; redness, swelling and pain around IV sites) and lesions in the mouth. Monitor the wound site and immunization status.
  - Administer antimicrobial, antiviral, and antifungal medications as prescribed.
  - Protect the child from sources of possible infection.
  - Use good hand hygiene.
  - Encourage the child and family to use good hand hygiene.
  - Encourage the child to avoid crowds while undergoing chemotherapy.
  - Screen visitors and staff for manifestations of infection.
  - Instruct the child to avoid fresh fruits and vegetables.
  - Avoid invasive procedures (injections, rectal temperatures, catheters). Apply pressure to puncture sites for 5 min.
  - Monitor for manifestations of bleeding.
  - Avoid aspirin and NSAIDs.
  - Administer filgrastim, a granulocyte colony-stimulating factor that stimulates WBC production, subcutaneously daily.
  - Monitor the child for headache, fever, and mild to moderate bone pain.
  - Administer epoetin alfa subcutaneously two to three times per week as prescribed to stimulate RBC formation.
  - Monitor blood pressure.
  - Administer oprelvekin subcutaneously daily as prescribed to stimulate platelet formation.
  - Encourage the use of a soft toothbrush.
  - Use gentle handling and positioning to protect from injury.
  - Organize care to provide for rest. Schedule rest periods.
- CLIENT EDUCATION Qpcc
  - Perform infection control procedures at home.
  - Provide support.

Anorexia, nausea, vomiting: Adverse effects of chemotherapy and radiation therapy

- NURSING ACTIONS
  - Avoid strong odors. Provide a pleasant atmosphere for meals.
  - Avoid offering the child's favorite foods during chemotherapy because they can develop an aversion to these foods.
  - Suggest and assist in selecting foods/fluids.
  - Provide small, frequent meals.
  - Administer antiemetics as prescribed, usually before meals.

Alteration in bowel elimination: Diarrhea is a result of radiation to the abdominal area. Some chemotherapeutic agents can cause constipation. If mobility and nutrition decrease, the child is more likely to develop constipation.

- NURSING ACTIONS
  - Provide meticulous skin care.
  - Provide a nutritious diet.
  - Determine if certain foods or drinks (high-fiber, lactose-rich) worsen the child's condition.
  - Monitor I&O and daily weight.

Mucositis and dry mouth

- NURSING ACTIONS
  - Provide a soft toothbrush and/or swabs.
  - Lubricate the child's lips.
  - Give soft, nonacidic foods. A pureed or liquid diet can be required.
  - Provide analgesics.
  - Avoid hydrogen peroxide and lemon glycerin swabs due to mucosal drying and irritation on eroded tissue.

- CLIENT EDUCATION ○PCC
  - Visit a dentist before therapy.
  - Use chlorhexidine mouth wash or salt rinses using ½ tsp table salt mixed with 1 tsp baking soda and 1 quart water.

Alopecia: Occurs with chemotherapy and radiation of the head and/or neck
- NURSING ACTIONS
  - Assess the child's feelings.
  - Discuss cutting long hair short.
  - Suggest wearing a disposable surgical cap for hair collection during heavy loss periods.
  - Use gentle shampoos. Gently brush the child's hair.
  - Avoid blow dryers and curling irons.
  - Suggest wearing a cotton hat or scarf.
- CLIENT EDUCATION ○PCC
  - Discuss the use of a wig, turbans, or hats.
  - Avoid blow dryers and curling irons.
  - Perform scalp hygiene.
  - Hair grows back in 3 to 6 months.

THERAPEUTIC PROCEDURES

Tumor debulking

PREOPERATIVE NURSING ACTIONS
- Avoid palpation of Wilms' tumor.
- Provide preoperative teaching to the child and family that includes length of surgery, where the child will recover, and what equipment will be in place (nasogastric tube, IV line, indwelling urinary catheter).

POSTOPERATIVE NURSING ACTIONS
- Monitor gastrointestinal activity (bowel sounds, bowel movements, distention, nausea, vomiting).
- Provide pain relief.
- Monitor vital signs and assess for any findings of infection.
- Encourage pulmonary hygiene.

INTERPROFESSIONAL CARE

- Social services can assist with access to medications and durable medical equipment if needed.
- A dietitian may be consulted for development of a diet plan.

COMPLICATIONS

- Metastasis
- Kidney failure
- Pancytopenia

Active Learning Scenario

A nurse is caring for a child who has an organ neoplasm. Use the ATI Active Learning Template: System Disorder to complete this item.

NURSING CARE: Describe seven actions.

INTERPROFESSIONAL CARE: Identify two potential referrals.

Active Learning Scenario Key

Using the ATI Active Learning Template: System Disorder
NURSING CARE
- If Wilms' tumor is suspected, do not palpate the abdomen.
- Use caution when handling or bathing the client to prevent trauma to the tumor site.
- Assess the child's and family's coping and support.
- Assess for developmental delays related to illness.
- Assess physical growth (height and weight).
- Provide education and support to the child and family regarding diagnostic testing, treatment plan, ongoing therapy, and prognosis.
- Monitor for findings of infection.
- Administer antibiotics as prescribed for infection.
- Keep the child's skin clean and dry.
- Provide oral hygiene.
- Provide age-appropriate diversional activities.
- Provide support to the child and family.

INTERPROFESSIONAL CARE
- Social services
- Dietitian

Ⓝ *NCLEX® Connection: Physiological Adaptation, Pathophysiology*

Application Exercises

1. A nurse is planning caring for a toddler who is hospitalized and has been diagnosed with a Wilms' tumor. Which of the following actions should the nurse plan to take?

    A. Palpate the child's abdomen to identify the size of the tumor.

    B. Monitor the child for hypertension.

    C. Teach the parents about dialysis.

    D. Obtain a 24-hr urine specimen from the child.

2. A nurse is teaching the parent of a child who has a Wilms' tumor. Which of the following statements should the nurse include in the teaching? (Select all that apply.)

    A. "Your child will need to have chemotherapy for 12 months."

    B. "Most children who have Wilms' tumors also have congenital anomalies."

    C. "Surgery is done usually within 48 hours of diagnosis."

    D. "Palpating the tumor could cause spread of the cancer."

    E. "Further treatments will start immediately after surgery."

3. A nurse is providing teaching to the parent of a child who has a neuroblastoma. Which of the following statements should the nurse include in the teaching? (Select all that apply.)

    A. "Chemotherapy and radiotherapy may be necessary for treatment."

    B. "Your child will need a bone marrow biopsy."

    C. "Your child will be paralyzed because of this tumor."

    D. "Most children are diagnosed around age 12."

    E. "Your child will need surgery for resection of the tumor."

4. A nurse is caring for a child who is receiving radiation following the surgical removal of a Wilm's tumor. Which of the following actions should the nurse take?

    A. Wash the radiation marks from the skin after each treatment.

    B. Cover the radiation site with snug, synthetic clothing.

    C. Instruct the caregiver to avoid using lotion on the site of radiation.

    D. Expose the radiation site to sunlight for 10 minutes a day.

Application Exercises Key

1. A. The child who has a Wilm's tumor is at risk for hypertension due to increased renin production. Pressure applied to the abdomen could rupture the encapsulated tumor; therefore, the nurse should not include palpating the toddler's abdomen in the plan of care.

    B. **CORRECT:** When generating solutions during the care of a child who has been hospitalized with a Wilm's tumor, the nurse should plan to monitor the child for hypertension.

    C. Wilms' tumor is usually unilateral leaving the child with one unaffected kidney; therefore, the nurse would not need to include teaching the parents about dialysis in the plan of care.

    D. A urinalysis, not a 24-hour urine is obtained for diagnostic evaluation of Wilms' tumor; therefore, the nurse should not include teaching about a 24 hour urine specimen in the plan of care.

    Ⓝ *NCLEX® Connection: Reduction of Risk Potential, Therapeutic Procedures*

2. C, D, E **CORRECT:** When taking action and teaching the parent of a child who has a Wilm's tumor, the nurse should include in the teaching that prompt removal of the tumor is best practice for treatment of Wilms' tumor; therefore, surgery to remove the tumor is usually performed within 48 hours of diagnosis. The nurse should also teach the parent that palpating the abdomen can cause rupture of the encapsulated tumor which can cause the cancer to spread. Additionally, the nurse should teach the parent that chemotherapy, and possibly radiation therapy, will begin immediately after surgery.

    A. The length of time the child will receive chemotherapy treatment depends on the stage of the tumor; therefore, the nurse should not teach the parent that the child will need chemotherapy for 12 months.

    B. About 10% of children who have Wilms' tumors have congenital anomalies; therefore, the nurse should not teach the parent that most children who have Wilm's tumors have congenital anomalies

    Ⓝ *NCLEX® Connection: Physiological Adaptation, Illness Management*

3. A, B, E **CORRECT:** When taking action and providing teaching to the parent of a child who has a neuroblastoma, the nurse should include in the teaching that chemotherapy and radiotherapy may be necessary for treatment, diagnostic testing includes a bone marrow biopsy, and resection of the tumor is the treatment of choice.

    C. Physical effects depend on the size and location of the tumor.

    D. Most cases occur before the age of 10 years, with a median age of 19 months.

    Ⓝ *NCLEX® Connection: Reduction of Risk Potential, Therapeutic Procedures*

4. A. The nurse should wash the site with lukewarm water being careful not to remove the skin markings.

    B. The child who is receiving radiation therapy should wear loose, cotton clothing, not snug, synthetic clothing

    C. **CORRECT:** When taking action during the care of a child who us receiving radiation following the surgical removal of a Wilm's tumor, the nurse should instruct the caregiver to avoid using lotion on the child's skin and site of radiation unless prescribed by the provider.

    D. The child who is receiving radiation therapy should have the site of radiation exposed to air; however, heat and sunlight should be avoided.

UNIT 2   SYSTEM DISORDERS
SECTION: NEOPLASTIC DISORDERS

CHAPTER 39 # Blood Neoplasms

Leukemia is the term for a group of malignancies that affect the bone marrow and lymphatic system. Peak onset in children is between ages 2 and 5 years. Leukemia is classified by the type of WBCs that becomes neoplastic and is commonly divided into two groups: acute lymphoblastic leukemia (ALL) and acute myeloid (AML). ALL is the most common childhood malignancy. Morphology, cytogenetic, chromosome and immunologic marker testing is used to further classify leukemia so that the most effective treatment is prescribed.

Leukemia causes an increase in the production of immature WBCs (leukoblasts) with neoplastic characteristics, which leads to infiltration of organs and tissues.

Bone marrow infiltration causes crowding of cells that would normally produce RBCs, platelets, and mature WBCs. Deficient RBCs cause anemia. Deficient mature WBCs (neutropenia) increase the risk for infection. Deficient platelets (thrombocytopenia) cause bleeding and bruising.

Infiltration of spleen, liver, and lymph nodes leads to tissue fibrosis. Infiltration of the CNS causes increased intracranial pressure. Other tissues can also be infiltrated (testes, prostate, ovaries, gastrointestinal tract, kidneys, and lungs).

ASSESSMENT

RISK FACTORS

- Leukemia is the most common cancer of childhood
- Male sex assigned at birth
- Non-Hispanic white Americans or Hispanic clients
- Family history of leukemia
- Children who have trisomy 21 (Down syndrome)

EXPECTED FINDINGS

History and physical assessment findings can reveal vague reports (anorexia, headache, fatigue).

PHYSICAL ASSESSMENT FINDINGS

- Low-grade fever
- Pallor
- Increased bruising and petechiae
- Listlessness
- Enlarged liver, lymph nodes, and joints
- Abdominal, leg, and joint pain
- Headache
- Vomiting and anorexia
- Unsteady gait
- Pain
- Enlarged kidneys and testicles
- Manifestations of increased intracranial pressure

LABORATORY TESTS

Complete blood count
- Anemia (low blood count)
- Thrombocytopenia (low platelets)
- Neutropenia (low neutrophils)
- Leukemic blasts (immature WBCs)
- Blood smear (immature WBC)

DIAGNOSTIC PROCEDURES

Bone marrow aspiration or biopsy analysis

The most definitive diagnostic procedure. If leukemia is present, the specimen will show prolific quantities of immature leukemic blast cells and protein markers indicating a specific type of leukemia.

NURSING ACTIONS

- Assist the provider with the procedure.
- Topical anesthetic (a eutectic mixture of local anesthetic cream) may be applied over the biopsy area 45 min to 1 hr prior to the procedure.
- Conscious sedation is induced using a general anesthetic (propofol).
- Positioning depends on the access site to be used (posterior or anterior iliac crest is most common; tibia may be used in children less than 18 months of age due to immaturity of the bone of the iliac crest).

POSTPROCEDURE

- Apply pressure to the site, then apply a pressure dressing.
- Assess vital signs frequently.
- Monitor for manifestations of bleeding and infection for 24 hr.

CLIENT EDUCATION: Understand proper procedure and postprocedure care.

Cerebrospinal fluid (CSF) analysis

CSF, obtained by lumbar puncture, is assessed to determine CNS involvement.

NURSING ACTIONS
- Assist the provider with the sterile procedure.
- A topical anesthetic cream may be applied over the biopsy area 1 hr prior to the procedure.
- Place the child in the side-lying position with the head flexed and knees drawn up toward the chest with their back arched, and assist in maintaining the position. Distraction can be required.
- Position the newborn upright with their head flexed forward.
- The child may be sedated.
- The provider will clean the skin and inject a local anesthetic.
- The provider will take pressure readings and collect three to five sterile test tubes of CSF.
- Pressure and an elastic or adhesive bandage will be applied to the puncture site after the needle is removed.
- Label specimens appropriately, and deliver them to the laboratory.
- Monitor the site for bleeding, hematoma, or infection.
- Monitor for manifestations of increased intracranial pressure (ICP) (increased blood pressure, decreased respirations, or changes in LOC).

CLIENT EDUCATION: Report manifestation such as headache, numbness and tingling of the lower extremities, and altered level of consciousness to the provider

Liver and kidney function studies

Used for baseline functioning before chemotherapy and also during therapy to monitor effectiveness.

CLIENT EDUCATION: Understand the length of time to receive results.

PATIENT-CENTERED CARE

NURSING CARE

- Provide emotional support to the child and family.
- Encourage peer contact if appropriate.
- Assess pain using an age-appropriate pain scale.
- Use pharmacological and nonpharmacological interventions to provide around-the-clock pain management.

MEDICATIONS

Chemotherapy

- The agents to be used depend on the type of leukemia, age, and whether leukemic cells are found in the cerebrospinal fluid.
- Common agents include vincristine, doxorubicin.
- The agent must be administered through a central line or port.

- Corticosteroids can be used as treatment for certain cancers and to minimize adverse effects of treatment.
- Goal of therapy is complete remission with less than 5% of blast cells present.
- Intrathecal methotrexate can be administered prophylactically to prevent CNS complications.

Chemotherapy is administered in different phases to treat leukemia.
- **Induction/remission therapy**: To achieve complete remission or less than 5% of leukemic cells in the bone marrow
- **Intensification therapy (consolidation)**: To destroy any remaining leukemic cells followed by a delayed intensification to prevent any resistant leukemic cells from emerging
- **Maintenance therapy**: To sustain the remission phase. Also requires frequent monitoring of CBC

NURSING ACTIONS
- Control nausea and vomiting with antiemetics prior to treatment. May be combined with dexamethasone.
- Manage adverse effects of treatment (myelosuppression).
- Assess for complications of adverse effects of chemotherapy.

CHEMOTHERAPY ADVERSE EFFECTS: REFER TO CHAPTER 38: ORGAN NEOPLASMS FOR ADVERSE EFFECTS OF CHEMOTHERAPY

CLIENT EDUCATION
- The use of steroid treatment can cause moon face and changes in skin and mood.
- Observe for manifestations of infection, skin breakdown, and nutritional deficiency.
- Notify treatment team immediately if the child develops a fever.
- Maintain good hygiene.
- Avoid individuals who have infectious diseases.
- Administer medications and provide nutritional support at home.
- Understand proper use of vascular access devices.
- Understand bleeding precautions and the management of active bleeding.

THERAPEUTIC PROCEDURES

Hematopoietic stem cell transplant (HCST)

HCST can be indicated for children who have AML during the first remission and for children who have ALL after a second remission.

Allogeneic transplant: The blood-forming stem cells generally are donated by another person.

NURSING ACTIONS
- Coordinate administration of high-dose chemotherapy and possible full-body radiation.
- Administer donor stem cells via IV infusion.
- Implement protective isolation. Qs
  - Private, positive-pressure room
  - At least 12 air exchanges/hr
  - HEPA filtration for incoming air
  - Respirator mask, gloves, and gowns
  - No dried or fresh flowers, and no potted plants

CLIENT EDUCATION: The child is at an increased risk for infection and bleeding until transfused stem cells grow.

Radiation therapy

NURSING ACTIONS
- Can be used for resistant CNS disorders.
- Assist with positioning.
- Provide support to the child and family.
- Manage adverse effects.

CLIENT EDUCATION
- Observe for adverse effects (fatigue, infection).
- Maintain adequate rest and a healthy diet.

INTERPROFESSIONAL CARE

Provide information regarding support services for the child and family.

COMPLICATIONS

Infection

Infection can be a complication of myelosuppression.

NURSING ACTIONS
- Provide the child with a private room. The room should be designed to allow for adequate air flow to reduce airborne pathogens.
- Restrict visitors and health personnel who have active illnesses.
- Adhere to strict hand hygiene.
- Assess potential sites of infections (oral ulcer, open cut), and monitor temperature.
- Administer antibiotics as prescribed after source of infection identified through chest radiographs; blood, stool, urine, and nasopharyngeal cultures.
- Encourage adequate protein and caloric intake.
- Monitor absolute neutrophil count (ANC).
- Use aseptic technique for all procedures.

CLIENT EDUCATION
- Understand infection control practices.
- Observe for manifestations of infection and call the provider if necessary.
- Avoid live vaccines while the immune system is depressed.

Hemorrhage

Bleeding (thrombocytopenia) can be a complication of myelosuppression.

NURSING ACTIONS
- Monitor for findings of bleeding: petechiae, ecchymoses, hematuria, bleeding gums, hematemesis, tarry stools.
- Avoid unnecessary skin punctures, and use surgical aseptic technique when performed. Apply pressure for 5 min to stop bleeding.
- Treat a nosebleed with cold and pressure.
- Administer platelet concentrates or platelet rich plasma as prescribed.
- Avoid obtaining temperatures rectally.
- No aspirin products.

CLIENT EDUCATION Qᴘᴄᴄ
- Understand the importance of and how to perform meticulous oral care to prevent gingival bleeding. Use a soft toothbrush, and avoid astringent mouthwashes.
- Take measures to control epistaxis (gentle pressure, packing the nostrils).
- Avoid activities that can lead to injury or bleeding.

CNS effects

Blindness, hydrocephalus, recurrent seizures

Kidney impairment

- Increased uric acid can obstruct renal tubules causing decreased excretion of chemotherapeutic agents.
- Administer allopurinol as prescribed to decrease uric acid production.

Testicular invasion

- Testicular involvement can occur

Anemia

Anemia can be a complication of myelosuppression.

NURSING ACTIONS
- Administer blood transfusions as prescribed.
- Allow for frequent rest periods.
- Administer oxygen therapy.
- Administer IV fluid replacement.

CLIENT EDUCATION: Be aware of foods high in iron. Qᴘᴄᴄ

Active Learning Scenario

A nurse is preparing to assist with a lumbar puncture. Use the ATI Active Learning Template: Diagnostic Procedure to complete this item.

DESCRIPTION OF THE PROCEDURE

NURSING INTERVENTIONS: Describe six.

POTENTIAL COMPLICATIONS: Identify two.

Application Exercises

1. A nurse is assessing a child who has leukemia. Which of the following should the nurse expect to find? (Select all that apply.)

   A. Hypothermia

   B. Anorexia

   C. Petechiae

   D. Erythema

   E. Unsteady gait

2. A nurse is planning care for an infant who is scheduled to have a lumbar puncture. Which of the following actions should the nurse include in the plan of care?

   A. Cleanse the thoracic area of the infant's back with an antiseptic solution.

   B. Apply a eutectic mixture of local anesthetic cream just before the procedure begins.

   C. Restrain the infant during the procedure to prevent movement.

   D. Position the infant with his head extended and chin raised.

3. A nurse is providing teaching to the parents of a child who has a new prescription for chemotherapy. Which of the following statements by the parents indicates understanding of the teaching?

   A. "My child should not be given any steroids while on chemotherapy."

   B. "My child will receive donor stem cells during chemotherapy."

   C. "I will need to monitor my child for infection and fever."

   D. "I should use clean technique when accessing my child's port."

4. A nurse is caring for a child who has thrombocytopenia. Which of the following actions should the nurse take? (Select all that apply.)

   A. Monitor for manifestations of bleeding.

   B. Administer routine immunizations.

   C. Obtain rectal temperatures.

   D. Avoid peripheral venipunctures.

   E. Limit visitors.

Application Exercises Key

1. B, C, E. **CORRECT:** When recognizing cues while assessing a child who has leukemia, the nurse should expect to find anorexia, petechiae, and an unsteady gait.
   A. The child who has leukemia will have a low-grade fever, not hypothermia.
   D. The child who has leukemia will exhibit pallor, not erythema.

   Ⓝ *NCLEX® Connection: Physiological Adaptation, Pathophysiology*

2. A. The lumbar area of the infant's back should be cleansed prior to the procedure.
   B. A local anesthetic cream should be applied 45 to 60 min prior to the procedure.
   C. **CORRECT:** When generating solutions for the care of an infant who is scheduled to have a lumbar puncture, the nurse should plan to implement measures that will reduces the infant's risk for injury such as restraining the infant during the procedure.
   D. The infant should be positioned with his neck flexed and chin to the chest.

   Ⓝ *NCLEX® Connection: Reduction of Risk Potential, Diagnostic Tests*

3. A. Children who are receiving chemotherapy my receive corticosteroids as an adjunct to treatment or to minimize adverse effects of treatment.
   B. Children receive donor stem cells during hematopoietic stem cells transplants, not during treatment with chemotherapy.
   C. **CORRECT:** When taking action and providing education to the parents of a child who has a new prescription for chemotherapy, the nurse should identify the statement, "I will need to monitor my child for infection and fever" as understanding of the teaching. Chemotherapy causes immunosuppression placing the child who is receiving treatment at a greater risk for infection.
   D. When accessing an implanted ventral venous access device, the parent should use aseptic technique, not clean technique.

   Ⓝ *NCLEX® Connection: Reduction of Risk Potential, System-Specific Assessments*

4. A, D. **CORRECT:** When taking actions during the care of a child who has thrombocytopenia, the nurse should recognize that the child who has thrombocytopenia is at risk for bleeding; therefore, the nurse should monitor for manifestations of bleeding and avoid peripheral venipunctures.
   B. The child who has thrombocytopenia is at risk for bleeding, and skin punctures should be avoided. Administering routine immunizations is not an appropriate action for the nurse to take.
   C. The child who has thrombocytopenia is at risk for bleeding and obtaining a rectal temperature could cause tissue injury.
   E. Limiting visitors protects the child from infection and is not an appropriate action to prevent bleeding.

   Ⓝ *NCLEX® Connection: Physiological Adaptation, Unexpected Response to Therapies*

Active Learning Scenario Key

Using the ATI Active Learning Template: Diagnostic Procedure

DESCRIPTION OF THE PROCEDURE: CSF is obtained to determine whether there is CNS involvement.

NURSING INTERVENTIONS
- Have the child empty their bladder.
- Apply a topical anesthetic 60 min before the procedure.
- Monitor the child if conscious sedation is used.
- Position the child in a side-lying position with the head flexed and knees drawn up toward the chest.
- Use distraction techniques if needed.
- Assist with the procedure.
- Apply pressure and an elastic bandage to the site after the needle is withdrawn.
- Label the specimens, and deliver them to the laboratory.
- Monitor for hematoma, bleeding, and infection.
- Keep the bed flat.
- Instruct the child to remain in a flat position for at least 30 min after the procedure.
- Encourage to drink full glass of fluid after the procedure to prevent spinal headache.

POTENTIAL COMPLICATIONS
- Spinal headache
- Hematoma
- Infection
- Bleeding

Ⓝ *NCLEX® Connection: Reduction of Risk Potential, Diagnostic Tests*

UNIT 2 SYSTEM DISORDERS
SECTION: NEOPLASTIC DISORDERS

CHAPTER 40 *Bone and Soft Tissue Cancers*

Malignant tumors in bone can originate from all tissues involved in bone growth, including osteoid matrix, blood vessels, and cartilage. Osteosarcoma usually occurs in the metaphysis of long bones, most often in the femur. Treatment frequently includes amputation or limb salvage procedure of the affected extremity as well as chemotherapy. Ewing's sarcoma (a primitive neuroectodermal tumor) occurs in the shafts of long bones and of trunk bones. Treatment includes surgical biopsy, intensive radiation therapy to tumor site, and chemotherapy, but not amputation. Prognosis depends on how quickly the disease is diagnosed and whether metastasis has occurred.

Soft tissue malignancies arise from undifferentiated cells in the soft tissues (muscles, tendons), in connective or fibrous tissue, or in blood or lymph vessels. These malignancies can begin in any area of the body. Rhabdomyosarcoma originates in skeletal muscle in any part of the body, but it most commonly occurs in the head and neck, with the orbit of the eye frequently affected. Treatment consists of surgical biopsy, local radiation therapy, and chemotherapy, rather than radical surgical procedures.

Children who undergo irradiation for malignancies in or near the pelvic area can experience sterilization and secondary cancers.

Bone Tumors

ASSESSMENT

RISK FACTORS

- Osteosarcoma usually peaks during adolescents and overlaps with growth spurts.
- More common in children who are males than females sex assigned at birth.
- Ewing's sarcoma occurs prior to 20 years of age and is more common in Caucasian clients.

EXPECTED FINDINGS

- Nonspecific bone pain that is often mistaken for an injury or growing pains
- Weakness, swelling, decreased movement, or limping
- Anemia, fever, or unexplained weight loss
- Inability to lift a heavy object

LABORATORY TESTS

CBC and other common tests can help rule out infection, iron deficiency anemia, and other possible causes of findings.

DIAGNOSTIC PROCEDURES

- X-rays, computed tomography (CT) scans, or magnetic resonance imaging (MRI) of the primary site
- Bone marrow biopsy
- CT of the chest and bone scans to evaluate metastasis

PATIENT-CENTERED CARE

NURSING CARE

- Use developmentally appropriate language when explaining the diagnosis and treatment.
- Allow the child time, usually several days, to prepare emotionally for surgery and chemotherapy. Qᴘᴄᴄ
- Avoid overwhelming the child with information.
- Provide emotional support for the child and family.
- Explain the possibility of sterilization to adolescents and caregivers, if indicated.

MEDICATIONS

Chemotherapy

Osteosarcoma
- Various agents used singly or in combination before and/or after surgery
- High-dose methotrexate with citrovorum factor rescue, doxorubicin, cisplatin, ifosfamide, and etoposide

Ewing's sarcoma: Vincristine, doxorubicin, and cyclophosphamide alternating with ifosfamide and etoposide

NURSING ACTIONS

- Control nausea and vomiting with antiemetics prior to treatment.
- Manage adverse effects of treatment.

CLIENT EDUCATION

- Observe for manifestations of infection, skin breakdown, and nutritional deficiency.
- Maintain good hygiene.
- Understand proper use of vascular access devices.
- Take bleeding precautions and properly manage active bleeding.

THERAPEUTIC PROCEDURES

Localized radiation therapy can be used in combination with chemotherapy and surgery.

NURSING ACTIONS

- Assist the child with positioning.
- Monitor for adverse effects.

CLIENT EDUCATION: Adhere to the course of therapy.

Surgical interventions

Surgical biopsy

- Tumor is biopsied under anesthesia to determine presence and/or tissue type of cancer.
- NURSING ACTIONS
  - Provide routine preoperative and postoperative care.
  - Provide for adequate pain relief.
  - Monitor wound for manifestations of infection.
  - Actions vary with extent and area of surgery, but nursing actions should include preprocedure and postprocedure assessments, including vital signs, medication for pain, and wound care as necessary.
- CLIENT EDUCATION: Educate the child and family regarding postprocedure care.

Limb salvage procedure for bone cancers

- Includes a course of chemotherapy to shrink the tumor and then total bone and joint replacement after the tumor and affected bone are removed.
- NURSING ACTIONS
  - Administer preoperative chemotherapy.
  - Assist with managing adverse effects.
  - Provide routine postoperative care.
  - Provide for adequate pain relief.
- CLIENT EDUCATION
  - Understand proper postoperative care.
  - Understand possible effects of preoperative chemotherapy (hair loss).

Limb amputation for bone cancer

- The child can receive chemotherapy both preoperatively and postoperatively.
- NURSING ACTIONS
  - Provide routine preoperative and postoperative care.
  - Provide emotional support.
  - Assess for the presence of phantom limb pain postoperatively, and medicate appropriately.
  - Work with the child and family to plan for issues (appropriate clothing to wear with prosthesis).

- CLIENT EDUCATION
  - Prepare the child for fitting of a temporary prosthesis, which can occur immediately after surgery. Qpcc
  - Cooperate with postoperative physical therapy.
  - Role-play issues that the child will need to deal with after discharge (talking to strangers who ask about the prosthesis).
  - The child's emotions (anger) are normal grief reactions after amputation, chemotherapy, and other treatments.

INTERPROFESSIONAL CARE

- Older children and adolescents can benefit from attending a support group for children who have cancer and/or have had amputations.
- Initiate a referral for mental health counseling to assist the child to resume normal activities.
- Initiate appropriate referrals to assist the child to resume normal activities (school attendance, physical activities).
- Initiate physical and occupational therapy referrals to start while in the hospital and to continue after discharge.

CLIENT EDUCATION

Follow up with the provider and community resources as instructed.

COMPLICATIONS

Skin desquamation

Either dry or moist, with permanent hyperpigmentation and possible damage to underlying structures

NURSING ACTIONS

- Assess the site frequently for infection.

CLIENT EDUCATION

- Prevent additional irritation to the site.
  - Use loose-fitting clothing.
  - Prevent exposure to sunlight or extremes of temperature.
- Maintain follow-up examinations.

Myelosuppression

Elimination of normal blood cells along with cancer cells is a risk with treatment by most chemotherapeutic agents. This can cause infection (reduced leukocytes), hemorrhage (reduced thrombocytes), and anemia (reduced red blood cells).

NURSING ACTIONS

- Evaluate laboratory data and assess for manifestations of complications.
  - Infection: elevated WBC and fever
  - Hemorrhage: blood in urine or stool, bruising, and petechiae
  - Anemia: fatigue and decreased hemoglobin/hematocrit

- Prevent infection.
  - Provide a private room when hospitalized.
  - Restrict staff/visitors that have infections.
  - Promote frequent hand hygiene by staff/visitors.
  - Avoid all live-virus vaccines during periods of immunosuppression. Qs
  - Ensure that household members are up-to-date on immunizations.
  - Provide a diet adequate in protein and calories.
- Prevent hemorrhage or injury from bleeding.
  - Use a strict aseptic technique for all invasive procedures.
  - Use gentle technique when providing mouth care.
  - Clean the perineal area carefully to prevent trauma, and avoid obtaining temperatures rectally.
  - Infuse platelets as prescribed.
- Prevent anemia or injury from anemia.
  - Provide rest periods as needed.
  - Infuse packed red blood cells as prescribed.

CLIENT EDUCATION: Practice strategies to recognize complications at home and to prevent injury from infection, hemorrhage, or bleeding.

Rhabdomyosarcoma

Most common soft tissue malignancy in children

ASSESSMENT

RISK FACTORS

Rhabdomyosarcoma occurs in children of all ages (but more commonly in children younger than 10 years of age) and is more common among Caucasians.

EXPECTED FINDINGS

- Can cause pain in local areas related to compression by the tumor (sore throat can occur with tumor of the nasopharynx)
- Possible absence of pain in some parts of the body (in the retroperitoneal area) until the tumor begins to obstruct organs

BASED ON AFFECTED AREA

- **CNS**: Impaired cranial nerve function, stiffness in the neck, decreased heart rate and respiratory rate
- **Orbit**: unilateral proptosis, ecchymosis of conjunctiva, strabismus
- **Nasopharynx**: stuffy nose, pain, nasal obstruction, epistaxis, palpable neck nodes, visible mass (late)
- **Paranasal sinuses**: nasal obstruction, pain, discharge, sinusitis, swelling
- **Middle ear**: chronic otitis media, pain, sanguinopurulent discharge, facial paralysis
- **Retroperitoneal area**: usually no findings, abdominal mass, pain, intestinal or genitourinary obstruction
- **Perineum**: visible superficial mass, bowel or bladder obstruction
- **Extremity**: pain, palpable fixed mass, lymph node enlargement

DIAGNOSTIC PROCEDURES

- CT scans or MRI of the primary site
- Biopsy of tumor is possible
- CT of the chest, bone scans, bone marrow biopsy, and lumbar puncture to evaluate metastasis

PATIENT-CENTERED CARE

NURSING CARE

- Use developmentally appropriate language when explaining the diagnosis and treatment.
- Allow the child time, usually several days, to prepare emotionally for surgery and chemotherapy.
- Avoid overwhelming the child with information.
- Provide emotional support for the parents and child.

MEDICATIONS

Chemotherapy

Vincristine, actinomycin D, cyclophosphamide, ifosfamide, topotecan, irinotecan, and doxorubicin for about 1 year

THERAPEUTIC PROCEDURES

Localized radiation therapy

Radiation therapy may be used in combination with chemotherapy and surgery.

Surgical interventions

Surgical biopsy
Tumor is biopsied under anesthesia to determine presence and/or tissue type of cancer.

INTERPROFESSIONAL CARE

- Older children and adolescents can benefit from attending a support group for children who have cancer.
- Initiate a referral for mental health counseling to assist the child to resume normal activities.
- Initiate physical and occupational therapy referrals to start while in the hospital and to continue after discharge.

CLIENT EDUCATION

Perform follow-up care.

CARE AFTER DISCHARGE: Community services: Initiate appropriate referrals to assist the child to resume normal activities (school attendance, physical activities).

COMPLICATIONS

- Skin desquamation
- Myelosuppression

Active Learning Scenario

A nurse is teaching a guardian of a child who has bone cancer and is receiving chemotherapy about myelosuppression. Use the ATI Active Learning Template: System Disorder to complete this item.

NURSING CARE: Describe two actions related to each of the following areas.

- Evaluating laboratory data to assess for complications
- Preventing infection
- Preventing hemorrhage or injury from bleeding
- Preventing anemia or injury from anemia

Application Exercises

1. A nurse is caring for a child who is being evaluated for osteosarcoma. Which of the following manifestations should the nurse expect the child to report?
   A. Pain
   B. Discoloration of the skin
   C. Abdominal mass
   D. Easy bruising

2. A nurse is caring for a child following an above-the-knee amputation. Which of the following actions should the nurse take?
   A. Avoid discussing the amputation.
   B. Inform the child and caregivers that chemotherapy will not be need after surgery.
   C. Prepare the child for a prosthesis fitting.
   D. Maintain the affected limb in the dependent position.

3. A nurse is providing home care information to the parents of a child who is receiving chemotherapy. Which of the following information should the nurse include in the teaching? (Select all that apply.)
   A. Manifestations of infection
   B. Bleeding precautions
   C. Hand hygiene
   D. Homeschooling
   E. Airborne precautions

4. A nurse is assessing a child who has rhabdomyosarcoma of the nasopharynx. Which of the following manifestations should the nurse expect to find? (Select all that apply.)
   A. Enlarged neck lymph nodes
   B. Pain
   C. Sinusitis
   D. Epistaxis
   E. Strabismus

Application Exercises Key

1. A. **CORRECT:** When caring for a child who is being evaluated for osteosarcoma, the nurse should expect the child to report bone pain. The child may also report weakness, swelling, decreased movement, limping, weight loss, and the inability to lift a heavy object. The child and family may also report an unexplained weight loss.
   B. Discoloration of the skin is not an expected finding of osteosarcoma.
   C. Abdominal mass is not an expected finding of osteosarcoma.
   D. Easy bruising is not an expected finding not an expected finding of osteosarcoma.

2. A. The loss of a limb entails a grieving process; therefore, the nurse should encourage discussion to facilitate grieving, not avoid discussing the amputation.
   B. Chemotherapy may be needed after the amputation; therefore, the nurse should not inform that child and caregivers that chemotherapy will not be needed after the surgery.
   C. **CORRECT:** When taking action during the care of a child following an above-the-knee amputation, the nurse should recognize that a prosthesis is fitted soon after surgery; therefore, the nurse should prepare the child for a prosthesis fitting to help the child cope with the transition.
   D. The affected limb should be elevated for the first 24 hours after surgery to decrease swelling; therefore, the nurse should not maintain the affected limb in a dependent position.

   Ⓝ NCLEX® Connection: *Reduction of Risk Potential, Potential for Complications from Surgical Procedures and Health Alterations*

3. A. **CORRECT:** When taking action and providing home care information to the parents of a child who is receiving chemotherapy, the nurse should recognize that chemotherapy destroys healthy WBCs, which increases the risk of infection; therefore, the nurse should provide information regarding manifestations of infection and how to perform proper hand hygiene.
   B. **CORRECT:** The nurse should also recognize that chemotherapy destroys healthy platelets, which increases the risk of bleeding; therefore, the nurse should also provide information on bleeding precautions.
   C. **CORRECT:** When taking action and providing home care information to the parents of a child who is receiving chemotherapy, the nurse should recognize that chemotherapy destroys healthy WBCs, which increases the risk of infection; therefore, the nurse should provide information regarding manifestations of infection and how to perform proper hand hygiene.
   D. Children who are receiving chemotherapy can continue to attend school following recommendations of the provider. Homeschooling should not be included in the teaching.
   E. Children who are receiving chemotherapy are at an increased risk for infection. However, they do not need to be placed on airborne precautions.

   Ⓝ NCLEX® Connection: *Psychosocial Integrity, Therapeutic Procedures*

4. A, B, D. **CORRECT:** When recognizing cues during the assessment of a child who has rhabdomyosarcoma of the nasopharynx, the nurse should expect to find enlarged neck lymph nodes, pain, and epistaxis.
   C. Sinusitis is a manifestation of rhabdomyosarcoma of the paranasal sinuses.
   E. Strabismus is a manifestation of rhabdomyosarcoma of the orbital area.

   Ⓝ NCLEX® Connection: *Physiological Adaptation, Pathophysiology*

Active Learning Scenario Key

Using the ATI Active Learning Template: System Disorder

NURSING CARE
- Evaluating laboratory data to assess for complications
  - Infection: elevated WBC and fever
  - Hemorrhage: blood in urine or stool, bruising, and petechiae
  - Anemia: fatigue and decreased hemoglobin/hematocrit
- Preventing infection
  - Provide a private room when hospitalized.
  - Restrict staff/visitors who have infections.
  - Promote frequent hand hygiene by staff/visitors.
  - Avoid all live-virus vaccines during periods of immunosuppression.
  - Ensure that household members are up-to-date on immunizations.
  - Provide a diet adequate in proteins and calories.
- Preventing hemorrhage or injury from bleeding
  - Use a strict aseptic technique for all invasive procedures.
  - Use gentle technique when providing mouth care.
  - Clean the perineal area carefully to prevent trauma, and avoid obtaining temperatures rectally.
  - Infuse platelets as prescribed.
- Preventing anemia or injury from anemia
  - Provide rest periods as needed.
  - Infuse packed red blood cells as prescribed.

Ⓝ NCLEX® Connection: *Physiological Adaptation, Pathophysiology*

When reviewing the following chapters, keep in mind the relevant topics and tasks of the NCLEX outline, in particular:

Health Promotion and Maintenance

DEVELOPMENTAL STAGES AND TRANSITIONS:
Compare the client's development to expected age/developmental stage and report any deviations.

HEALTH SCREENING
Perform health history/health and risk assessment.

Apply knowledge of pathophysiology to health screening.

HEALTH PROMOTION/DISEASE PREVENTION
Plan and/or participate in community health education.

Educate the client on actions to promote/maintain health and prevent disease.

Physiological Adaptation

ALTERATIONS IN BODY SYSTEMS
Assess adaptation of a client to health alteration, illness, and/or disease.

Apply knowledge of nursing procedures, pathophysiology, and psychomotor skills when caring for a client who has an alteration in body systems.

Promote client progress toward recovery from an alteration in body systems.

PATHOPHYSIOLOGY: Identify pathophysiology
related to an acute or chronic condition.

MEDICAL EMERGENCIES: Apply knowledge of nursing
procedures and psychomotor skills when caring for a client experiencing a medical emergency.

Reduction of Risk Potential

POTENTIAL FOR ALTERATIONS IN BODY SYSTEMS
Educate client on methods to prevent complications associated with activity level/diagnosed illness/disease.

Apply knowledge of pathophysiology to monitoring for complications.

THERAPEUTIC PROCEDURES: Monitor the client
before and after a procedure/surgery.

CHAPTER 41 *Burns*

Thermal, cold, chemical, electrical, and radioactive agents can cause burns, which result in cellular destruction of the skin layers and underlying tissue. The type and severity of the burn affect the treatment plan.

Thermal burns occur when there is exposure to flames, hot surfaces, or hot liquids. Chemical burns occur when there is exposure to a caustic agent (acid, alkali, or organic compound). Cleaning agents used in the home and industrial setting cause chemical burns.

Electrical burns occur when an electrical current passes through the body. This type of burn can result in severe damage, including loss of organ function, tissue destruction with the subsequent need for amputation of a limb, and cardiac and respiratory arrest.

HEALTH PROMOTION AND DISEASE PREVENTION

- Provide adequate supervision.
- Establish a safe play area.
- Keep hot liquids, electrical cords, and dangling objects out of reach.

ASSESSMENT

RISK FACTORS

- Abuse, neglect, or lack of supervision
- Developmental growth of the child

EXPECTED FINDINGS

SUBJECTIVE DATA
- Type of burning agent (dry heat, moist heat, chemical, electrical, ionizing radiation)
- Duration of contact
- Area of the body in which the burn occurred
- Younger children have deeper injuries due to thinner skin. Children less than 2 years old have a higher mortality due to decreased protein stores and immature renal and immune functioning
- Extent, depth, and severity of injury

PHYSICAL ASSESSMENT FINDINGS (41.1)

41.1 Stages of burns*

	FIRST-DEGREE	SECOND-DEGREE		THIRD-DEGREE	FOURTH-DEGREE
	Superficial	*Superficial partial thickness*	*Deep partial thickness*	*Full thickness*	*Deep full thickness*
DAMAGE	Damage to epidermis	Damage to the entire epidermis Dermal elements are intact	Damage to the entire epidermis and some parts of the dermis Sweat glands and hair follicles remain intact	Damage to the entire epidermis and dermis and possible damage to the subcutaneous tissue Nerve endings, hair follicles, and sweat glands are destroyed	Damage to all layers of the skin that extends to muscle, fascia, and bones
APPEARANCE	Pink to red in color with no blisters Blanches with pressure	Painful, moist, red in color with blisters, mild to moderate edema, and no eschar Blanches with pressure	Mottled, red to white in color, with blisters and moderate edema Blanches with pressure	Red to tan, black, brown, or waxy white in color Dry, leathery appearance No blanching	Color variable Dull and dry Charring Possible visible ligaments, bone, or tendons
SENSATION/ HEALING	Painful Heals within 3 to 7 days No scarring	Painful Heals in less than 21 days Variable amounts of scarring Sensitive to temperature changes, exposure to air, and light touch	Painful Sensitive to temperature changes and light touch Healing time can extend beyond 21 days Scarring is likely	As burn heals, painful sensations return and severity of pain increases Heals within weeks to months Scarring is present Autografting is required	No pain is present Heals within weeks to months Scarring is present Autografting is required Amputation possible

*This can vary depending on the child's skin tone and severity of burn.

EXTENT OF INJURY

Total body surface area (TBSA)

- Age-related charts determine the extent of injury to body surface, which is expressed in percentages.
- Infants' skin is thin, so injury is likely to be deeper.

Severity grading system (41.2)

Classification

The severity of the injury depends on the child’s age, causative agent, body area involved, and the extent and depth of the burn.

Minor: treated in outpatient setting

Moderate: treated in a hospital with expertise in burn care

Major: requires medical services of a burn center

LABORATORY TESTS

MAJOR BURNS: CBC, blood electrolytes, BUN, ABGs, random glucose levels, liver enzymes, urinalysis

PATIENT-CENTERED CARE

NURSING CARE

Emergency care (on-site)

- Priority action is to stop the burning process.
  - Position the child horizontally and roll in a rug or blanket to extinguish the fire. (If rug or blanket is not available, roll the child over slowly.)
  - Remove clothing or jewelry that can conduct heat.
  - Apply tepid water soaks or run water over the injury (major burns) Do not use ice.
  - Flush burns caused by liquid chemicals with a large volume of water. While wearing gloves, brush dry chemicals from the skin, before flushing with a large volume of water.
- Assess the child's condition (maintain airway patency).
- Cover burn injury with clean dry cloth to prevent contamination (do not apply ointment without medical evaluation).

- Provide warmth for child as indicated (prevent hypothermia depending on extent of burn injury).
- Transport child to receive evaluation of burn injury by provider or ED depending on extent of injury.
- Provide reassurance to child and family.

Minor burns

- If necessary, child is seen in a health care facility for medical care.
- Cleanse with mild soap and tepid water (avoid excess friction).
- Removing blisters is controversial.
- Use antimicrobial ointment.
- Apply clean dressing.
  - Nonadherent: fine-mesh gauze
  - Hydrocolloid: occlusive dressing
- Provide warmth as needed (to prevent hypothermia).
- Administer mild analgesia (acetaminophen).
- Check immunization status. Administer tetanus vaccine if it has been more than 5 years since last immunization.
- Educate the family to avoid using greasy lotions or butter on burns.
- Educate the family to monitor for manifestations of infection.

Major burns

PHASES OF BURN MANAGEMENT

Acute (emergent/resuscitative): focuses on managing shock and preventing respiratory complications

Management: focuses on preventing infections and closing the burn wound in a timely manner

Rehabilitative: occurs after closure of burn wound, preventing complications from scarring

- Maintain airway and ventilation (priority action) QEBP
  - Provide humidified 100% supplemental oxygen as prescribed.
  - Assess monitor respirations and oxygen saturation level.
  - Check ABGs and carbon monoxide level.
  - Prepare to intubate if needed (Monitor for findings of air hunger, nasal flaring, grunting, or signs of respiratory distress).
  - Prepare for child for escharotomy (full thickness chest burns) this will promote ventilation.
- Provide and monitor fluid replacement therapy
  - Fluid replacement is important during the first 24 hr.

41.2 Severity grading system

	MINOR	MODERATE	MAJOR
Partial-thickness burns	Less than 10% of TBSA	10% to 20% of TBSA	Greater than 20% of TBSA
Full-thickness burns	Usually outpatient Can require 1- to 2-day admission	Admission to hospital, preferably one with expertise in burn care	Admission to a burn center

From Vaccarro P., Trofino, R.: Care of the patient with minor to moderate burns. In Trofino R., editor: Nursing care of the burn-injured patient, Philadelphia, 1991, Davis. Adopted by the American Burn Association

- Initiate IV access with large-bore catheter. Multiple access points can be necessary.
- Monitor vital signs.
- Maintain cardiac output.
- Obtain a baseline weight and monitor daily weights.
- Insert indwelling urinary catheter for monitoring of output.
- Ensure child receives correct fluid requirements (this is calculated by using several formulas such as Parkland's).
- Isotonic crystalloid solutions (lactated Ringer's) are used during the early stage of burn recovery.
- Colloid solutions (albumin or plasma) may be used after the first 24 to 48 hr of burn recovery.
- Monitor capillary refill and level of consciousness to determine sufficient hydration. QEBP
- Maintain urine output of 0.5 to 1 mL/kg/hr if the child weighs less than 30 kg (66 lb).
- Maintain urine output of 30 mL/hr if the child weighs more than 30 kg (66 lb).
- Be prepared to administer blood products as prescribed.
- Monitor for manifestations of shock and notify the provider of findings.
- Alterations in sensorium (confusion)
  - Increased capillary refill
  - Spiking fever
  - Mottled or cool extremities
  - Weak peripheral pulses
  - Tachycardia
  - Tachypnea
  - Decreased urine output
- Manage pain.
  - Establish ongoing monitoring of pain and effectiveness of pain management.
  - Avoid IM or subcutaneous injections.
  - Administer prescribed IV opioid analgesics (morphine sulfate, midazolam, and fentanyl).
  - Monitor for respiratory depression when using opioid analgesics. Qs
  - Administer pain medications prior to dressing changes or procedures.
  - Use nonpharmacologic methods for pain control (guided imagery, music therapy, therapeutic touch) to enhance the effects of analgesics and promote improved pain management.
- Prevent infection.
  - Follow standard precautions when performing wound care.
  - Restrict plants and flowers due to the risk of contact with pseudomonas.
  - Change position frequently to prevent contractures and prolonged pressure.
  - Limit visitors.
  - Use reverse isolation if prescribed.
  - Monitor for manifestations of infection, and report to the provider.
  - Use client-designated equipment (blood pressure cuffs and thermometers).
  - Administer tetanus toxoid if indicated.
  - Administer antibiotics if infection is present.

- Provide nutritional support.
  - Increase caloric intake to meet increased metabolic demands and prevent hypoglycemia.
  - Increase protein intake to prevent tissue breakdown and promote healing.
  - Provide enteral therapy feedings if prescribed for proper nutrition and to provide nourishment to bowels.
  - Insert NG tube for stomach decompression if indicated.
- Restore mobility.
  - Maintain correct body alignment, splint extremities, and facilitate position changes to prevent contractures.
  - Maintain active and passive range of motion.
  - Assist with ambulation as soon as the child is stable.
  - Apply pressure dressings to prevent contractures and scarring.
  - Closely monitor areas at high risk for pressure injury (heels, sacrum, back of head).
- Provide psychological support.
  - Provide developmentally appropriate support for the child.
  - Assist with coping.
  - Use family-centered approach.
  - Make referrals as needed.

THERAPEUTIC MANAGEMENT

MEDICATIONS

Topical agents

Silver sulfadiazine (inhibits the growth of bacteria), mafenide acetate, santyl, bacitracin
- Use with second- and third-degree burns.
- Apply to cleansed, debrided area.
- Wear sterile gloves for application.

Topical prepackaged mesh gauze dressings

Nanocrystalline film of pure silver, hydrofiber with ionic silver, silver silicone foam, glucosaminoglycan hydrogel
- Used for second-degree burns
- Protects wound and provides comfort
- Increases rate of healing
- Reduces frequency of dressing changes

Morphine sulfate

Analgesia

NURSING ACTIONS
- Administer IV. May provide medication prior to dressing changes.
- Monitor for respiratory depression.
- Monitor pain relief.

CLIENT EDUCATION: Perform safety precautions needed with opioid administration.

Midazolam, fentanyl, propofol, and nitrous oxide

Sedation and analgesia

NURSING ACTIONS
- Administer IV just prior to the start of a procedure.
- Monitor the need for sedation.
- Monitor pain relief.

CLIENT EDUCATION: Perform safety precautions needed with opioid administration.

Nitrous oxide/oxygen mixture

Short-term analgesic gas.

NURSING ACTIONS
- Self-administered by the child
- Useful for relieving anxiety and increasing pain threshold during procedures

Wound care

NURSING ACTIONS
- Premedicate as prescribed prior to wound care.
  - Administer analgesics.
  - Administer hydroxyzine or diphenhydramine for pruritus.
- Remove previous dressings.
- Assess for odors, drainage, and discharge.
- Cleanse the wound as prescribed.
- Prepare child for debridement if needed.
  - Provide analgesic prior to procedure
  - Involves the removal of non-vital tissue
  - Prepare child for hydrotherapy
    - Cleanses the burn and causes the separation of eschar
    - Performed by showering or immersion (once or twice daily)

Skin coverings (grafting)

- Methods
  - **Open:** use of a topical antimicrobial medication, burn wound is uncovered
  - **Exposure:** burn wound is open to air
  - **Modified:** use of antimicrobial medication or applied to thin gauze or net secured to the burn wound
  - **Occlusive:** antimicrobial medication is impregnated in gauze or applied directly to wound; multiple gauze placed over primary layer that is secured with a gauze or net

Temporary skin coverings may be used to promote healing of large burns. Requires repeated surgical application.
- **Allograft (homograft):** Skin from humans that is used for partial and full thickness burn wounds. Rejection can occur 14 days after application.
- **Xenograft:** Obtained from animals (porcine/pigs) for partial-thickness burn wounds. It does not vascularize but provides pain control while the burn heals.
- **Synthetic skin coverings:** (hydrocolloids, transparent adhesives) Used for partial-thickness burn wounds.
- **Artificial skin:** A biologic product that allows the dermis to regenerate, used for partial- and full-thickness burns (healing is faster).

Permanent skin coverings may be the treatment of choice for burns covering large areas of the body.
- **Autografts:** tissue obtained from an undamaged area of the child's own skin
- **Sheet graft:** Sheet of skin from donor site is used to cover the wound
- **Mesh graft:** Sheet of skin is removed from donor site and placed in a mesher so skin graft has small slits in it; allows graft to cover larger areas of burn wound

Cultured epithelium: Epithelial cells cultured for use when grafting sites are limited

NURSING ACTIONS FOR GRAFTING
- Do not change graft site dressing. Only change if prescribed.
- Provide wound care to the donor site as prescribed.
- Administer analgesics as prescribed.
- Monitor for infection before and after skin coverings or grafts are applied.
  - Monitor dressings for fluids, drainage, and odor.
  - Monitor for excessive pain.
- Monitor for fever.

CLIENT EDUCATION: Report evidence of infection.

INTERPROFESSIONAL CARE

Refer to services (nutrition, child life, social support, respiratory therapy, occupational/physical therapy, individual and family counseling) as prescribed.

CLIENT EDUCATION QTC

- The child should continue to perform range-of-motion exercises and to work with a physical therapist to prevent contractures.
- Assess the wound for infection and perform wound care.
- Perform age-appropriate safety measures for the home (covering electrical outlets, supervising children when in the bath, keeping irons out of reach of children, teaching the dangers of playing with matches). Qs
- Avoid sun exposure between 1000 and 1400, wear protective clothing, and apply sunscreen to prevent sunburn.
- Expected delays in growth and weight for up to three years post burn injury.
- Increased risk of bone remodeling.

CARE AFTER DISCHARGE
- Initiate a referral for home health services.
- Initiate a referral to occupational therapy for evaluation of the home environment and assistance to relearn how to perform ADLs.
- Initiate a referral to social services for community support services.

COMPLICATIONS

Inhalation injury

Direct thermal injury
- Occurs with burns to the face and lips. Damage occurs to the tracheobronchial tree after inhalation of heated gases and toxic chemicals produced during combustion.
- Can be delayed 24 to 48 hr.
- Findings include wheezing, increased secretions, hoarseness, wet rales in the lungs, singed nasal hairs, laryngeal edema, and carbonaceous secretions.

Carbon monoxide injury
- Occurs when incident takes place in an enclosed area.
- Findings include mucosal erythema and edema followed by sloughing of the mucosa.

NURSING ACTIONS: Maintain airway and ventilation and provide 100% oxygen as prescribed.

Hypertrophic scarring

Scar tissue can result from the deposit of collagen as healing occurs

NURSING ACTIONS
- Apply uniform pressure to scar area.
- Child may require custom fitted pressure garments.
- Continue physical therapy.
- Apply hydroxyzine or diphenhydramine if prescribed for itching.
- Massage scars as indicated and apply moisturizers to scars as prescribed.

Pulmonary problems

Include edema, bacterial pneumonia, aspiration, embolus, and pulmonary insufficiency.

NURSING ACTIONS
- Maintain airway via intubation, sometimes tracheostomy.
- Administer oxygen as prescribed.

Wound sepsis

Burn wounds are a medium for bacteria growth.

NURSING ACTIONS
- Monitor and report findings immediately.
- Initial sign of sepsis is disorientation.
- Monitor for other findings: spiking fever, decreased bowel sounds, hyperglycemia, thrombocytopenia, abdominal distension, diarrhea, leukopenia.

Application Exercises

1. A nurse is caring for a client who has a superficial partial-thickness burn. Which of the following actions should the nurse take?
   - A. Administer IV infusion of 0.9% sodium chloride.
   - B. Apply ice to burn.
   - C. Clean the affected area using a soft-bristle brush.
   - D. Administer acetaminophen.

2. A nurse is caring for a child who has a major full thickness burn and is experiencing severe pain. Which of the following actions should the nurse implement to manage this child's pain?
   - A. Administer morphine sulfate IV.
   - B. Administer meperidine IM.
   - C. Administer acetaminophen PO.
   - D. Administer hydrocodone PO.

3. A nurse is assessing a child who has major burns and suspected shock. Which of the following findings should the nurse expect? (Select all that apply.)
   - A. Altered sensorium
   - B. Increased body temperature
   - C. Decreased capillary refill time
   - D. Decreased urine output
   - E. Slow respirations

4. A nurse is caring for an adolescent who has a moderate burn. Which of the following actions should the nurse take?
   - A. Maintain immobilization of the affected area.
   - B. Expose affected area to the air.
   - C. Encourage a high protein and high calorie diet.
   - D. Implement droplet precautions.

5. Sort the following types of skin coverings into Temporary or Permanent.
   - A. Allograft
   - B. Artificial
   - C. Autograft
   - D. Cultured epithelium
   - E. Mesh graft
   - F. Sheet graft
   - G. Synthetic
   - H. Xenograft

Active Learning Scenario

A nurse is teaching a newly licensed nurse about manifestations of burns. Use the ATI Active Learning Template: Basic Concept to complete this item.

UNDERLYING PRINCIPLES: List the depth, appearance, sensation, and healing of first-, second-, third-, and fourth-degree burns.

Active Learning Scenario Key

Using the ATI Active Learning Template: Basic Concept

UNDERLYING PRINCIPLES

Superficial (first-degree)
- Damage to the epidermis
- Pink to red in color with no blisters
- Blanches with pressure
- Painful
- Heals within 3 to 7 days with no scarring

Superficial partial thickness (second-degree)
- Damage to the entire epidermis with intact dermal elements
- Moist
- Red in color with blisters
- Blanches with pressure
- Mild to moderate edema
- No eschar
- Painful
- Sensitive to temperature changes and light touch
- Heals in less than 21 days with variable scarring

Deep partial thickness (second-degree)
- Damage to the entire epidermis and some parts of the dermis
- Sweat glands and hair follicles remain intact
- Mottled
- Red to white in color with blisters
- Blanches with pressure
- Moderate edema
- Painful
- Sensitive to temperature changes and light touch
- Healing can go beyond 21 days with scarring

Full thickness (third degree)
- Damage to the entire epidermis and dermis with possible damage to the subcutaneous tissue
- Nerve endings, hair follicles, and sweat glands are destroyed
- Red to tan, black, brown, or waxy white in color
- Dry, leathery appearance
- No blanching
- As burn heals, painful sensations return and severity of pain increases
- Heals within weeks to months
- Scarring is present
- Grafting is required

Deep full thickness (fourth-degree)
- Damage to all layers of the skin that extends to the muscle, tendons, and bones.
- Color variable, dull, and dry with charring
- Possible visible ligaments, bone, or tendons
- No pain is present
- Heals within weeks to months
- Scarring is present and grafting is required
- Amputation possible

Ⓝ *NCLEX® Connection: Physiological Adaptation, Pathophysiology*

Application Exercises Key

1. A. An IV infusion of 0.9% sodium chloride is not indicated for superficial partial thickness burn but for a child who has major burn injury.
   B. The application of ice can cause vasoconstriction and further tissue damage.
   C. The burn is cleaned by irrigating with tepid water. The use of a soft bristle brush can cause friction and further tissue damage.
   D. **CORRECT:** A superficial partial thickness burn involves damage to the epidermis and can be very painful for the child. Therefore, the nurse should administer an analgesic such as acetaminophen to promote comfort.

   Ⓝ *NCLEX® Connection: Physiological Adaptation, Illness Management*

2. A. **CORRECT:** A full thickness burn extends to the dermis and epidermis and possibly the subcutaneous layer of the skin and the child may experience severe pain. A narcotic analgesic such as morphine is indicated to manage the child's pain. It is administered intravenously.
   B. Meperidine can be given however, the Intramuscular is avoided because this can cause more pain for the child.
   C. Acetaminophen can be administered for minor burns and mild pain.
   D. Ibuprofen is only administered if the child has no active bleeding.

   Ⓝ *NCLEX® Connection: Pharmacological and Parenteral Therapies, Pharmacological Pain Management*

3. A, B, D. **CORRECT:** Findings for shock include altered sensorium, increased body temperature, and decreased urine output.
   C, E. Other findings include increased capillary refill and increased respirations as the body compensates for decreased perfusion.

   Ⓝ *NCLEX® Connection: Physiological Adaptation, Hemodynamics*

4. A. Active and passive range of motion of the affected area is recommended to prevent contractures.
   B. Dressings should be applied to the burned area to prevent infection.
   C. **CORRECT:** The nurse should encourage the adolescent to consume a high protein and high calorie diet because this will promote healing and meet the metabolic requirements to maintain homeostasis.
   D. Droplet precautions are not indicated for a child who has a condition that is spread by air droplets such as influenza.

   Ⓝ *NCLEX® Connection: Physiological Adaptation, Pathophysiology*

5. **TEMPORARY:** A, B, G, H; **PERMANENT:** C, D, E, F

   Temporary skin grafts include allografts, xenografts, synthetic skin grafts, and artificial skin grafts.
   Permanent skin grafts include allografts, sheet grafts, cultured epithelium, and mesh grafts.

CHAPTER 42

Complications of Infants

It is essential for a nurse to immediately identify complications and implement appropriate interventions for complications of newborns and infants. Providing ongoing emotional support parents or caregivers is also imperative to the plan of care.

Complications include phenylketonuria (PKU), meningocele, necrotizing enterocolitis (NEC), respiratory distress syndrome (RDS), congenital hypothyroidism, substance-exposed infants, hyperbilirubinemia, chromosomal abnormalities, neonatal seizures, complications of premature infants, newborn sepsis, and plagiocephaly.

Phenylketonuria (PKU)

PKU is an inherited metabolic disorder in which the newborn lacks the enzyme phenylalanine hydroxylase. This enzyme converts phenylalanine, an essential amino acid, into tyrosine. The lack of this enzyme leads to the accumulation of phenylalanine in the newborn's bloodstream and tissues, which causes cognitive impairment. PKU accounts for 1:10,000 births in the US.

The key to prevention of PKU in newborns is identification of clients in their reproductive years who have the disorder. These clients must adhere to strict dietary guidelines from 3 months before conception throughout pregnancy. Failure to follow strict dietary guidelines during pregnancy can result in fetal complications such as microcephaly, cognitive impairment, and heart defects. All newborns are screened for PKU within 2 days following birth to allow the newborn to ingest a source of protein. Immediate identification and providing the newborn with dietary restrictions, significantly decreases the occurrence of cognitive impairment.

ASSESSMENT

RISK FACTORS

PKU is inherited as an autosomal recessive trait. Clients who have PKU or who have had a child who has PKU can undergo genetic testing to determine the risk of PKU in future children.

EXPECTED FINDINGS

- Growth failure
- Frequent vomiting
- Irritability
- Musty odor to urine
- Microcephaly
- Heart defects
- Blue eyes, very fair skin, light blonde hair

LABORATORY TESTS

Newborn metabolic screen: Blood spot analysis is performed on all newborns within 2 days following birth to allow for early identification of PKU.
- Expected reference range of phenylalanine in newborns is 0.5 to 1 mg/dL.
- Some states require a repeat newborn metabolic screen when the newborn is 1 to 2 weeks of age.

Guthrie test: Confirms diagnosis when blood spot analysis is positive.

PATIENT-CENTERED CARE

NURSING CARE

Nursing care focuses on dietary intake.
- Initiate dietary restrictions as soon as PKU is diagnosed, or within 7 to 10 days of birth.
- Provide the newborn on a formula low in phenylalanine.
  - Intake should be 20 to 30 mg phenylalanine per kilogram of body weight per day.
  - Monitor phenylalanine level (should be less than 8 mg/dL).
- Encourage the client to breastfeed in moderation if desired. Breastmilk contains phenylalanine, so breastfeeding exclusively might not be possible.
- Monitor the newborn for findings of PKU.
- Provide parents with support and education.
  - Consult with a registered dietitian.
  - Provide referrals to support groups.

THERAPEUTIC MANAGEMENT

- Dietary restrictions
  - Newborns can be breastfed in moderation. If formula feeding, will require a formula low in phenylalanine.
  - Limit intake of foods high in phenylalanine (meats, eggs, milk). Encourage foods low in phenylalanine potatoes, lettuce, peas, bananas.
- Sapropterin can be prescribed to decrease phenylalanine levels.
  - Administer orally.
  - May require frequent monitoring of phenylalanine levels.
- Monitor laboratory findings.
  - Hemoglobin (monitor for anemia)
  - Phenylalanine (evaluate effectiveness of therapy)

COMPLICATIONS

ASSESSMENT FINDINGS OF COMPLICATIONS

- Cognitive impairment (can be severe)
- Hyperactivity
- Unexpected behavior (erratic, fright reactions, biting arm, head banging)
- Disorientation
- Spasticity or catatonic-like positions
- Seizures

Meningocele/ Myelomeningocele

Meningocele and myelomeningocele are neural tube defects (NTD) that are present at birth and affect the CNS and spine. These defects occur when the neural tube fails to close during the third to fourth week of embryonic development. These defects are also classified as spina bifida.

Meningocele is the protrusion of a sac-like cyst that contains meninges and spinal fluid.

Myelomeningocele is the protrusion of a sac-like cyst that contains meninges, spinal fluid, and a portion of the spinal cord and nerves.

ASSESSMENT

RISK FACTORS

- Use of medications or illicit substances during pregnancy
- Malnutrition during pregnancy ⓈSDoH
- Insufficient intake of folic acid during pregnancy
- Exposure to radiation or chemicals during pregnancy
- Prepregnancy obesity, diabetes mellitus, hyperthermia, or low levels of vitamin B12
- Previous birth of neonate who had a neural tube defect

EXPECTED FINDINGS

PHYSICAL ASSESSMENT FINDINGS

- Protrusion of a sac-like cyst midline of the spine: Cysts are most commonly found in the lumbar or lumbosacral area.
- Sensory and/or neuromotor dysfunction
  - Type and severity of dysfunction dependent on location of defect
  - Observe lower extremities for movement and response to stimuli
- Potential constant dribbling of urine and loss of feces
- Possible limb deformities

DIAGNOSTIC TESTS

MATERNAL TESTING DURING PREGNANCY

- Elevated alpha-fetoprotein levels in maternal blood
- Chorionic villi sampling
- Amniocentesis
- Ultrasound

NEWBORN TESTING

- MRI
- Ultrasound
- CT scan
- Neurologic evaluation

PATIENT-CENTERED CARE

NURSING CARE

- Assess for infant-parent attachment.
- Assess the cyst.
- Perform routine newborn assessments.
- Assess neurologic status.
- Obtain accurate measurements of output.
- Assess fontanels, and monitor head circumference.

THERAPEUTIC PROCEDURES

Closure of the meningocele/myelomeningocele sac

Done as soon as possible to prevent complications due to injury or infection

PREOPERATIVE NURSING ACTIONS

- Prepare the family for the newborn's surgery (within 24 to 72 hr after birth).
- Protect the sac from injury.
- Place the infant in a radiant warmer, without clothing.
- Apply a sterile, moist non-adhering dressing with 0.9% sodium chloride on the cyst, re-wetting as needed to prevent drying.
- Inspect the cyst closely for leakage of fluid or manifestations of irritation.
- Assess for manifestations of infection (fever, irritability, and lethargy).
- Administer IV antibiotics as prescribed.
- Avoid measuring temperatures rectally.
- Avoid putting pressure on the sac.

POSTOPERATIVE NURSING ACTIONS

- Monitor vital signs.
- Monitor I&O.
- Monitor weight.
- Assess for manifestations of infection.
- Provide pain management as prescribed.
- Assess for leakage of CSF.
- Maintain the newborn in a prone position until other positions are prescribed.
- Resume oral feedings.
- Provide range of motion (ROM) to extremities.
- Assess fontanels for bulging.
- Measure head circumference.

CLIENT EDUCATION

- Provide education to the parents on postoperative home care.
- Depending on degree of the newborn's disability, teach the parents ROM techniques.

ONGOING CARE

- Assess skin integrity, head circumference, and bowel and bladder functioning.
- Assess for allergies (latex).
- Assess cognitive and motor development.
- Monitor for infections.
- Address concerns with body image.
- Offer support to family.
- Assist the client with independence throughout lifespan.
- Assist the family with obtaining medical equipment/services.

INTERPROFESSIONAL CARE

Neurosurgery, neurology, urology, orthopedics, physical therapy, occupational therapy, and social services may be consulted.

COMPLICATIONS

Skin pressure injury

Caused by prolonged pressure on one area

NURSING ACTIONS

- Monitor skin for breakdown.
- Reposition frequently to prevent pressure on bony prominences.
- Monitor skin under splints and braces.

CLIENT EDUCATION: Teach parents to monitor skin integrity.

Latex allergy

The infant can have a high risk of allergy to latex. Allergy responses range from urticaria to wheezing, which can progress to anaphylaxis.

NURSING ACTIONS

- Assist with testing for allergy.
- Reduce exposure to latex. Qs

CLIENT EDUCATION

- Avoid exposing the infant to latex.
- Be aware of household items that can contain latex (disposable diapers, cleaning gloves, water toys).
- Observe for manifestations of an allergic reaction and report them to the provider.
- Understand proper use of epinephrine.

Increased intracranial pressure

Caused by shunt malformation or hydrocephalus

MANIFESTATIONS: High-pitched cry, lethargy, vomiting, bulging fontanels and/or widening cranial suture lines, increased head circumference

NURSING ACTIONS

- Prepare for surgery for shunt or shunt revision.
- Use gentle movements when performing ROM exercises.
- Minimize environmental stressors (noise, lights, frequent visitors).
- Assess and manage pain.

CLIENT EDUCATION: Observe for manifestations of shunt malfunction and hydrocephalus and report them to the provider.

Bladder issues

Urinary diversion may be performed to manage bladder dysfunction (either spasticity or flaccidity).

NURSING ACTIONS

- Monitor for manifestations of bladder dysfunction.
- Monitor for manifestations of bladder infection.
- Monitor for bleeding.
- Prepare the newborn and family for surgery if necessary.
- Teach the parents how to care for the stoma (vesicostomy) if applicable.

Orthopedic issues

Corrections of associated potential problems (clubfoot, scoliosis, and other malformations of the feet and legs)

NURSING ACTIONS

- Monitor for manifestations of infection.
- Administer pain medications.
- Prepare the newborn and family for surgery if needed.
- Provide cast care if cast is present.
- Monitor for neurologic deficits.

CLIENT EDUCATION

- Observe for manifestations of infection.
- Understand proper cast and splint care.

Necrotizing enterocolitis (NEC)

NEC is an inflammatory disease of the gastrointestinal mucosa caused by ischemia or hypoxia. Ischemia results in death of mucosal cells leading to necrotic patches that interfere with digestion.

ASSESSMENT

RISK FACTORS

- Prematurity
- Respiratory distress syndrome
- Polycythemia
- Exchange transfusion
- Intrauterine growth restriction
- Shock
- Asphyxia
- Receiving enteral feedings
- Pre-existing infection
- GI vascular compromise
- Immature GI host defense

EXPECTED FINDINGS

PHYSICAL ASSESSMENT FINDINGS
- Abdominal distention
- Gastric residuals
- Bloody stools
- Periods of apnea begin or worsen
- Hypotension
- Lethargy
- Poor feeding
- Decreased urinary output

LABORATORY TESTS

- CBC with differential
- ABGs
- Coagulation studies
- Blood cultures
- Electrolytes

DIAGNOSTIC PROCEDURES

Abdominal x-rays
- Sausage-shaped dilation of intestine
- Marked distention of intestine
- Characteristic "soapsuds" appearance of the intestinal wall due to air infiltration
- Free air in abdominal cavity if perforation has occurred

PATIENT-CENTERED CARE

NURSING CARE

- Treatment begins with prevention. Withhold feedings for 24 to 48 hr from newborns who suffered birth asphyxia.
- Initiate feeding with breast milk, which has a protective effect against the development of NEC.
- Discontinue all feedings at first manifestation of NEC.
- Administer IV or TPN to rest the GI tract.
- Insert an NG tube for abdominal decompression.
- Administer IV antibiotics as prescribed.
- Handle the abdomen carefully to prevent intestinal perforation.
- Measure abdominal girth just above the umbilicus every 4 to 8 hr.
- Assist with serial abdominal x-rays every 4 to 6 hr.
- Monitor vital signs.
- Perform all routine newborn assessments.
- Prepare the newborn and family for surgical intervention, if indicated.
  - Removal of necrotized portion of bowel.
  - Temporary colostomy is a possibility.
  - Facilitate bonding.

COMPLICATIONS

- Short-bowel syndrome (disorder of absorption)
- Colonic stricture with possible obstruction
- Fat malabsorption
- Failure to thrive

Respiratory distress syndrome (RDS)

RDS occurs as a result of surfactant deficiency in the lungs and is characterized by poor gas exchange and ventilatory failure. Surfactant is a phospholipid that assists in alveoli expansion. Surfactant keeps alveoli from collapsing and allows gas exchange to occur. Atelectasis (collapsing of a portion of lung) increases the work of breathing. As a result, respiratory acidosis and hypoxemia can develop.

- Complications from RDS are related to oxygen therapy and mechanical ventilation.
  - Pneumothorax
  - Pneumomediastinum
  - Retinopathy of prematurity
  - Bronchopulmonary dysplasia
  - Infection
  - Intraventricular hemorrhage

ASSESSMENT

RISK FACTORS

- Preterm gestation
- Perinatal asphyxia (meconium staining, cord prolapse, nuchal cord)
- Maternal diabetes mellitus
- Premature rupture of membranes
- Maternal use of barbiturates or narcotics close to birth
- Cesarean birth
- Multifetal pregnancy
- Cold stress
- Sepsis
- Airway obstruction
- Hypoglycemia

EXPECTED FINDINGS

PHYSICAL ASSESSMENT FINDINGS
- Tachypnea (respiratory rate greater than 60/min)
- Nasal flaring
- Expiratory grunting
- Retractions
- Labored breathing with prolonged expiration
- Fine crackles on auscultation
- Cyanosis
- Unresponsiveness, flaccidity, and apnea with decreased breath sounds (manifestations of worsened RDS)

LABORATORY TESTS

- Culture and sensitivity of the blood, urine, and cerebrospinal fluid
- Blood glucose

DIAGNOSTIC PROCEDURES

- ABGs reveal hypercapnia (excess of carbon dioxide in the blood) and respiratory or mixed acidosis.
- Chest x-ray

PATIENT-CENTERED CARE

NURSING CARE

- Suction the newborn's mouth, trachea, and nose as needed. Qs
- Maintain thermoregulation.
- Provide mouth and skin care.
- Maintain adequate oxygenation, prevent lactic acidosis, and avoid the toxic effects of oxygen.
- Decrease environmental stimuli.

THERAPEUTIC MANAGEMENT

RESPIRATORY SUPPORT

- Ventilation: use of a ventilator controls force of air delivery
- Oxygen therapy: can be prescribed to administer by mask, cannula, continous positive airway pressure (CPAP), assistive ventilation with positive end expiratory pressure (PEEP)
- Nitric oxide: administration causes pulmonary vasodilation

SUPPORTIVE CARE

- Prevent hypothermia (keep newborn warm)
- Provide hydration and nutrition (IV fluids, gavage feedings, glucose)

MEDICATIONS

Beractant, poractant alfa, calfactant

Classification: Lung surfactant

Intended effect: It is prescribed for newborns who are premature and have RDS. It restores surfactant and improves respiratory compliance.

NURSING ACTIONS

- Perform a respiratory assessment including ABGs, respiratory rhythm, and rate and color before and after administration of agent.
- Provide suction to the newborn prior to administration of the medication.
- Assess endotracheal tube placement.
- Avoid suctioning of the endotracheal tube for 1 hr after administration of the medication.

Congenital hypothyroidism

Congenital hypothyroidism occurs due to an absent or nonfunctioning thyroid gland in a newborn. Thyroid hypofunction can be caused by maternal iodine deficiency or maternal antithyroid medications during pregnancy.

- Findings might not appear until 3 months of age in a formula-fed infant and 6 months of age in a breastfed infant.
- Early diagnosis is crucial due to severe progressive physical and cognitive dysfunction that will occur if left untreated.

ASSESSMENT

RISK FACTORS

- Assigned sex at birth: female
- Low birth weight or birth weight greater than 4.5 kg (4,500 g)
- Maternal low iodine levels during pregnancy

EXPECTED FINDINGS

PHYSICAL ASSESSMENT FINDINGS

- Sleeping excessively
- Enlarged tongue
- Respiratory difficulty
- Poor sucking
- Cool, dry skin on extremities
- Jaundice
- Subnormal temperature, respiratory rate and pulse
- Short, thick neck
- Hypotonia with decreased deep tendon reflexes
- Abdominal distention and constipation

LABORATORY TESTS

- Newborn metabolic screen: blood spot analysis performed within 2 days of birth
- T3, T4, and TSH levels
- Blood lipid levels

DIAGNOSTIC PROCEDURES

- X-rays to evaluate bone growth
- Ultrasound of thyroid

PATIENT-CENTERED CARE

NURSING CARE

- Monitor vital signs and weight.
- Monitor respiratory status.
- Assess for feeding difficulties.
- Treatment is administration of synthetic thyroid hormone (sodium levothyroxine).
  - Administer medication as prescribed.
  - Medication must be taken indefinitely.
- Administer supplemental vitamin D to support rapid bone growth.
- Monitor thyroid levels (T3, T4 and TSH).

CLIENT EDUCATION: Understand the importance of proper medication administration.

Substance-exposed infants

Maternal substance use during pregnancy consists of any use of alcohol or drugs. Intrauterine drug exposure can cause anomalies, neurobehavioral changes, and evidence of withdrawal in the neonate. These changes depend on the specific drug or combination of drugs used, dosage, route of administration, metabolism and excretion by the mother and her fetus, timing of exposure, and length of exposure.

- Substance withdrawal in the newborn occurs when the mother uses drugs that have addictive properties during pregnancy. This includes illicit substances, heroin, opiates, alcohol, tobacco, methadone, and prescription medications.
- Fetal alcohol spectrum disorder (FASD) is an umbrella term used to describe the range of clinical effects that can occur because of maternal alcohol intake. Fetal alcohol syndrome (FAS) refers specifically to children who exhibit the most severe manifestations of FASD including atypical facial features, growth restriction, and neurodevelopmental deficits as well as a confirmed history of maternal alcohol consumption.
- Newborns who have FAS are at risk for specific congenital physical defects, along with long-term complications.
  - Feeding problems
  - Central nervous system dysfunction (learning disabilities, low IQ, seizures)
  - Behavioral difficulties (hyperactivity [ADHD])
  - Language abnormalities
  - Delayed growth and development
  - Poor maternal-newborn bonding

ASSESSMENT

RISK FACTORS

- Maternal use of substances prior to knowing they are pregnant
- Maternal substance use and addiction

EXPECTED FINDINGS

PHYSICAL ASSESSMENT FINDINGS

Monitor the neonate for neonatal abstinence syndrome (NAS) and neonatal opioid withdrawal syndrome (NOWS) and increased wakefulness using the neonatal abstinence scoring system that assesses for and scores the following.

- **CNS**: increased wakefulness, a high-pitched, shrill cry, incessant crying, irritability, tremors, hyperactive with an increased Moro reflex, increased deep-tendon reflexes, increased muscle tone, abrasions and/or excoriations on the face and knees, and convulsions
- **Metabolic, vasomotor, and respiratory**: nasal congestion with flaring, frequent yawning, skin mottling, tachypnea greater than 60/min, sweating, and temperature greater than 37.2° C (99° F) or temperature greater than 38.3° C (101° F)
- **Gastrointestinal**: poor feeding, regurgitation (projectile vomiting), diarrhea, and excessive, uncoordinated, and constant sucking

Heroin withdrawal

Neonatal opioid withdrawal syndrome (NOWS): Low birth weight and small for gestational age (SGA), decreased Moro reflexes (rather than increased), jittery, hyperactive, and hypothermia or hyperthermia. The infant has a shrill persistent cry.

Methadone withdrawal

Neonatal opioid withdrawal syndrome (NOWS): Increased incidence of seizures, sleep pattern disturbances, higher birth weights, and higher risk of sudden unexpected infant death (SUID).

Cocaine exposure

- Infant can appear normal or exhibit neurologic problems at birth. Newborn can exhibit neurobehavioral depression or excitability.
- High-pitched cry, abnormal sleep patterns, excessive sucking, hypertonicity, tremors, irritability, inability to console, and poor tolerance to changes in routine.

Marijuana exposure

Associated with a decrease in newborn birth weight and length, fetal growth

Methamphetamine withdrawal

Small head circumference, SGA, agitation, vomiting, rapid respiratory rate, bradycardia or tachycardia, jitteriness, sleep pattern disturbances, emotional disturbances, and delayed growth and development

Fetal alcohol spectrum disorder

- Craniofacial features include microcephaly, small eyes with epicanthal folds, and short palpebral fissures, thin upper lip, flat midface and indistinct philtrum
- Lack of stranger anxiety and appropriate judgment skills
- Many vital organ anomalies (limb defect and heart defects, including ventricular septal defects)

- Prenatal and postnatal growth restriction
- Developmental delays and neurologic abnormalities
- IQ deficit
- Diminished fine motor skills
- Attention deficit disorder

Tobacco exposure

Prematurity, low birth weight, increased risk for SUID, increased risk for bronchitis, pneumonia, and developmental delays

LABORATORY TESTS

Blood tests should be done to differentiate between neonatal substance withdrawal and central nervous system irritability.
- CBC
- Blood glucose
- Calcium
- Electrolytes
- Drug screen of urine or meconium to reveal the agent used by the mother
- Hair analysis

DIAGNOSTIC PROCEDURES

Chest x-ray for FASD to rule out congenital heart defects

PATIENT-CENTERED CARE

NURSING CARE

Nursing care for maternal substance use and neonatal effects or withdrawal include the following in addition to normal newborn care.
- Perform a neonatal abstinence scoring system assessment, as prescribed.
- Elicit and assess reflexes.
- Monitor the ability to feed and digest intake.
- Monitor fluids and electrolytes with skin turgor, mucous membranes, fontanels, and I&O.
- Observe the newborn's behavior.

MEDICATIONS

Phenobarbital

CLASSIFICATION: Anticonvulsant

INTENDED EFFECT: It is prescribed to decrease CNS irritability and control seizures for newborns who are susceptible to seizures.

NURSING ACTIONS
- Assess IV site frequently.
- Check for any medication incompatibilities.
- Decrease environmental stimuli.
- Cluster cares for newborns to minimize stimulation.
- Swaddle the newborn to reduce self-stimulation and protect the skin from abrasions.
- Monitor and maintain fluids and electrolytes.

- Administer frequent, small feedings of high-calorie formula. The newborn can require gavage feedings.
- Elevate the newborn's head during and following feedings, and burp the newborn to reduce vomiting and aspiration. Qs
- Try various nipples to compensate for a poor suck reflex.
- Have suction available to reduce the risk for aspiration.
- For newborns who are addicted to cocaine, avoid eye contact. Use vertical rocking and a pacifier.
- Consult lactation services to evaluate whether breastfeeding is desired or contraindicated to avoid passing narcotics in breast milk. Methadone is not contraindicated during breastfeeding.
- Prevent infection.
- Initiate a consult with child protective services.
- Morphine and clonidine may be administered to decrease central nervous system irritability.

CLIENT EDUCATION
- Refer the mother to a drug and/or alcohol treatment center.
- Discuss the importance of SUID prevention activities due to the increased rate in newborns of mothers who used methadone.

Hyperbilirubinemia

Hyperbilirubinemia is an elevation of blood bilirubin levels resulting in jaundice. Jaundice normally appears in the head (especially the sclera and mucous membranes), and then progresses down the thorax, abdomen, and extremities.

Jaundice can be either physiologic or pathologic
- **Physiologic jaundice** is considered benign (resulting from normal newborn physiology of increased bilirubin production due to the shortened lifespan and breakdown of fetal RBCs and liver immaturity). The newborn with physiological jaundice has no other manifestations and shows evidence of jaundice after 24 hr of age.
- **Hemolytic disease of the newborn (HDN)**, or pathologic jaundice, is a result of an underlying disease. HDN appears before 24 hr of age. In the term newborn, normal unconjugated bilirubin levels are 0.2 to 1.4 mg/dL. Levels must exceed 5 mg/dL before jaundice is observed. HDN is usually caused by a blood group incompatibility or isoimmunization.

Kernicterus (bilirubin encephalopathy): When certain pathologic conditions exist in addition to increased bilirubin levels, the newborn has an increased permeability of the blood–brain barrier to unconjugated bilirubin. The newborn has the potential for irreversible brain damage. It is a neurologic syndrome caused by bilirubin depositing in brain cells. Survivors can experience neurologic damage, cerebral palsy, seizures and display cognitive impairment, ADHD, delayed or abnormal motor movement, behavioral disorders, perceptual problems or sensorineural hearing loss.

ASSESSMENT

RISK FACTORS

Pathologic hyperbilirubinemia
- Blood bilirubin level in the high-risk zone on the hour-specific nomogram
- Rh or ABO incompatibility with positive direct Coombs test
- Cephalohematoma or significant bruising
- Appearance of jaundice within 24 hr of birth
- Ineffective, difficult breastfeeding
- Gestational age 35 to 36 weeks
- Sibling who has jaundice
- Hereditary hemolytic disease
- East Asian or Asian-American race

EXPECTED FINDINGS

PHYSICAL ASSESSMENT FINDINGS
- Yellowish tint to skin, sclera, and mucous membranes and nails.
- To verify jaundice, press the newborn's skin on the cheek or abdomen lightly with one finger. Then release pressure, and observe the skin color for yellowish tint as the skin is blanched.
- Note the time of jaundice onset to distinguish between physiologic and pathologic jaundice.
- Assess the underlying cause by reviewing the maternal prenatal, family, and newborn history.
- Hypoxia, hypothermia, hypoglycemia, and metabolic acidosis can increase the risk of brain damage despite lower blood levels of bilirubin.

FINDINGS OF KERNICTERUS
- Very yellowish skin
- Lethargy
- Hypotonic
- Poor feeding
- Decreased activity
- High-pitched cry
- Temperature instability

LABORATORY TESTS

- An elevated blood bilirubin level can occur (direct and indirect bilirubin). Monitor bilirubin level until it returns to normal. Use of hour-specific blood bilirubin levels to predict newborns at risk for hyperbilirubinemia is the gold standard for monitoring newborns greater than 35 weeks gestation. Q͟EBP
- Assess maternal and newborn blood type to determine whether there is a presence of ABO incompatibility. This occurs if the newborn has blood type A or B, and the mother is type O.
- Review Hgb and Hct.
- A direct Coombs test reveals the presence of antibody-coated (sensitized) Rh-positive RBCs in the newborn.
- Check electrolyte levels for dehydration from phototherapy.

DIAGNOSTIC PROCEDURES

Transcutaneous bilirubin level is a noninvasive method to measure a newborn's bilirubin level.

PATIENT-CENTERED CARE

NURSING CARE

- Observe the skin and mucous membranes for jaundice.
- Monitor vital signs with careful attention to temperature.
- Set up phototherapy if prescribed.
  - Maintain an eye mask over the newborn's eyes for protection of corneas and retinas.
  - Keep the newborn undressed with the exception of a diaper.
  - Avoid applying lotions or ointments to the skin because they absorb heat and can cause burns.
  - Remove the newborn from phototherapy every 4 hr, and unmask the newborn's eyes, checking for inflammation or injury.
  - Reposition the newborn every 2 hr to expose all body surfaces to the phototherapy lights and prevent pressure sores.
  - Check the lamp energy with a photometer per facility protocol.
  - Turn off the phototherapy lights before drawing blood for testing.
- Observe for effects of phototherapy.
  - Bronze discoloration: not a serious complication
  - Maculopapular skin rash: not a serious complication
  - Development of pressure areas
  - Dehydration (poor skin turgor, dry mucous membranes, decreased urinary output)
  - Elevated temperature
- Encourage the parents to hold and interact with the newborn when phototherapy lights are off.
- Monitor elimination and daily weights for evidence of dehydration.
- Check the newborn's axillary temperature every 4 hr during phototherapy because temperature can become elevated.
- Feed the newborn early and frequently, every 3 to 4 hr. This will promote bilirubin excretion in the stools.
- Encourage continued breastfeeding of the newborn. Supplementation with donor breast milk or formula may be prescribed.

CLIENT EDUCATION: Observe for the rebound effect; bilirubin initially rises after treatment is discontinued but resolves without additional intervention.

THERAPEUTIC MANAGEMENT

Phototherapy is the primary treatment for hyperbilirubinemia. It is prescribed if a newborn's blood bilirubin is in the high-risk zone on the hour-specific blood bilirubin nomogram. Phototherapy converts bilirubin into a soluble form that can be excreted in the stool and urine. Q͟EBP

Newborn sepsis

Infection can be contracted by the newborn before, during, or after birth. Newborns are more susceptible to micro-organisms due to their limited immunity and inability to localize infection. The infection can spread rapidly into the bloodstream.

Newborn sepsis is the presence of micro-organisms or their toxins in the blood or tissues of the newborn during the first month after birth. Manifestations of sepsis are subtle and can resemble other diseases. The nurse often notices them during routine care of the newborn.

Organisms frequently responsible for newborn infections include *Staphylococcus aureus*, *S. epidermidis*, *Escherichia coli*, *Haemophilus influenzae*, group beta-hemolytic streptococcus, *Klebsiella*, and *Pseudomonas*.

Prevention of infection and newborn sepsis starts perinatally with maternal screening for infections, prophylactic interventions, and the use of sterile and aseptic techniques during birth. Prophylactic antibiotic treatment of the eyes of all newborns and appropriate umbilical cord care also help to prevent newborn infection and sepsis.

ASSESSMENT

RISK FACTORS

- Nosocomial exposure in the NICU
- Premature birth
- Prolonged rupture of membranes
- Maternal infection (cytomegalovirus, herpes, hepatitis, and human immunodeficiency virus)
- Invasive procedures (IV lines and ET tubes)
- TPN
- Congenital anomalies
- Diminished immune response

EXPECTED FINDINGS

PHYSICAL ASSESSMENT FINDINGS
- Temperature instability (hypothermia common)
- Suspicious drainage (eyes, umbilical stump)
- Poor feeding pattern (weak suck, decreased intake)
- Vomiting and diarrhea
- Poor weight gain
- Abdominal distention
- Large residual if feeding by gavage
- Apnea, retractions, grunting, cyanosis, and nasal flaring
- Decreased oxygen saturation
- Color changes (pallor, jaundice, and petechiae)
- Tachycardia or bradycardia
- Tachypnea or apnea
- Low blood pressure
- Irritability and seizure activity
- Poor muscle tone and lethargy

LABORATORY TESTS

- CBC
- Blood, urine, and cerebrospinal fluid cultures and sensitivities
- Positive blood cultures, indicates the presence of infection/sepsis
- Chemical profile shows a fluid and electrolyte imbalance

PATIENT-CENTERED CARE

NURSING CARE

- Assess infection risks (review maternal health record).
- Monitor for findings of opportunistic infection.
- Monitor vital signs continuously.
- Monitor I&O and daily weight.
- Monitor fluid and electrolyte status.
- Restrict any visitors with infections.
- Obtain specimens (blood, urine, stool) to assist in identifying the causative organism.
- Initiate and maintain IV therapy as prescribed to administer electrolyte replacements, fluids, and medications.
- Administer medications as prescribed (broad-spectrum antibiotics prior to cultures being obtained).
- Initiate and maintain respiratory support as needed.
- Assess IV site for evidence of infection.
- Provide newborn care to maintain temperature.
- Maintain standard precautions.
- Clean and sterilize all equipment to be used.

CLIENT EDUCATION
- Understand infection control.
  - Use clean bottles and nipples for each feeding.
  - Discard any unused formula.
  - Demonstrate and supervise proper hand hygiene.
  - Demonstrate infection control measures.
  - Ensure adequate rest for newborn, and decrease physical stimulation.
  - Provide emotional support to the family. Q**PCC**

Plagiocephaly

Plagiocephaly is an acquired condition that occurs from cranial molding in infancy. The infant's head becomes asymmetric or oblique in shape due to flattening of the occiput. Plagiocephaly is attributed to the supine sleep position, as its occurrence has increased significantly since the Safe to Sleep campaign of infants sleeping on their backs was initiated to help prevent SUID.

- The key to prevention of plagiocephaly is to provide education on the importance of tummy time, which is allowing the infant to lie in the prone position for 3 to 5 minutes, 2 to 3 times each day. Parents should also alternate the infant's head position each night to avoid persistent pressure on the occiput.
- Treatment for plagiocephaly includes physical therapy and the wearing of a customized helmet to reshape the skull.

ASSESSMENT

RISK FACTORS

- Placing the infant in the supine sleep position
- Torticollis

EXPECTED FINDINGS

PHYSICAL ASSESSMENT FINDINGS
- Oblique shape of head
- Asymmetrical skull and facial features
- Flattened occiput
- Frontal and parietal bossing
- Prominent cheekbone
- Anterior displacement of an ear
- Possible decreased range of motion in neck if torticollis present

PATIENT-CENTERED CARE

NURSING CARE

- Refer parents to physical therapy for neck exercises.
- Assist parents in the proper use of the skull–molding helmet.

CLIENT EDUCATION

- Understand the importance of daily "tummy time" when infant is awake.
- Limit the time the infant is in a car seat, bouncer, or swing.
- Understand the importance of alternating the infant's head position during sleep.
- Continue to place infant in the supine position for sleep.

42.1 Case Study

Scenario Introduction

Malaya is a registered nurse on a mother-baby unit who is caring for Josh Stewart. Josh was born 4 days ago at 36 weeks' gestation via a spontaneous, uncomplicated vaginal birth. He weighed 2835 grams (6 lbs 4 oz). Josh was discharged from the hospital after 48 hours and his mother was instructed to bring him back to the unit today for a serum bilirubin. Malaya has reviewed Josh's medical record and noted that upon discharge he was breastfeeding. He was voiding and stooling and had an 8% weight loss. Both Josh and his mother had a blood type of O+.

Scene 1

Malaya: Hello, Mrs. Stewart. My name is Malaya and I will be caring for your baby today. How have you both been doing since you were discharged?

Mrs. Stewart: We have been ok. Breastfeeding has seemed harder than it was while I was here in the hospital, but I think we are getting the hang of it.

Malaya provides Mrs. Stewart some additional breastfeeding education and encouragement. Malaya also learns that Josh has been having 3-4 wet diapers a day but has only had 2 bowel movements since discharge. Malaya leaves the room to gather the supplies needed to obtain blood for the bilirubin level.

Scene 2

Malaya: Ok, Mrs. Stewart. I have everything that I need to draw the blood for the bilirubin test. Would you like to breastfeed Josh while I perform the heelstick? That will provide some comfort and pain relief for him during the procedure.

Mrs. Stewart: Yes! Anything to make him feel better, and it is time for him to eat anyway.

Malaya obtains the blood sample, labels the collection tube and transports the tube to the laboratory.

Scene 3

Malaya has received the results is calling the pediatrician to report the bilirubin level.

Malaya: Dr. Konz, this is Malaya, I am calling you with the bilirubin results for Josh Stewart, a 4 day old newborn who was birthed at 36 weeks of gestation. He was discharged 48 hours after birth. His mother was instructed to return to the unit today to have his bilirubin checked. At 96 hours old, his bilirubin level is 16 mg/dL. He is breastfeeding and voiding well, but has only had 2 bowel movements since discharge. He has maintained his discharge weight of 2608 g (5 lb 12 oz), which was an 8% weight loss. He does have yellowing of the mucous membranes as well as his face and chest.

Scenario Conclusion

Based on Josh's serum bilirubin level and Malaya's report to Dr. Konz, she provides Malaya with a prescription to initiate phototherapy on Josh and to redraw his serum bilirubin level in 6 hours.

Case Study Exercises

1. After reviewing Josh's medical record, which of the following findings should Malaya identify as risk factors for hyperbilirubinemia? (Select all that apply.)

   A. Blood type

   B. Gestational age

   C. Feeding method

   D. Delivery type

2. Malaya is preparing to provide teaching to Josh's mother about phototherapy. Which of the following information should be included in the teaching?

   A. Phototherapy helps the newborn excrete bilirubin from their system.

   B. Lotion will need to be applied to the newborn's skin every 2 hours during phototherapy.

   C. A t-shirt and diaper will be worn during phototherapy.

   D. The newborn will need to be repositioned every 4 hours during phototherapy.

COMPLICATIONS

- There is no evidence that positional plagiocephaly leads to permanent cognitive or neurologic damage.
- Torticollis, or tightening of the sternocleidomastoid muscle on one side of the neck, can develop. Physical therapy can successfully treat torticollis within 4 to 8 weeks.

Newborn seizures

Newborn seizures are usually a manifestation of a serious underlying disease. The most common cause for newborn seizures is hypoxic–ischemic encephalopathy (HIE), or cellular damage due to a hypoxic perinatal episode.
- Newborn seizures are divided into four subtypes: clonic, tonic, myoclonic, and subtle.
- Newborn seizures can be difficult to identify due to subtle manifestations. Seizures must be differentiated from normal newborn jitteriness and tremors. Newborns typically exhibit oral movements, oculomotor deviations and apnea during seizure activity.

ASSESSMENT

RISK FACTORS

Metabolic: Hyperglycemia, hypoglycemia, PKU, hypocalcemia, hypomagnesemia

Toxic: Uremia, kernicterus

Prenatal infection: Toxoplasmosis, syphilis, cytomegalovirus, herpes, hepatitis

Postnatal infection: Bacterial or viral meningitis, sepsis, brain abscess

Trauma during birth: Hypoxia, intracranial hemorrhage, subarachnoid or subdural hemorrhage, intraventricular hemorrhage

Miscellaneous: Degenerative disease, narcotic withdrawal, stroke (fetal, perinatal, or neonatal), benign familial newborn seizures

EXPECTED FINDINGS

Findings vary based on type of seizure.
- **Clonic:** Slow rhythmic jerking movements; one to three movements per second
- **Focal:** Involves face, or upper or lower extremities on one side of the body; can involve neck or trunk; newborn is conscious during seizure
- **Multifocal:** Can migrate randomly from one part of the body to another; movements can start at different times

Tonic: Extension, stiffening movements
- **Generalized:** Extension of all limbs; upper limbs maintain a stiffly flexed position
- **Focal:** Sustained posturing of one limb; asymmetric posturing of trunk or neck

Subtle: Most common in premature newborns, often overlooked
- Horizontal eye deviation, repetitive blinking, fluttering of eyelids, staring
- Sucking or other oral/buccal/tongue movements
- Arm movements resembling swimming or rowing
- Leg movements resembling pedaling
- Apnea is common

Myoclonic: Rapid jerks that involve flexor muscle groups
- **Focal:** Involves upper extremity flexor muscles; no changes in EEG
- **Multifocal:** Asynchronous twitching of several parts of the body; no changes in EEG
- **Generalized:** Bilateral jerks of upper and lower limbs; associated with EEG discharges

LABORATORY TESTS

- Blood glucose levels
- Blood electrolytes
- CSF analyzed for blood, protein, glucose and cultured

DIAGNOSTIC PROCEDURES

- Electroencephalogram (EEG): continuous video EEG is gold standard for diagnosis Q EBP
- CT scan
- Ultrasound
- Echoencephalography

PATIENT-CENTERED CARE

NURSING CARE

- Early recognition of seizure activity.
- Monitor vital signs.
- Continue routine newborn assessments.
- Administer antiseizure medications as prescribed.
- Administer medications as prescribed for the underlying cause.
- Respiratory support if hypoxia present.
- Encourage infant–parent bonding.

CLIENT EDUCATION
- Be aware of newborn's status and treatment plan.
- Understand home medications and safe administration.

Complications of the preterm newborn

The preterm infant is a newborn who is birthed alive before the completion of the 37th week of gestation. Preterm infants are further divided into two groups: late preterm (born between 34 and 37 6/7 weeks gestation) and early preterm (born between 24- and 34-weeks of gestation). The exact cause of preterm labor and birth is unknown. Early recognition and treatment of preterm labor is an important part of nursing care and maternal education.

- All preterm infants need additional care at birth to improve both short- and long-term outcomes. Preterm infants are more prone to complications (hypoglycemia, respiratory distress syndrome, sepsis, congenital anomalies, and death).
- Nursing care of the preterm infant focuses on cardiorespiratory support, thermoregulation, and early recognition and intervention of complications.

ASSESSMENT

RISK FACTORS

- Maternal low socioeconomic level
- Maternal poor nutritional status during pregnancy
- Lack of prenatal care
- Multiple pregnancies
- Gestational hypertension
- Placental problems
- Previous preterm birth
- Maternal smoking, alcohol, or drug use during pregnancy
- Maternal age younger than 20 years
- Maternal infection
- Premature rupture of membranes
- Premature separation of the placenta
- Closely spaced pregnancies

EXPECTED FINDINGS

PHYSICAL ASSESSMENT FINDINGS
- Head large in proportion to chest
- Thin skin with visible veins
- Lanugo abundant over body
- Vernix caseosa
- Few or no sole creases
- Ear cartilage soft and pliable
- Poor suck/swallow reflex
- Hypotonicity
- Males: testicles undescended and few rugae on the scrotum
- Females: prominent clitoris and labia minora
- Respiratory difficulty (nasal flaring, retractions, grunting)
- Frequent periods of apnea
- Temperature instability
- Hypoglycemia
- Weak, high-pitched cry

LABORATORY TESTS

- CBC
- ABGs
- Blood glucose
- Blood cultures
- Electrolytes
- Urinalysis
- Bilirubin

PATIENT-CENTERED CARE

NURSING CARE

- Facilitate bonding with parents and siblings.
- Weigh daily or as condition warrants.
- Monitor respiratory status.
  - RDS is common due to lack of surfactant.
  - Supplemental oxygen or assisted ventilation are often required.
  - Episodes of apnea are common.
  - Continuously monitor oxygen saturation and respiratory rate.
  - Assess breath sounds for crackles, wheezing, and stridor.
- Monitor temperature.
  - Provide external source of warmth as condition warrants.
  - Prevent heat loss through conduction, convection, radiation, and evaporation.
  - Maintain a neutral thermal environment.
- Monitor cardiac status.
  - Assess heart rate and rhythm.
  - Monitor for murmurs.
  - Monitor skin color for cyanosis, mottling, and pallor.
  - Monitor blood pressure using the appropriate size cuff.
  - Monitor peripheral pulses and capillary refill times.
- Monitor gastrointestinal status.
  - Assess for abdominal distention.
  - Monitor for regurgitation and gastric residuals.
  - Monitor bowel sounds.
  - Monitor amount, color, and consistency of stools.
  - Monitor blood glucose level.
- Monitor genitourinary status.
  - Assess genitalia.
  - Monitor urine for amount, color, and pH.
- Monitor neurologic-musculoskeletal status.
  - Assess motor activity.
  - Assess reflexes (Moro, grasp, Babinski, sucking, and others as condition warrants).
  - Assess head circumference and fontanels.
  - Provide the amount of stimuli appropriate for gestation age. (Early preterm infants require low environmental stimuli and minimal interruptions in sleep.)

- Monitor skin.
  - Monitor for areas of redness, irritation, blisters, abrasions, or discoloration. Pay special attention to areas where monitoring equipment, IVs, or other equipment comes in contact with the skin.
  - Assess skin turgor and texture.
  - Assess for birthmarks, rashes, and lesions.
  - Assess IV sites for manifestations of infection or infiltration. Qs

CLIENT EDUCATION
- Visit the newborn and call for updates when unable to visit.
- Express feelings.
- Continue breastfeeding (pump breasts until the newborn is able to latch onto breasts.)
- Understand treatment plan, equipment, and monitors.
- Utilize resources of support as needed.

COMPLICATIONS

Possible sequelae from preterm birth and subsequent treatment

Anemia of prematurity

- Delay cord clamping at birth if possible, to maintain maximum RBC level.
- Minimize blood draws, and document amount of blood drawn.
- Transfuse blood as prescribed.

Retinopathy of prematurity

- Immature blood vessels in retina constrict when exposed to high concentration of oxygen.
- Retina can detach, causing blindness.
- PO$_2$ levels greater than 100 mm Hg greatly increase risk of retinal damage.
- Continuous monitoring of oxygen saturation levels is necessary.

Acute bilirubin encephalopathy

- Brain cells are more susceptible to damage from high bilirubin levels.
- Provide phototherapy or exchange transfusion as prescribed.

Persistent patent ductus arteriosus

- Pulmonary hypertension from lack of surfactant prevents ductus from closing.
- Administer IV fluids cautiously.
- Administer indomethacin as prescribed to cause closure of ductus.
- Educate parents about possibility of surgical closure if ductus does not close.

Periventricular/intraventricular hemorrhage

- Most common in very low birth weight infants.
- Causes include rapid change in blood pressure (from hypoxia, IV infusions, or a pneumothorax).
- Prognosis for Grades I & II is good. Prognosis more guarded for grades III & IV.
- Hydrocephalus can develop as a long-term effect of hemorrhage.

INTRAVENTRICULAR HEMORRHAGE GRADES
- Grade I: Bleeding in a small area of one ventricle
- Grade II: Greater amount of bleeding, possibly multiple ventricle involvement
- Grade III: Extensive bleeding causing ventricle enlargement
- Grade IV: Extensive bleeding, including into brain tissue surrounding ventricles

Necrotizing enterocolitis

- Hypoxia leads to death of mucosal cells in the intestine.
- Causes abdominal distention, bleeding in stools, and temperature instability. Perforation is possible.
- Temporary colostomy can be necessary.

Chromosomal abnormalities

- Genetic disorders are passed from one generation to the next due to a disorder in a gene or chromosome. Genetic disorders can occur at the moment of fusion of sperm and egg or earlier, during meiotic division of the egg or sperm. Up to 50% of miscarriages are due to chromosomal disorders.
- Mendelian laws are the principles of genetic inheritance of disease.
  - **Homozygous**: Two healthy genes for a like trait
  - **Heterozygous**: One healthy gene and one unhealthy gene for a like trait
- Different types and characteristics of genetic disorders and inheritance include autosomal dominant, autosomal recessive, X-linked dominant, X-linked recessive, mitochondrial, and multifactorial.
- Provide education and support to parents who seek genetic counseling. Nurses also play an important role in supporting parents to make an informed decision about pregnancy and future reproductive options.

ASSESSMENT

RISK FACTORS

- Parent who has existing genetic disorder or inborn error of metabolism
- Previous child born with a genetic disorder or inborn error of metabolism
- Previous stillbirth
- A close relative with a genetic disorder or inborn error of metabolism
- Parents who are closely related
- Parent who is a known carrier of a genetic disorder
- Woman older than 35 or man older than 55 at time of conception
- Exposure to infectious or environmental toxins (cytomegalovirus, radiation, chemicals)

MODES OF INHERITANCE

Autosomal dominant

Huntington's disease, Marfan syndrome
- Males and females equally affected.
- Children of affected parent have 50% chance of being affected.
- Expression of these genes can be very minor to severe and debilitating.

Autosomal recessive

Cystic fibrosis, phenylketonuria, galactosemia, Tay-Sachs disease, sickle cell
- Males and females equally affected.
- Both males and females can be carriers.
- Carrier parents have 25% chance of having an affected child with each pregnancy.
- Carrier parents have 50% chance of having a carrier child with each pregnancy.

Sex-linked: X-linked dominant

Hypophosphatemic vitamin D-resistant rickets, incontinentia pigmenti
- All males and females who have the gene are affected.
- All daughters of an affected man have the disorder and a 50% chance of passing the defective gene to her children.
- Affected males do not transmit the defective gene to their sons.

Sex-linked: X-linked recessive

Hemophilia types A and B, Duchenne muscular dystrophy, fragile X syndrome
- Most affected persons are male; affected females are very rare.
- Parents of affected children do not have the disorder.

Mitochondrial

Leigh syndrome, Kearns-Sayre syndrome
- Male carriers cannot pass the disorder to any children.
- Female carriers will pass disorder to 100% of their children.
- Inherited solely from cytoplasm of egg.

Multifactorial (complex)

Neural tube defects, cleft lip and palate, pyloric stenosis, many congenital heart defects, diabetes mellitus type 1, pyloric stenosis
- Have a higher than usual occurrence in some families, but no specific mode of inheritance identified
- Can occur from multiple gene combinations and environmental influence

Autosomal aneuploidies

- The uneven division (nondisjunction) of a cell leading to an uneven number of chromosomes
- Frequently leads to one extra or one too few chromosomes in a cell

Trisomy 21 (Down syndrome)
- Most frequently occurring chromosomal disorder
- Broad, flat nose
- Epicanthal fold
- Protruding tongue
- Short neck with extra pad of fat
- Hypotonicity
- Low set ears
- Fifth finger curved inward
- Single palmar crease
- Mild to moderate cognitive deficits
- Cardiac anomalies common
- Altered immune system

Trisomy 18 (Edwards syndrome)
- Severe cognitive deficits
- SGA
- Low-set ears, small jaw
- Misshapen fingers and toes
- Rocker-bottom feet
- Most die in infancy

Trisomy 13 (Patau syndrome)
- Severe cognitive deficits
- Midline body disorders: cleft lip/palate, cardiac defects, abnormal genitalia
- Microcephaly
- Eyes small or missing

Klinefelter syndrome: Male who has an extra X chromosome
- Characteristics not noticeable until puberty
- Testes remain small leading to sterility
- Gynecomastia
- Elongated lower limbs

Turner syndrome: Female who has only one functional X chromosome
- Short stature
- Small, nonfunctioning ovaries leading to sterility
- No secondary sex characteristics develop at puberty except pubic hair
- Neck webbed and short
- Mild learning disabilities to severe cognitive deficits

DIAGNOSTIC TESTS AND PROCEDURES

- DNA analysis of parents prior to conception
- Newborn screening

TESTS DURING PREGNANCY
- Blood AFP level (elevated in the presence of a NTD; decreased in the presence of chromosomal abnormality)
- Chorionic villus sampling
- Amniocentesis
- Ultrasonography

PATIENT-CENTERED CARE

NURSING CARE

- Obtain a complete family history.
- Perform physical assessment of parents for any abnormalities.
- Refer for genetic screening.
- Provide emotional support and guidance. ○PCC
- Refer to support groups.
- Perform physical examination of newborn for any abnormalities.
- Monitor affected infants closely, including cardiac and respiratory status, and feeding difficulties.

COMPLICATIONS

Short- and long-term complications vary based on type of chromosomal abnormality and the severity of its effects.

CLIENT EDUCATION
- Be aware of expected outcomes for infant.
- Observe for manifestations and report to the provider if necessary.

Application Exercises

1. A nurse is providing preconception teaching with a client who has phenylketonuria (PKU). Which of the following information should the nurse include in the teaching?

   A. Follow a low-phenylalanine diet once pregnancy is confirmed.

   B. The disorder can cause cognitive impairment in newborns.

   C. Increase intake of dietary proteins prior to conception.

   D. The client will require a cesarean section birth due to the likelihood of having a fetus with macrosomia.

2. A nurse is reviewing the medical record of a newborn who has necrotizing enterocolitis (NEC). Which of the following findings is a risk factor for NEC?

   A. Macrosomia

   B. Transient tachypnea of the newborn (TTN)

   C. Maternal gestational hypertension

   D. Gestational age 36 weeks

3. A nurse is assessing an infant who has congenital hypothyroidism. Which of the following manifestations should the nurse expect to find? (Select all that apply.)

   A. Hypertonicity

   B. Cool extremities

   C. Short neck

   D. Tachycardia

   E. Hyperreflexia

4. A nurse is teaching the parent of a newborn how to treat the newborn's plagiocephaly. Which of the following statements by the parent indicates an understanding of the teaching?

   A. "I should put my baby to sleep on the belly during her afternoon nap."

   B. "I will monitor my baby for manifestations of neurologic damage."

   C. "I should change which side of the head my baby sleeps on every night."

   D. "I should allow my baby to sleep in an infant swing."

Active Learning Scenario

A nurse is planning care for a newborn who has a myelomeningocele. What actions should the nurse include in the plan of care? Use the ATI Active Learning Template: System Disorder to complete this item.

NURSING CARE: Include nursing actions before and after surgery for a newborn who has a myelomeningocele.

Case Study Exercises Key

1. A. Newborns who are birthed prematurely, or before 37 weeks of gestation, are at a greater risk due to immature hepatic function as well as difficulties associated with prematurity and breastfeeding.
   B. **CORRECT:** When recognizing cues while reviewing the medical record, Malaya should have identified that a gestational age of 36 weeks as well as breastfeeding are risk factors for hyperbilirubinemia.
   C. **CORRECT:** When recognizing cues while reviewing the medical record, Malaya should have identified that a gestational age of 36 weeks as well as breastfeeding are risk factors for hyperbilirubinemia.
   D. Newborns who are breastfeed are at a greater risk due to decreased fluid and caloric intake until a mature milk supply is established.

   Ⓝ *NCLEX® Connection: Health Promotion and Maintenance, Health Promotion/Disease Prevention*

2. A. **CORRECT:** When generating solutions while preparing to teach the newborns mother about phototherapy, the nurse should include that phototherapy converts bilirubin into a form that can be more easily excreted through stool and urine thus lowering serum bilirubin levels

   Ⓝ *NCLEX® Connection: Physiological Adaptation, Medical Emergencies*

Active Learning Scenario Key

Using the ATI Active Learning Template: System Disorder
NURSING CARE

Preoperative
- Protect the sac.
- Place the infant in a radiant warmer, without clothing.
- Apply sterile, moist non-adhering dressing saturated with 0.9% sodium chloride. Re-wet as needed.
- Assess cysts for findings of fluid leak or infection.
- Administer prescribed antibiotics.
- Avoid measuring temperature rectally.
- Prepare the parents for the newborn's surgery.

Postoperative
- Monitor vital signs.
- Monitor I&O.
- Assess the surgical site for redness, edema, and drainage.
- Provide pain management.
- Assess for leakage of CSF.
- Maintain prone position until other positions are prescribed.

Ⓝ *NCLEX® Connection: Safety and Infection Control, Accident/Error/Injury Prevention*

Application Exercises Key

1. A. A client who has PKU should follow a low-phenylalanine diet for at least 3 months prior to conception and throughout the pregnancy.
   B. **CORRECT:** When taking action and providing preconception education to a client who has PKU, the nurse should include in the teaching that if the client does not follow a low-phenylalanine diet, congenital heart defects can occur.
   C. A client who has PKU should decrease dietary intake of protein prior to conception.
   D. A client who has PKU is at no higher risk of fetal macrosomia and will not require a cesarean birth.

   Ⓝ *NCLEX® Connection: Physiological Adaptation, Medical Emergencies*

2. A. Macrosomia does not place a newborn at risk for NEC.
   B. TTN does not place a newborn at risk for NEC.
   C. Maternal gestational hypertension does not place a newborn at risk for NEC.
   D. **CORRECT:** When reviewing the chart of a newborn who has NEC, the nurse should identify that preterm birth places a newborn at risk for NEC; therefore, a gestational age of 36 weeks is a risk factor for NEC.

   Ⓝ *NCLEX® Connection: Physiological Adaptation, Medical Emergencies*

3. B, C. **CORRECT:** When recognizing cues during the assessment of an infant who has congenital hypothyroidism, the nurse should expect the infant to have cool extremities and a short neck.
   A. Hypertonicity is not an expected finding in an infant who has congenital hypothyroidism.
   D. Tachycardia is not an expected finding in an infant who has congenital hypothyroidism.
   E. Hyperreflexia is not an expected finding in an infant who has congenital hypothyroidism.

   Ⓝ *NCLEX® Connection: Physiological Adaptation, Medical Emergencies*

4. A. A newborn who has plagiocephaly should not be placed in the prone position to sleep. The nurse should provide education on the importance of tummy time, which is allowing the infant to lie in the prone position for 3 to 5 minutes a day, 2 to 3 times each day.
   B. Plagiocephaly has not been found to cause permanent cognitive of neurological damage.
   C. **CORRECT:** When evaluating the outcomes of teaching to the parent of a newborn who has plagiocephaly, the nurse should identify that the statement, "I should change which side of the head my baby sleeps on every night" as an indication of understanding.
   D. A newborn who has plagiocephaly should not be allowed to sleep in an infant swing.

   Ⓝ *NCLEX® Connection: Reduction of Risk Potential, Diagnostic Tests*

UNIT 3   OTHER SPECIFIC NEEDS

CHAPTER 43 *Pediatric Emergencies*

In caring for children, nurses often deal with emergent care situations that require rapid assessment and intervention and offer opportunities for parent and community education.

Respiratory Emergencies

Respiratory insufficiency: Increased work of breathing with mostly adequate gas exchange or hypoxia with acidosis

Respiratory failure: Inability to maintain adequate oxygenation of the blood

Apnea
- Cessation of respirations for more than 20 seconds
- Can be associated with hypoxemia or bradycardia
- Can be central or obstructive

Respiratory arrest: Complete cessation of respirations

Airway obstruction: Can be due to aspiration of a foreign body

ASSESSMENT

RISK FACTORS
- Infants and toddlers
- Primary inefficient gas exchange due to cerebral trauma, brain tumor, toxicity, asphyxia, or CNS infection
- Obstructive lung disease caused by aspiration, infection, tumor, anaphylaxis, laryngospasm, or asthma
- Restrictive lung disease resulting from cystic fibrosis, pneumonia, or respiratory distress syndrome

EXPECTED FINDINGS
- History of illnesses (chronic or acute)
- History of events leading to respiratory emergency
- Allergies

EARLY INDICATIONS OF RESPIRATORY DISTRESS
- Restlessness
- Tachypnea
- Tachycardia
- Diaphoresis
- Nasal flaring
- Retractions
- Grunting
- Dyspnea
- Wheezing

ADVANCED HYPOXIA
- Bradypnea
- Bradycardia
- Peripheral or central cyanosis
- Stupor
- Coma

INDICATIONS OF CHOKING
- Universal choking sign (clutching neck with hands)
- Inability to speak
- Weak, ineffective cough
- High-pitched sounds or no sound
- Dyspnea
- Cyanosis

LABORATORY TESTS

Arterial blood gases (ABGs)

DIAGNOSTIC PROCEDURES

Chest x-rays

PATIENT-CENTERED CARE

NURSING CARE
- Follow the American Heart Association (AHA) guidelines for CPR for respiratory and cardiac arrest.
- Follow the facility's protocol for activating the rapid response team. Ⓠ EBP
- Use current basic life support and advanced cardiac life support guidelines for neonates and for pediatric clients.
- Position to maintain patent airway. Monitor respiratory status. Monitor vital signs.
- Administer oxygen as prescribed.
- Suction as needed.
- Prepare for intubation if needed.
- Use a calm approach with the child and family.
- Administer medications, IV fluids, and emergency medications as prescribed.
- Keep the family informed of the child's status.

Obstructed airway
- Follow the AHA guidelines for a choking child.
- For infants, use a combination of back blows and chest thrusts.
- For children and adolescents, use abdominal thrusts.
- Remove any visual obstruction or large debris from the mouth, but do not perform blind finger sweep.
- Place the recovered child (one who resumes breathing) into the recovery position (side-lying position with legs bent at knees for stability).

CLIENT EDUCATION
- Observe for manifestations of respiratory distress.
- Learn CPR.
- Teach the family about strategies to prevent respiratory emergencies (recognizing choking hazards for toddlers).

Drowning

Asphyxiation while child is submerged in fluid can occur in any standing body of water that is at least 1 inch deep (bathtub, toilet, bucket, pool, pond, lake).

- Submersion injury (near-drowning) incidents are those in which children have survived for 24 hr after being submerged in fluid.
- Families should be taught preventive measures. Qs

ASSESSMENT

RISK FACTORS

- Children ages 1 to 4 years
- Swimming (can be overconfident or lack ability)
- Inadequate supervision or unattended in bathtub, pools
- Not wearing life jackets when in water
- Diving
- Child maltreatment

EXPECTED FINDINGS

- History of event including location and time of submersion
- Type and temperature of the fluid
- Respiratory assessment (see respiratory emergencies)
- Body temperature (hypothermia)
- Bruising, spinal cord injury, or other physical injuries

LABORATORY TESTS

ABGs

DIAGNOSTIC PROCEDURES

Chest x-rays

PATIENT-CENTERED CARE

NURSING CARE

Based on degree of cerebral insult

- Administer oxygen, can need mechanical ventilation.
- Monitor vital signs.
- Administer medications, IV fluids, and emergency medications as prescribed.
- Provide chest physiotherapy.
- Monitor for complications that can occur 24 hr after incident (cerebral edema, respiratory distress).
- Use a calm approach with the child and family.
- Keep the family informed of the child's status.

CLIENT EDUCATION

- Lock toilet seats when their child is at home.
- Do not leave the child unattended in the bathtub.
- Even a small amount of water can lead to accidental drowning.
- Do not leave the child unattended in a swimming pool, even if the child can swim.
- Make sure private pools are fenced with locked gates to prevent children from wandering into the pool area.
- Provide life jackets when boating.

Brief Resolved Unexplained Event

Formerly called apparent life-threatening event (ALTE). A brief resolved unexplained event (BRUE) is a sudden event where the infant exhibits apnea, change in color, change in muscle tone, and level of consciousness.

ASSESSMENT

RISK FACTORS

- Gastroesophageal reflux
- Respiratory infections
- Seizure
- Urinary tract infection (UTI)
- Sepsis
- Metabolic disorders
- Neurologic disorders
- Airway anatomy anomaly

EXPECTED FINDINGS

- Description of the event by the observer
- CPR efforts provided
- Maternal history

EVENT: Apnea can be present during event.
- Change in color: pallor, redness, cyanosis
- Change in muscle tone: hypotonia
- Choking, gagging, coughing

LABORATORY TESTS

Blood cultures

Urinalysis: UTI

CBC

Blood glucose

Electrolytes

DIAGNOSTIC PROCEDURES

Electrocardiogram

Magnetic resonance imaging

Sleep study

PATIENT-CENTERED CARE

NURSING CARE

- Prepare the infant and family for testing.
- Monitor the infant for recurrent events.
- Encourage the family to learn CPR.

CLIENT TEACHING: Use an apnea monitor, if prescribed.

Sudden unexpected infant death

- Sudden unexpected infant death (SUID), formerly called sudden infant death syndrome (SIDS) is the sudden, unexpected death of an infant, with or without an identified cause, occurring during the first year of life.
- Preventive measures should be taught to families.

ASSESSMENT

RISK FACTORS

- Maternal smoking during pregnancy
- Secondhand smoke
- Co-sleeping with parent or adult
- Nonstandard bed (sofa, soft bedding, water beds, pillows)
- Prone or side-lying sleeping
- Low birth weight
- Prematurity
- Twin or multiple birth
- Low Apgar scores
- Viral illness
- Family history of SIDS
- Poverty
- Heart rhythm abnormalities

EXPECTED FINDINGS

- History of events prior to discovery of infant
- History of illnesses
- Pregnancy and birth history
- Presence of risk factors

PATIENT-CENTERED CARE

NURSING CARE

- Provide support.
- Allow the infant's family an opportunity to express feelings.
- Plan a home health visit to follow a death.
- Refer to support groups, counseling, or community groups.

CLIENT TEACHING: Teach the family how to reduce the risks of SUID.
- Place the infant on the back for every sleep. Qs
- Avoid exposure to tobacco smoke.
- Prevent overheating.
- Use a firm, tight-fitting mattress in the infant's crib.

- Remove pillows, quilts, and stuffed animals from the crib during sleep.
- Ensure that the infant's head is kept uncovered during sleep.
- Offer pacifier at naps and night.
- Encourage breastfeeding.
- Avoid co-sleeping. Recommend infant sleep on separate surface in their parents' room, close to the parents' bed for first 6 months.
- Maintain immunizations up to date.
- Provide education on the importance of tummy time, which is allowing the infant to lie in the prone position for 3 to 5 minutes, 2 to 3 times each day.

Poisoning

- Ingestion of or exposure to toxic substances.
- Preventive measures should be taught to families.

ASSESSMENT

RISK FACTORS

- Children younger than 6 years of age
- Improperly stored medications, household chemicals, and hazardous substances
- Exposure to plants, cosmetics, and heavy metals, which are potential sources of toxic substances
- Lead ingestion from lead-based paint, soil contamination

EXPECTED FINDINGS

Information regarding poisonous agent
- Name and location
- Amount ingested
- Time of ingestion

Specific poisons

Physical response depends on specific poison. QEBP

Acetaminophen
- **0 to 24 hr after ingestion:** Nausea, vomiting, sweating, and pallor
- **24 to 72 hr after ingestion:** Improvement in condition; may report right upper quadrant pain
- **72 hr to 96 hr (hepatic stage):** Pain in upper right quadrant, confusion, stupor, jaundice, and coagulation disturbances. Greatest risk for death.
- **Final stage:** Gradual recovery

Acetylsalicylic acid (aspirin)
- **Acute toxicity:** Nausea, vomiting, disorientation, , tachypnea, tinnitus, oliguria, lightheadedness, and seizures
- **Chronic toxicity:** Subtle version of acute manifestations, bleeding tendencies, dehydration, and seizures more severe than acute poisoning

Supplemental iron

- I**nitial period (30 min to 6 hr after ingestion):** Vomiting, hematemesis, diarrhea, gastric pain, and bloody stools
- **Latency period (6 to 24 hr after ingestion):** Improvement of condition
- **Systemic toxicity period (6 to 72 hr after ingestion):** metabolic acidosis, hyperglycemia, bleeding, fever, shock, and possible death
- **Hepatic injury period (12 to 96 hr after ingestion):** Coma, elevated AST and ALT, hypoglycemia, jaundice
- **Recovery period (2 to 8 weeks):** Repair of intestinal mucosa. Possible GI scarring and obstruction.

Hydrocarbons: Gasoline, kerosene, lighter fluid, paint thinner, turpentine

- Gagging, choking, coughing, nausea, and vomiting
- Lethargy, weakness, tachypnea, cyanosis, grunting, and retractions

Corrosives: Household cleaners, batteries, denture cleaners, bleach

- Pain and burning in mouth, throat, and stomach
- Edematous lips, tongue, and pharynx with white mucous membranes
- Vomiting with hemoptysis
- Drooling
- Anxiety
- Shock

Lead

- **Low-dose exposure:** Distractibility, impulsiveness, hyperactivity, hearing impairment, and mild intellectual difficulty
- **High-dose exposure:** Cognitive delays varying in severity, blindness, paralysis, coma, seizures, and death
- **Other manifestations:** Kidney impairment, impaired calcium function, and anemia

LABORATORY TESTS

- Blood lead
- CBC with differential
- ABGs
- Blood iron
- Blood acetaminophen
- Liver function tests
- Blood alcohol and toxicology screening

PATIENT-CENTERED CARE

NURSING CARE

- Depends on the poison ingested
- Monitor for ongoing changes.
- Terminate exposure.
- Provide cardiorespiratory support as needed.
- Notify local or regional poison control center.
- Administer IV fluids as prescribed.
- Provide cardiac monitoring.
- Monitor vital signs and oxygen saturation.

- Monitor I&O.
- Administer antidote if indicated.
- Assist with gastric decontamination if indicated.
  - Activated charcoal
  - Gastric lavage
  - Increasing bowel motility
  - Syrup of ipecac is contraindicated for routine poison control treatment
- Keep the family informed of the child's condition.

Interventions for specific substances

Acetaminophen: N–acetylcysteine given orally

Acetylsalicylic acid

- Activated charcoal
- Sodium bicarbonate
- Oxygen and ventilation
- Vitamin K
- Hemodialysis for severe cases

Supplemental iron

- Emesis or lavage
- Chelation therapy using deferoxamine mesylate

Hydrocarbons (gasoline, kerosene, lighter fluid, paint thinner, turpentine)

- Do not induce vomiting
- Intubation with cuffed endotracheal tube prior to any gastric decontamination
- Treatment of chemical pneumonia

Corrosives (household cleaners, batteries, denture cleaners, bleach)

- Airway maintenance
- NPO
- No attempt to neutralize acid (corrosive)
- Do not induce vomiting
- Analgesics for pain

Lead: Chelation therapy using calcium EDTA (calcium disodium versenate)

CLIENT EDUCATION

POISON PREVENTION

- Keep toxic agents out of reach of children. Q**s**
- Lock cabinets containing potentially harmful substances.
- Do not take medication in front of children.
- Discard unused medications.
- When giving a child medication, do not say it is candy.
- Use non–mercury thermometers.
- Eliminate lead–based paint in the environment.
- Encourage hand hygiene prior to eating.
- Do not store food in lead–based containers.

COMPLICATIONS

Cognitive impairments

Varies with degree of anoxic insult or lead levels in blood

NURSING ACTIONS
- Provide prevention measures to families.
- Routine screening for lead levels at 1, 2, and 3 years of age.
- Provide case management for children who have elevated lead levels.
- Make appropriate referrals (community nurse, teacher, early intervention).

Active Learning Scenario

A nurse is teaching a group of caregivers about prevention of sudden infant death syndrome (SUID). What should the nurse include in the teaching? Use the ATI Active Learning Template: System Disorder to complete this item.

NURSING CARE: Identify at least seven methods to reduce the risk of SUID.

Active Learning Scenario Key

Using the ATI Active Learning Template: System Disorder
NURSING CARE: Methods to reduce the risk of SUID
- Place the infant on the back for sleep.
- Avoid exposure to tobacco smoke.
- Prevent overheating.
- Use a firm, tight-fitting mattress in the infant's crib.
- Remove pillows, quilts, and sheepskins from the crib during sleep.
- Ensure that the infant's head is kept uncovered during sleep.
- Offer pacifier at naps and night.
- Encourage breastfeeding.
- Avoid co-sleeping.
- Maintain immunizations up to date.

Ⓝ *NCLEX® Connection: Psychosocial Integrity, Abuse or Neglect*

Application Exercises

1. A nurse is caring for a child who is experiencing respiratory distress. Which of the following findings are early manifestations of respiratory distress? (Select all that apply.)
   - A. Bradypnea
   - B. Peripheral cyanosis
   - C. Tachycardia
   - D. Diaphoresis
   - E. Restlessness

2. A nurse in a community center is providing an in-service to a group of parents on management of airway obstructions in toddlers. Which of the following responses by one of the caregivers indicates understanding? (Select all that apply.)
   - A. "I will push on my child's abdomen."
   - B. "I will hyperextend my child's head to open the airway."
   - C. "I will use my finger to check my child's mouth for objects."
   - D. "I will place my child in my car and take them to the closest emergency facility."

3. A nurse in the emergency department is admitting an infant who experienced a brief resolved unexplained event. Which of the following prescriptions by the provider should the nurse anticipate?
   - A. Echocardiogram
   - B. Urinalysis
   - C. Arterial blood gases
   - D. Sputum culture

4. A nurse is providing teaching to a caregiver about acetaminophen poisoning. Which of the following information should the nurse include in the teaching?
   - A. Nausea begins 24 hr after ingestion.
   - B. Pallor can appear as early as 2 hr after ingestion.
   - C. Jaundice will appear in 12 hr if the child is toxic.
   - D. Children can have 4 g/day of acetaminophen.

5. A nurse in the emergency department is caring for a child whose parent reports that the child has swallowed paint thinner. The child is lethargic, gagging, and cyanotic. Which of the following actions should the nurse take?
   - A. Induce vomiting with syrup of ipecac.
   - B. Insert a nasogastric tube, and administer activated charcoal.
   - C. Prepare for intubation with a cuffed endotracheal tube.
   - D. Administer chelation therapy using deferoxamine mesylate.

1. C, D, E. **CORRECT:** When analyzing cues during the care of a child who is experiencing respiratory distress, the nurse should identify tachycardia, diaphoresis, and restlessness as early manifestations of respiratory distress.
   A. Bradypnea is an advanced manifestation of respiratory distress.
   B. Cyanosis is an advanced manifestation of hypoxia.

Ⓝ *NCLEX® Connection: Health Promotion and Maintenance, Health Promotion/Disease Prevention*

2. A. **CORRECT:** When taking action and providing education to a group of parents on management of airway obstruction in toddlers, the nurse should include using abdominal thrusts to clear an obstructed airway and listening over the child's mouth for sounds of breathing.
   B. The nurse should teach the caregiver to position the child with the chin elevated, rather than hyperextended, to open the airway.
   C. Finger sweeps to check for an impaired airway are not performed because this action can cause an object to be pushed further down into the toddler's throat, causing injury. Teach the caregivers to attempt to clear the child's airway according to AHA guidelines and to call 911.
   D. Attempting to independently transport the child to an emergency facility delays treatment.

Ⓝ *NCLEX® Connection: Physiological Adaptation, Illness Management*

3. A. An electrocardiogram, not an echocardiogram, should be anticipated by the nurse.
   B. **CORRECT:** When generating solutions during the admission of an infant who experienced a brief resolved unexplained event, the nurse should anticipate a prescription for a urinalysis to rule out a urinary tract infection.
   C. ABGs are not routinely performed for an infant who experienced a brief resolved unexplained event.
   D. A blood culture, not a sputum culture, is obtained to assess for bacterial or viral infections.

Ⓝ *NCLEX® Connection: Physiological Adaptation, Alterations in Body Systems*

4. A. Nausea is a manifestation that begins within the first 24 hr after ingestion. Jaundice will appear in 72 hr to 96 hr.
   B. **CORRECT:** When taking actions and providing education to a caregiver about acetaminophen poisoning, the nurse should include that pallor can appear as early as 2 hr after ingestion.
   C. The maximum dose of acetaminophen in children 2 to 5 years of age is 720 mg/day.
   D. In children 6 to 12 years of age, it is 2.6 g/day.

Ⓝ *NCLEX® Connection: Physiological Adaptation, Illness Management*

5. A. Inducing vomiting with syrup of ipecac is contraindicated as a poison control measure.
   B. Activated charcoal is indicated for acetylsalicylic acid poisoning.
   C. **CORRECT:** When taking action during the care of a child who has swallowed paint thinner and is lethargic, gagging, and cyanotic, the nurse should prepare the child for intubation with a cuffed endotracheal tube. Treatment for poisoning with hydrocarbons includes intubation to protect the airway before proceeding with gastric decontamination.
   D. Chelation therapy is indicated for lead poisoning.

Ⓝ *NCLEX® Connection: Physiological Adaptation, Alterations in Body Systems*

UNIT 3   OTHER SPECIFIC NEEDS

CHAPTER 44 *Psychosocial Issues of Infants, Children, and Adolescents*

Nurses care for pediatric clients who have psychosocial issues, as well as physical illness. Psychosocial issues (depression) can occur as a result of a physical illness, be independent from physical illness, or be the cause for somatic manifestations (pain due to maltreatment). It is important that the nurse be familiar with various psychosocial issues to ensure the child receives appropriate screenings, referrals and treatment.

Depression

- Difficult to detect and often overlooked in school-aged children because children have limitations in expressing their feelings.
- Findings must be present for 1 year to diagnose major depressive disorder in children and adolescents.

ASSESSMENT

RISK FACTORS

- Family history
- Traumatic event

EXPECTED FINDINGS

- Sad facial expressions
- Tendency to remain alone
- Withdrawn from family, friends, and activities
- Fatigue
- Tearful/crying
- Ill feeling
- Feelings of worthlessness
- Weight loss or gain
- Alterations in sleep
- Lack of interest in school, drop in performance in school
- Statements regarding low self-esteem
- Hopelessness
- Suicidal ideation
- Constipation

PATIENT-CENTERED CARE

NURSING CARE

- Plan care that is individualized.

- Obtain health history and growth and development information.
- Assess for substance use.
- Assess for actual or potential risk to self (including a suicide plan, lethality of the plan, and the means to carry out the plan).
- Assist with coping strategies.
- Encourage peer group discussions, mentoring, and counseling.
- Interview the child.

MEDICATIONS

Tricyclic antidepressants or selective serotonin reuptake inhibitors (SSRIs)

Trazodone, sertraline, paroxetine, bupropion, venlafaxine

NURSING ACTIONS
- Monitor for adverse effects.
- Monitor for suicidal ideation.

CLIENT EDUCATION
- Observe for adverse effects.
- Therapeutic effectiveness can take up to 2 weeks.
- Do not abruptly discontinue the medication.

COMPLICATIONS

Suicide

EXPECTED FINDINGS
- Monitor carefully for verbal and nonverbal clues. It is essential to ask the client if they are thinking of suicide. This will not give the client the idea.
- Suicidal comments usually are made to someone that the client perceives as supportive.
- Comments or signals can be overt (direct) or covert (indirect).
  - Overt comment: "There is just no reason for me to go on living."
  - Covert comment: "Everything is looking pretty grim for me."
- Determine the client's suicide plan.
  - Does the client have a plan?
  - How lethal is the plan?
  - Can the client describe the plan exactly?
  - Does the client have access to the intended method?
  - Has the client's mood changed? A sudden change in mood from sad and depressed to happy and peaceful can indicate a client's intention to commit suicide.

PHYSICAL FINDINGS: Lacerations, scratches, and scars that could indicate previous attempts at self-harm

Posttraumatic stress disorder

Develops following a traumatic or catastrophic event

ASSESSMENT

RISK FACTORS

- Potential genetic predisposition
- Traumatic incident
- Repeated trauma
- Mental health disorder
- Natural disaster
- Sexual assault
- Witness to homicide, suicide or another violent act

EXPECTED FINDINGS

INITIAL RESPONSE
- Lasts a few minutes to 2 hr
- Increased stress hormones (fight or flight)
- Psychosis

SECOND PHASE
- Lasts approximately 2 weeks
- Period of calm (feeling of numbness, denial)
- Defense mechanisms decrease

THIRD PHASE (COPING)
- Extends 2 to 3 months
- Client gets worse instead of better.
- Depression, phobias, anxiety, conversion reactions, repetitive movements, flashbacks, or obsessions

PATIENT-CENTERED CARE

NURSING CARE

- Refer to psychotherapy services.
- Monitor for behavior changes/problems.
- Assist the client and family with coping strategies.
- Allow the client and family to express their feelings.
- Prevent or reduce long-term effects.

MEDICATIONS

Selective norepinephrine reuptake inhibitors may be used on an individual basis.

Attention-Deficit/ Hyperactivity Disorder

- Inattentiveness, hyperactivity, and impulsiveness usually revealed prior to age 7.
- Common in childhood and can persist into adulthood.
- A child must meet diagnostic criteria for diagnosis of attention-deficit hyperactivity disorder (ADHD).
  - Manifestations are present between the ages of 4 and 18 years.
  - Manifestations are present in more than one setting.
  - Evidence of social or academic impairment.
  - Six or more findings from a category are present (inattention or hyperactivity-impulsivity).

ASSESSMENT

RISK FACTORS

- Can be a familial tendency
- Exposure to toxins or medicines
- Chronic otitis media, meningitis, or head trauma

EXPECTED FINDINGS

INATTENTION
- Failing to pay close attention to detail or making careless mistakes
- Blocking incoming stimuli
- Difficulty sustaining attention
- Does not seem to listen
- Failing to follow through on instructions
- Difficulty organizing activities
- Avoiding or disliking activities that require mental effort for a period of time (reading)
- Losing things
- Easily distracted
- Forgetfulness

HYPERACTIVITY
- Fidgeting
- Failing to remain seated
- Inappropriate running
- Difficulty engaging in quiet play
- Seeming to be busy all the time
- Talking excessively

IMPULSIVITY
- Blurting out responses before questions are asked
- Difficulty waiting turns
- Interrupting often
- Striking out, biting, shouting

PATIENT-CENTERED CARE

NURSING CARE

- Obtain medical, developmental, or behavioral history.
- Use behavioral checklists with adaptive scales.
- Use a calm, firm, respectful approach with the child.
- Use modeling to demonstrate acceptable behavior.
- Obtain the child's attention before giving directions. Provide short and clear explanations.
- Set clear limits on unacceptable behaviors and be consistent.
- Plan physical activities through which the child can use energy and obtain success.
- Focus on the child's and family's strengths, not just the problems.
- Support the parents' efforts to remain hopeful.
- Provide a safe environment for the child and others.
- Provide the child with specific positive feedback when expectations are met.
- Identify issues that result in power struggles.
- Assist the child in developing effective coping mechanisms.
- Encourage the child to participate in a form of group, individual, or family therapy.
- Assist the family with behavioral strategies.
  - Positive reinforcement
  - Rewards for good behavior
  - Age-appropriate consequences
- Assist the family with modification of the environment to help the child become successful.
  - Structured environment
  - Charts to assist with organization
  - Decreasing stimuli in the environment
  - Consistent study area
  - Modeling positive behaviors
  - Using steps when assigning chores
  - Using pastel colors
- Assist with appropriate classroom placement in the school.
  - Collaborate with the school nurse.
  - Allow more time for testing.
  - Place in classroom that has order and consistent rules.
  - Offer verbal instruction combined with visual cues.
  - Plan academic subjects in the morning.
  - Include regular breaks.
  - Provide for small classroom settings or work groups.

MEDICATIONS

Methylphenidate, dextroamphetamine

Psychostimulant, which increases dopamine and norepinephrine levels

NURSING ACTIONS
- Gradually increase dose to reach therapeutic results.
- Give last dose of the day prior to 1800 to prevent insomnia.
- Monitor for adverse effects, including insomnia, anorexia, nervousness, hyper/hypotension, tachycardia, and anemia.

- Avoid caffeine.
- Store properly. The medication has potential for misuse by others.
- Tricyclic antidepressants are used as adjunct therapy to treat insomnia.

Atomoxetine

Selective norepinephrine reuptake inhibitor

NURSING ACTIONS
- Gradual increase in dose to reach therapeutic results.
- Monitor for adverse effects (suicidal ideation).

Autism Spectrum Disorder

Complex neurodevelopmental disorders with spectrum of behaviors affecting an individual's ability to communicate and interact with others in a social setting.

ASSESSMENT

RISK FACTORS

- Possible genetic component
- Exact cause unknown

EXPECTED FINDINGS

- Delays in at least one of the following
  - Social interaction
  - Social communication
  - Imaginative play prior to age 3 years
- Distress when routines are changed
- Unusual attachments to objects
- Inability to start or continue conversation
- Using gestures instead of words
- Delayed or absent language development
- Grunting or humming
- Inability to adjust gaze to look at something else
- Not referring to self correctly
- Withdrawn, labile mood
- Lack of empathy
- Decreased pain sensation
- Spending time alone rather than playing with others
- Avoiding eye contact
- Withdrawal from physical contact
- Heightened or lowered senses
- Not imitating actions of others
- Minimal pretend play
- Exhibiting repetitive movements
- Typical IQ less than 70

PATIENT-CENTERED CARE

NURSING CARE

- Assist with screening assessment tools, such as the Checklist for Autism in Toddlers (CHAT) or Pervasive Developmental Disorders Screening Test.
- Refer to early intervention, physical therapy, occupational therapy, and speech and language therapy.
- Assist with behavior modification program.
  - Promote positive reinforcement.
  - Increase social awareness.
  - Teach verbal communication.
  - Decrease unacceptable behaviors.
  - Set realistic goals.
  - Structure opportunities for small successes.
  - Set clear rules.
- Decrease environmental stimulation.
- Assist with nutritional needs.
- Introduce the child to new situations slowly.
- Monitor for behavior changes.
- Encourage age-appropriate play.
- Communicate at an age-appropriate level (brief and concrete).
- Provide support to the family.
- Encourage support groups.

MEDICATIONS

Used on an individual basis to control aggression, anxiety, hyperactivity, irritability, mood swings, compulsions, and attention problems.
- SSRIs can decrease aggression.
- Antipsychotics and melatonin can help with insomnia.

Intellectual Disability

- Previously called mental retardation

ASSESSMENT

RISK FACTORS

- Familial, social, environmental, organic or other unknown causes
- Infections (congenital rubella, syphilis)
- Fetal alcohol syndrome
- Chronic lead ingestion
- Trauma to the brain
- Gestational disorders
- Pre-existing disease (Down syndrome, mental health disorders, microcephaly, hydrocephaly, metabolic disorders, cerebral palsy)

EXPECTED FINDINGS

- Can range from mild to severe
- Delayed developmental milestones
- Inability to reason or problem solve

EARLY MANIFESTATIONS

- Abnormal eye contact
- Feeding difficulties
- Language difficulties
- Fine and gross motor delays
- Decrease alertness
- Unresponsive to contact
- Reduced response to name
- Decreased response to social cues
- Echolalia
- Clients "lose" milestones between 15 to 30 months (Autism regression)

PATIENT-CENTERED CARE

NURSING CARE

- DSM-5-TR used to diagnose
- Determine the child's deficiency.
- Care and teaching should be individualized to the client's needs.
- Make appropriate referrals (early intervention program, social work, speech therapy, physical therapy, and occupational therapy).
- Add visual cues with verbal instruction.
- Give one-step instructions.
- Assist the family in teaching the child self-cares.
- Assist the family in promoting development.
- Encourage play.
- Assist the family with selecting activities and toys.
- Assist with communication skills.
- Encourage social activities.

Failure to Thrive

Inadequate growth resulting from the inability to obtain or use calories required for growth. It is usually described in an infant or child who falls below the fifth percentile for weight (and possibly for height) or who has persistent weight loss. Failure to thrive (FTT) can be classified according to the cause:
- Inadequate caloric intake (incorrect formula prep, breastfeeding difficulties, or excessive juice consumption)
- Inadequate absorption (cystic fibrosis, celiac or Crohn's disease)
- Increased metabolism (hyperthyroidism)
- Defective utilization (Down syndrome)

ASSESSMENT

RISK FACTORS

- Preterm birth with low birth weight or intrauterine growth restriction
- Parental neglect, lack of parental knowledge, or disturbed maternal-child attachment
- Poverty
- Health or childrearing beliefs
- Family stress
- Feeding resistance

ORGANIC CAUSES: Cerebral palsy, chronic kidney failure, congenital heart disease, hyperthyroidism, cystic fibrosis, celiac disease, hepatic disease, Down syndrome, prematurity, and gastroesophageal reflux

EXPECTED FINDINGS

- Less than the fifth percentile on the growth chart for weight
- Malnourished appearance
- Poor muscle tone, lack of subcutaneous fat
- No fear of strangers
- Minimal smiling
- Decreased activity level
- Withdrawal behavior
- Developmental delays
- Feeding disorder
- Wide-eyed gaze, absent eye contact
- Stiff or flaccid body

PATIENT-CENTERED CARE

NURSING CARE

Child may need to be removed from guardians' care in order to evaluate carefully and receive therapy.

- Obtain a nutritional history.
- Observe parent-child interactions.
- Obtain accurate baseline height and weight. Observe for low weight, malnourished appearance, and manifestations of dehydration.
- Weigh the child daily without clothing or a diaper.
- Maintain I&O and calorie counts as prescribed.
- Establish a routine for eating that encourages usual times, duration, and setting.
- Reinforce proper positioning, latching on, and timing for children who are breastfed.
- Provide 24 kcal/oz formula as prescribed.
- Provide high-calorie milk supplements for children.
- Administer multivitamin supplements including zinc and iron.
- Limit juice to 4 oz/day.
- Provide developmental stimulation.
- Nurture the child (rocking and talking to the child).
- Encourage caregivers to do the following.
  - Maintain eye contact and face-to-face posture during feedings.
  - Talk to the infant while feeding.
  - Burp the infant frequently.
  - Keep the environment quiet and avoid distractions.
  - Be persistent, remaining calm during 10 to 15 min of food refusal.
  - Introduce new foods slowly.
  - Never force the infant to eat.

CLIENT EDUCATION

- Recognize and respond to the infant's cues of hunger.
- Mix formula properly according to provided step-by-step written instructions.

COMPLICATIONS

Extreme malnourishment

Nursing actions: Prepare the client and parents for tube feedings or IV therapy.

Maltreatment of Infants and Children

Maltreatment of infants and children is attributed to a variety of predisposing factors, which include parental, child, and environmental characteristics. Child maltreatment can occur across all economic and educational backgrounds and racial/ethnic/religious groups.

Maltreatment of children is made of several specific types of behaviors.

- **Physical:** causing pain or harm to a child (shaken baby syndrome, fractures, factitious disorder imposed on another)
- **Sexual:** occurring when sexual contact takes place without consent, whether or not the victim is able to give consent (includes any sexual behavior toward a minor and dating violence among adolescents)
- **Emotional:** humiliating, threatening, or intimidating a child (includes behavior that minimizes an individual's feelings of self-worth)
- **Neglect:** includes failure to provide the following.
  - Physical care: feeding, clothing, shelter, medical or dental care, safety, education
  - Emotional care and/or stimulation to foster normal development: nurturing, affection, attention

ASSESSMENT

RISK FACTORS

CAREGIVER CHARACTERISTICS
- Young age
- Having a partner unrelated to the child
- Social isolation
- Low-income situation
- Lack of education
- Low self-esteem
- Lack of parenting knowledge
- Substance use disorder
- History of having been abused
- Lack of support systems

CHARACTERISTICS OF THE CHILD
- Child 1-year-old or younger is at greater risk due to the need for constant attention and increased demands of caregiving.
- Infants and children who are unwanted, hyperactive, or who have physical or mental disabilities are at risk due to their increased demands and need for constant attention.
- Premature infants are at risk due to the possible failure of parent-child bonding at birth.

ENVIRONMENTAL CHARACTERISTICS
- Chronic stress
- Divorce, alcohol or substance use disorder, poverty
- Unemployment, inadequate housing, crowded living conditions
- Substitute caregivers

EXPECTED FINDINGS

WARNING INDICATORS OF MALTREATMENT
- Physical evidence of maltreatment
- Vague explanation of injury
- Other injuries discovered that are not related to the original client concern
- Delay in seeking care
- Statement of possible abuse from a caregiver or client
- Inconsistencies between the caregiver's report and the child's injuries
- Inconsistency between nature of injury and developmental level of the child
- Repeated injuries requiring emergency treatment
- Inappropriate responses from the parents or child

Physical neglect
- Failure to thrive, malnutrition
- Lack of hygiene
- Frequent injuries
- Delay in seeking health care
- Dull affect
- School absences
- Self-stimulating behaviors

Physical maltreatment
- Bruises, welts in various stages of healing
- Bruising in a non-mobile client
- Multiple fractures at different stages of healing
- Burns
- Fractures
- Lacerations
- Fear of parents
- Lack of emotional response/reaction
- Superficial relationships
- Withdrawal
- Aggression

Emotional neglect and abuse
- Failure to thrive
- Eating disorder
- Enuresis
- Sleep disturbances
- Self-stimulating behaviors
- Withdrawal
- Lack of social smile (infant)
- Extreme behaviors
- Delayed development
- Attempts suicide
- Caregiver behaviors: rejecting, isolating, terrorizing, ignoring, verbally assaulting, or over pressuring the child

Sexual abuse defined as the employment, use, persuasion, or inducement of a child to engage in any sexually explicit conduct. Examples include pedophilia, prostitution, incest, molestation, and pornography.
- Bruises, lacerations
- Bleeding of genitalia, anus, or mouth
- Sexually transmitted infection
- Difficulty walking or standing
- UTI
- Regressive behavior
- Withdrawal
- Personality changes
- Bloody, torn, or stained underwear
- Unusual body odor

Abusive head trauma (ART) or shaken baby syndrome: Shaking can cause intracranial hemorrhage. Caregiver's frustrations with persistent crying can lead to this.
- Can have no external manifestations of injury
- Vomiting, poor feeding, and listlessness
- Respiratory distress
- Bulging fontanels
- Retinal hemorrhages
- Seizures
- Posturing
- Alterations in level of consciousness
- Apnea
- Bradycardia
- Blindness
- Unresponsiveness
- Bruising in an infant before 6 months of age, should be deemed suspicious by the nurse.

LABORATORY TESTS

CBC, urinalysis, and other tests that assess for sexually transmitted infections or bleeding

DIAGNOSTIC PROCEDURES

Depend upon the assessment findings and injuries.
- Radiograph
- Computed tomography or magnetic resonance imaging scan

PATIENT-CENTERED CARE

NURSING CARE

- Identify maltreatment as soon as possible. Conduct detailed history and physical examination.
- The nursing priority is to have the child removed from the abusive situation.
- Mandatory reporting is required of all health care providers, including suspected cases of child maltreatment. There are civil and criminal penalties for not reporting.
- Assess for unusual bruising on the abdomen, back, and buttocks. Document thoroughly with size, shape, and color. Use diagrams to represent location.

- Assess the mechanism of injury, which might not be congruent with the physical appearance of the injury. Many bruises at different stages of healing can indicate ongoing beatings.
- Observe for bruises or welts in the shape of a belt buckle or other objects.
- Observe for burns that appear glove- or stocking-like on hands or feet, which can indicate forced immersion into boiling water. Small, round burns can be caused by lit cigarettes. Document detailed descriptions of all findings.
- Note fractures that have unusual features (forearm spiral fractures) which could be caused by twisting the extremity forcefully. The presence of multiple fractures is suspicious.
- Check the child for head injuries. Assess the child's level of consciousness, making sure to note equal and reactive pupils. Monitor for nausea/vomiting.
- Clearly and objectively document information obtained in the interview and during the physical assessment.
- Photograph and detail all visible injuries, if possible, including measuring devices to show size of injuries.
- Conduct the interview with the client and guardians individually.
- Be direct, honest, and professional.
- Use language the child understands.
- Be understanding and attentive.
- Client circumstances are case-sensitive, and referrals are made to always keep the client safe. When applicable, explain the process if a referral is made to child or adult protective services.
- Assess safety and reduce danger for the victim.
- Use open-ended questions that require a descriptive response. These questions are less threatening and elicit more relevant information.
- Provide support for the child and parents.
- Demonstrate behaviors for child-rearing with the parents and child.
- Provide consistent care to the child.
- Avoid asking the child probing questions.
- Promote self-esteem.
- Assist with alleviating feelings of shame and guilt.
- Assist the child with grieving the loss of parents, if indicated.
- Discharge can begin once legal determination of placement has been decided.

INTERPROFESSIONAL CARE

Initiate appropriate referrals for social services.

Bullying

Physical, verbal, or emotional abuse that is repetitive by a person to another person with intent to establish power and dominance with intimidation. This could be with or without face-to-face contact.

SETTINGS: school, playground, bus, texting, or online

ASSESSMENT

RISK FACTORS

PERPETRATORS OF BULLYING BEHAVIOR
- Male sex
- Depression
- Decreased academic performance
- Decreased social involvement with peers
- Exposure to spouse or partner violence
- Conduct problems
- Criminal acts
- Dropping out of school

RECIPIENTS OF BULLYING BEHAVIOR
- Low self-esteem
- Loneliness
- Somatic reports
- Anxiety
- Depression

PATIENT-CENTERED CARE

CLIENT EDUCATION
- Observe for manifestations and be inquisitive.
- Obtain support from the family.
- Refer to counseling and bully prevention programs.
- Follow procedures for investigating and reporting.
- Refer for mental health evaluation because bullying can be an early indication of mental health disorders.

Active Learning Scenario

A nurse is teaching a group of caregivers about abusive head trauma (AHT) or shaken baby syndrome What manifestations should be included in this presentation? Use the ATI Active Learning Template: Basic Concept to complete this item.

UNDERLYING PRINCIPLES: Include seven manifestations.

Active Learning Scenario Key

Using the ATI Active Learning Template: Basic Concept
UNDERLYING PRINCIPLES
- Vomiting, poor feeding, and listlessness
- Respiratory distress
- Bulging fontanels
- Retinal hemorrhages
- Seizures
- Posturing
- Alterations in level of consciousness
- Apnea
- Bradycardia

Ⓝ *NCLEX® Connection: Physiological Adaptation, Illness Management*

Application Exercises

1. A nurse is caring for a child who has a depressive disorder. List 3 clinical manifestations the nurse should expect.

2. A nurse is teaching a parent about posttraumatic stress disorder (PTSD). Which of the following information should the nurse include in the teaching? (Select all that apply.)

   A. Children who have PTSD can benefit from psychotherapy.

   B. A manifestation of PTSD is psychosis.

   C. Personality disorders are a complication of PTSD.

   D. There are six stages of PTSD.

   E. PTSD develops following a traumatic event.

3. A nurse is teaching the parent of a child about risk factors for attention-deficit/hyperactivity disorder (ADHD). Which of the following should the nurse include in the teaching?

   A. Formula-feeding as an infant

   B. History of head trauma

   C. History of postterm birth

   D. Child of a single parent

4. A nurse is providing instruction to the teacher of a child who has attention-deficit/hyperactivity disorder (ADHD). Which of the following classroom strategies should the nurse include in the teaching? (Select all that apply.)

   A. Eliminate testing.

   B. Allow for regular breaks.

   C. Combine verbal instruction with visual cues.

   D. Establish consistent classroom rules.

   E. Increase stimuli in the environment.

5. A nurse is teaching a group of parents about characteristics of infants who have failure to thrive. Which of the following characteristics should the nurse include in the teaching?

   A. Intense fear of strangers

   B. Increased risk for childhood obesity

   C. Inability to form close relationships with siblings

   D. Developmental delays

Application Exercises Key

1. The nurse should recognize a child who has depressive disorders could exhibit the following manifestation weight loss or gain, low self-esteem, alterations in sleep patterns, sad facial expressions, withdrawn from family, friends, and activities, fatigue, tendencies to remain alone, feeling of worthlessness, hopelessness, lack of interest in school, drop in school performance, and suicidal ideations

   Ⓝ NCLEX® Connection: Health Promotion and Maintenance, Health Screening

2. A, B, D. **CORRECT:** The nurse should teach the guardian about posttraumatic stress disorder (PTSD) to include children who have PTSD should be referred to psychotherapy to assist with resolution of the traumatic event. The child often has psychosis that can be related to the traumatic event. PTSD develops following a traumatic event (assault, serious injury, or a life-threatening episode).

   C. Personality disorders are not a complication of PTSD.

   E. PTSD has three stages: the initial response, and second and third phase.

   Ⓝ NCLEX® Connection: Reduction of Risk Potential, Therapeutic Procedures

3. A. Being formula-fed as an infant is not a risk factor for the development of ADHD.

   B. **CORRECT:** The nurse should discuss risk factors for attention-deficit/hyperactivity disorder (ADHD) which include a history of head trauma

   C. History of a post-term birth is not a risk factor for the development of ADHD.

   D. Being the child of a single parent does not increase the risk of development of ADHD.

   Ⓝ NCLEX® Connection: Reduction of Risk Potential, Therapeutic Procedures

4. B, C, D. **CORRECT:** The nurse should include the following strategies for a teacher of a child who has attention-deficit/hyperactivity disorder (ADHD): allow for regular breaks will assist the client who has ADHD to focus on the required tasks, combining verbal instructions with visual cues will assist the client who has ADHD with learning information, providing consistent classroom rules will assist the client who has ADHD to become successful. Also, allowing for added time when testing can assist the client who has ADHD to be successful.

   A. Allowing for added time when testing can assist the client who has ADHD to be successful.

   E. Stimuli in the environment distract the client who has ADHD, so it should be decreased.

   Ⓝ NCLEX® Connection: Physiological Adaptation, Pathophysiology

5. A. They do not exhibit an intense fear of strangers or are not at an increases risk for childhood obesity, nor do they have an inability to form close relationships..

   B. They do not exhibit an intense fear of strangers or are not at an increases risk for childhood obesity, nor do they have an inability to form close relationships..

   C. They do not exhibit an intense fear of strangers or are not at an increases risk for childhood obesity, nor do they have an inability to form close relationships.

   D. **CORRECT:** The nurse should include the following information when teaching a group of guardians about characteristics of infants who have failure to thrive developmental delays due to decreased nutritional intake which if needed for brain development.

   Ⓝ NCLEX® Connection: Health Promotion and Maintenance, Health Screening

References

Academy of Nutrition and Dietetics. (2021). *Do's and don'ts for baby's first foods.* https://www.eatright.org/food/nutrition/eating-as-a-family/dos-and-donts-for-babys-first-foods

Agrawal, S. & Khazaeni, B. (2021, July 18). *Acetaminophen toxicity.* StatPearls. https://www.ncbi.nlm.nih.gov/books/NBK441917/

Alamarat, Z. & Hasbun, R. (2020). Management of acute bacterial meningitis in children. *Infection and drug resistance, 13,* 4077–4089. https://doi.org/10.2147/IDR.S240162

American Academy of Pediatrics (2022). *Breastfeeding recommendations.* https://www.cdc.gov/breastfeeding/recommendations/index.htm

American Academy of Pediatrics. (2019, March 15). *Swim lessons: When to start & what parents should know.* Healthychildren.org. https://www.healthychildren.org/English/safety-prevention/at-play/Pages/Swim-Lessons.aspx

American Academy of Pediatrics. (2022). *Back to sleep, tummy to play.* https://www.healthychildren.org/English/ages-stages/baby/sleep/Pages/Back-to-Sleep-Tummy-to-Play.aspx

American Academy of Pediatrics. (2022). *Policy statement: Breastfeeding and the use of human milk.* https://doi.org/10.1542/peds.2022-057988

American Academy of Pediatrics. (2022). *Starting solid foods.* https://www.healthychildren.org/English/ages-stages/baby/feeding-nutrition/Pages/Starting-Solid-Foods.aspx

Anand, S. & Lotfollahzadeh, S. (2021). *Epispadias.* StatPearls.

Asim, M., Alkadi, M. M., Asim, H., & Ghaffar, A. (2019). Dehydration and volume depletion: How to handle misconceptions. *World Journal of Nephrology, 8*(1), 23–32

Asthma and Allergy Foundation of America. (2018). *Asthma diagnosis. Asthma and Allergy Foundation of America.* https://www.aafa.org/asthma-diagnosis/

Asthma and Allergy Foundation of America. (n.d.). *Lung function tests to diagnose asthma.* https://www.aafa.org/lung-function-tests-diagnose-asthma.aspx

Avital, O. & Karakashian, A. (2019). *Kidney injury, acute, in children [Review of kidney injury, acute, in children].* CINAHL Information Systems.

Beck, L., Bomback, A. S., Choi, M. J., Holzman, L. B., Langford, C., Mariani, L. H., Somers, M. J., Trachtman, H., & Waldman, M. (2013). KDOQI US Commentary on the 2012 KDIGO clinical practice guideline for glomerulonephritis. *American Journal of Kidney Diseases, 62*(3), 403–441. https://doi.org/10.1053/j.ajkd.2013.06.002

Berman, A., Snyder, S., & Frandsen, G. (2021). *Kozier & Erb's fundamentals of nursing: Concepts, process, and practice* (11th ed.) Pearson.

Boling, B. & Karakashian, A. (2018). *Renal failure, chronic, in children: Therapy – transplantation and dialysis [Review of renal failure, chronic, in children: Therapy – transplantation and dialysis].* CINAHL Information Systems.

Boys and Girls Club of America. (n.d.). *Workforce readiness: Building tomorrow's leaders, innovators and problem-solvers.* https://www.bgca.org/programs/career-development

Caple, C. (2018). *Major burns overview: Managing the pediatric patient with [Review of major burns overview: Managing the pediatric patient with].* CINAHL Information Systems.

Centers for Disease Control and Prevention. (2019, July 22). *Type and duration of precautions recommended for selected infections and conditions.* https://www.cdc.gov/infectioncontrol/guidelines/isolation/appendix/type-duration-precautions.html#varicella

Centers for Disease Control and Prevention. (2020). *Influenza.* https://www.cdc.gov/flu/prevent/egg-allergies.htm

Centers for Disease Control and Prevention. (2020, December 31). *Rubella (German measles, three-day measles): For healthcare professionals.* https://www.cdc.gov/rubella/hcp.html

Centers for Disease Control and Prevention. (2020, November 5). *Measles (Rubeola): Transmission of measles.* https://www.cdc.gov/measles/transmission.html

Centers for Disease Control and Prevention. (2020, September 9). *Vaccine safety: Hepatitis A vaccine.* https://www.cdc.gov/vaccinesafety/vaccines/hepatitis-a-vaccine.html

Centers for Disease Control and Prevention. (2021). *Birth-18 years immunization schedule.* https://www.cdc.gov/vaccines/schedules/hcp/imz/child-adolescent.html

Centers for Disease Control and Prevention. (2021). *When, what, and how to introduce solid foods.* https://www.cdc.gov/nutrition/infantandtoddlernutrition/foods-and-drinks/when-to-introduce-solid-foods.html

Centers for Disease Control and Prevention. (2021, April 13). *Hib vaccine recommendations.* https://www.cdc.gov/vaccines/vpd/hib/hcp/recommendations.html

Centers for Disease Control and Prevention. (2021, April 28). *Chickenpox (Varicella): For healthcare professionals.* https://www.cdc.gov/chickenpox/hcp/index.html

Centers for Disease Control and Prevention. (2021, August 24). *When, what, and how to introduce solid foods.* https://www.cdc.gov/nutrition/infantandtoddlernutrition/foods-and-drinks/when-to-introduce-solid-foods.html

Centers for Disease Control and Prevention. (2021, August 6). *Vaccine information statements (VISs): MMR (Measles, mumps, rubella) VIS.* https://www.cdc.gov/vaccines/hcp/vis/vis-statements/mmr.html

Centers for Disease Control and Prevention. (2021, December 10). *Flu vaccine and people with egg allergies.* https://www.cdc.gov/flu/prevent/egg-allergies.htm

Centers for Disease Control and Prevention. (2021, December 13). *COVID-19 vaccines for children and teens.* https://www.cdc.gov/coronavirus/2019-ncov/vaccines/recommendations/children-teens.html

Centers for Disease Control and Prevention. (2021, June 16). *Nucleic acid amplification tests (NAATs).* https://www.cdc.gov/coronavirus/2019-ncov/lab/naats.html

Centers for Disease Control and Prevention. (2021, March 5). *Virus classification.* https://www.cdc.gov/norovirus/lab/virus-classification.html

Centers for Disease Control and Prevention. (2021, November 16). *HPV vaccine recommendations.* https://www.cdc.gov/vaccines/vpd/hpv/hcp/recommendations.html

Centers for Disease Control and Prevention. (2021, October 15). *Vaccine information statements (VISs). Hepatitis A VIS.* https://www.cdc.gov/vaccines/hcp/vis/vis-statements/hep-a.html

Centers for Disease Control and Prevention. (2021, September 9). *Vaccine safety: Measles, mumps, rubella (MMR) vaccine.* https://www.cdc.gov/vaccinesafety/vaccines/mmr-vaccine.html

Centers for Disease Control and Prevention. (2022). *Frequently asked questions: What are the benefits of breastfeeding?* https://www.cdc.gov/breastfeeding/faq/index.htm#howlong

Centers for Disease Control and Prevention. (2022, February 17). *Child and adolescent immunization schedule.* https://www.cdc.gov/vaccines/schedules/hcp/imz/child-adolescent.html#appendix-hepa

Centers for Disease Control and Prevention. (2022, February 17). *Child and adolescent immunization schedule.* https://www.cdc.gov/vaccines/schedules/hcp/imz/child-adolescent.html#note-tdap

Centers for Disease Control and Prevention. (2022, July 5). *What is a developmental milestone?.* https://www.cdc.gov/ncbddd/actearly/milestones/index.html

Centers for Disease Control and Prevention. (2022, March 15). *Vaccine recommendations and guidelines of the ACIP: Contraindications and precautions.* https://www.cdc.gov/vaccines/hcp/acip-recs/general-recs/contraindications.html

Centers for Disease Control and Prevention. (2022, March 16). *Terms, definitions, and calculations used in CDC HIV surveillance publications.* https://www.cdc.gov/hiv/statistics/surveillance/terms.html

Centers for Disease Control and Prevention. (2022, March 4). *Guidance for antigen testing for SARS-CoV-2 for healthcare providers testing individuals in the community.* https://www.cdc.gov/coronavirus/2019-ncov/lab/resources/antigen-tests-guidelines.html

Centers for Disease Control and Prevention. (2022, May 24). *Stay up to date with your COVID-19 vaccines.* https://www.cdc.gov/coronavirus/2019-ncov/vaccines/stay-up-to-date.html

Children's Health Orange County. (2021, May). *Growth & development: 6 to 12 years (School age).* https://www.choc.org/primary-care/ages-stages/6-to-12-years/

Children's Hospital of Philadelphia. (2022). *Osteosarcoma (Bone cancer in children).* https://www.chop.edu/conditions-diseases/osteosarcoma-in-children

Cleveland Clinic. (2022). *Benefits of tummy time and how to do it safely: A few minutes a day can go a long way for your newborn.* https://health.clevelandclinic.org/3-benefits-of-tummy-time-for-newborns-how-to-do-it-safely/

Course Hero. (2019). *Piaget's theory of cognitive development.* Coursehero.com. https://www.coursehero.com/study-guides/wmopen-lifespandevelopment/cognitive-development-in-early-childhood/

DeVille, J. D., Song, E., & Ouellette, C. P. (2022, March 11). *COVID-19: Management in children.* UptoDate.

DeVille, J. D., Song, E., & Ouellette, C. P. (2022, March 11). *COVID-19: Clinical manifestation and diagnosis in children.* UptoDate.

deWit, S. C., Stromberg, H. K., & Dallred, C. V. (2021). *Medical-Surgical nursing: Concepts and practice* (4th ed.). Elsevier.

Drutz, J. E. (2021). *Acute pharyngitis in children and adolescents: Symptomatic treatment.* UptoDate.

Dudek, S. G. (2022). *Nutrition essentials for nursing practice* (9th ed.). Lippincott, Williams & Wolter.

Duryea, T. K. & Fleischer, D. M. (2022, March 17). *Patient education: Starting solid foods during infancy (Beyond the basics).* Uptodate.

Epilepsy Foundation. (2019, May). *Febrile seizures.* https://www.epilepsy.com/learn/types-seizures/febrile-seizures

Epilepsy Society. (2018). *Focal aware seizures (previously called simple partial seizures).* https://epilepsysociety.org.uk/about-epilepsy/epileptic-seizures/focal-aware-seizures

Farrell, S. E. (2021, October 5). *Acetaminophen toxicity clinical presentation.* https://emedicine.medscape.com/article/820200-clinical#b3

Fastle, R. K. & Bothner, J. (2020, October 8). *Lumbar puncture: Indications, contraindications, technique, and complications in children.* UptoDate.

Francis, L., DePriest, K., Wilson, M., & Gross, D. (2018). Child poverty, toxic stress, and social determinants of health: Screening and care coordination. *Online Journal of Issues in Nursing, 23*(3), 2. https://doi.org/10.3912/OJIN.Vol23No03Man02

Freedman, S. (2022, February 18). *Oral rehydration therapy.* UptoDate.

Gillam-Krakauer, M. & Mahajan, K. (2021, August 11). *Patent ductus arteriosus.* StatPearls. https://www.ncbi.nlm.nih.gov/books/NBK430758/

Heering, H. & Avital, O. (2018). *Enuresis, nocturnal: Behavioral interventions: Alarms [Review of enuresis, nocturnal: Behavioral interventions].* CINAHL Information Systems.

HIV.gov. (2021, December 30). *Recommendations for the use of antiretroviral drugs during pregnancy and interventions to reduce perinatal HIV transmission in the United States.* https://clinicalinfo.hiv.gov/en/guidelines/perinatal/diagnosis-hiv-infection-infants-and-children

Hockenberry, M. J., Wilson, D. & Rodgers, C. (2019). *Wong's nursing care of infants and children* (11th ed.). Elsevier.

Horrii, K. (2022, February 10). *Diaper dermatitis.* UptoDate. https://www.uptodate.com/contents/diaper-dermatitis

Immunize.org. (2020). *Rotavirus.* https://www.immunize.org/askexperts/experts_rota.asp

Inker, L. A., Astor, B. C., Fox, C. H., Isakova, T., Lash, J. P., Peralta, C. A., Kurella Tamura, M., & Feldman, H. I. (2014). KDOQI US commentary on the 2012 KDIGO clinical practice guideline for the evaluation and management of CKD. *American Journal of Kidney Diseases, 63*(5), 713–735. https://doi.org/10.1053/j.ajkd.2014.01.416

Kumar, A., Maini, K., & Sharma S. (2021, December 17). *Simple partial seizure.* StatPearls.

Laffel, L. & Svoren B. (2022, January 21). *Epidemology, presentation, and diagnosis of type 2 diabetes mellitus in children and adolescents.* UptoDate.

Levitsky, L. L. & Madhusmita, M. (2021, Oct 1). *Epidemology, presentation, and diagnosis of type 1 diabetes mellitus in children and adolescents.* UptoDate.

Levitsky, L. L. & Madhusmita, M. (2022, February 2). *Hypoglycemia in children and adolescents with type 1 diabetes mellitus.* UptoDate.

Lilley, L. L., Rainsforth Colllins, S., & Snyder, J. S. (2020). *Pharmacology and the nursing process* (9th ed.). Elsevier.

Marcella, E. (2019). The rule of '2': Teaching a simplified approach to behavioral urotherapy. *Urologic Nursing, 39*(3), 145. https://doi.org/10.7257/1053-816x.2019.39.3.145

MD Anderson Cancer Center. (2022). *Childhood osteosarcoma symptoms.* https://www.mdanderson.org/cancer-types/childhood-osteosarcoma/childhood-osteosarcoma-symptoms.html

MedlinePlus. (2022, August 02). *Brief resolved unexplained event-BRUE.* https://medlineplus.gov/ency/article/007683.htm

MedlinePlus. (2022, March 21). *Brain herniation.* https://medlineplus.gov/ency/article/001421.htm

Moore. (2018). *Allograft tissue safety and technology [Review of allograft tissue safety and technology].* Biologics in Orthopedic Surgery. https://doi.org/https://dx.doi.org/10.1016%2FB978-0-323-55140-3.00005-9

National Institute of Child Health and Human Development. (2022). *Babies need tummy time.* https://safetosleep.nichd.nih.gov/safesleepbasics/tummytime#way

National Library of Medicine. (2017, September 1). *Fosamprenavir.* https://www.ncbi.nlm.nih.gov/books/NBK548011/

Office of Disease Prevention and Health Promotion. (n.d.a.). *Reduce the proportion of children with a parent or guardian who has served time in jail-SDOH-05.* Healthy People 2030. U.S. Department of Health and Human Services. https://health.gov/healthypeople/objectives-and-data/browse-objectives/social-and-community-context/reduce-proportion-children-parent-or-guardian-who-has-served-time-jail-sdoh-05

Office of Disease Prevention and Health Promotion. (n.d.b.). *Reduce the proportion of people living in poverty-SDOH-01.* Healthy People 2030. U.S. Department of Health and Human Services. https://health.gov/healthypeople/objectives-and-data/browse-objectives/economic-stability/reduce-proportion-people-living-poverty-sdoh-01

Office of Disease Prevention and Health Promotion. (n.d.c.). *Health care access and quality.* Healthy People 2030. U.S. Department of Health and Human Services. https://health.gov/healthypeople/objectives-and-data/browse-objectives/health-care-access-and-quality

Office of Disease Prevention and Health Promotion. (n.d.d.). *Education access and quality.* Healthy People 2030. U.S. Department of Health and Human Services. https://health.gov/healthypeople/objectives-and-data/browse-objectives/education-access-and-quality

Ogbru, O. (n.d.). *Amprenavir.* Medicinenet.

Pagana, K. D., Pagana, T. J., & Pagana, T. N. (2022). *Mosby's manual of diagnostic and laboratory tests* (7th ed.). Elsevier.

Parmar, M. (2021). *Hemolytic-uremic syndrome medication [Review of hemolytic-uremic syndrome medication].* Medscape.

Potter, P. A., Perry, A. G., Stockert, P. A., & Hall, A. M. (2021). *Fundamentals of nursing* (10th ed.). Elsevier.

Redondo, M. J., Libman, I., Maahs, D. M., Lyons, S. K., Sacaco, M., Reusch, J., Rodriguez, H., & DiMegllo, L. A. (2021, February). *The evolution of hemoglobin A1c targets for youth with type 1 diabetes: Rationales and supporting evidence. Diabetes Care, 44*(2), 301-312.

Rivera, D. M. (11, November 2020). *Pediatric HIV infection workup.* https://emedicine.medscape.com/article/965086-workup#c15

Runde, T. J. & Nappe, T. M. (2021, July 14). *Salicylates toxicity.* StatPearls.

Safe Kids Worldwide. (2022). *Pedestrian safety tips: Teach kids how to walk safely.* Safekids.org. https://www.safekids.org/tip/pedestrian-safety-tips

Sanvistores, T. & Mendez, M.D. (2021). *Types of parenting styles and effects on children.* StatPearls.

Schroeder, M. K., Juul, K. V., Mahler, B., Nørgaard, J. P., & Rittig, S. (2017). Desmopressin use in pediatric nocturnal enuresis patients: is there a sex difference in prescription patterns?. *European Journal of Pediatrics, 177*(3), 389-394. https://doi.org/10.1007/s00431-017-3074-x

Schub, T. (2018). *Burns in children [Review of burns in children].* CINAHL Information Systems.

Schub, T. (2018). *Hemolytic uremic syndrome [Review of hemolytic uremic syndrome].* CINAHL Information Systems.

Selewski, D. T., Askenazi, D. J., Kashani, K., Basu, R. K., Gist, K. M., Harer, M. W., Jetton, J. G., Sutherland, S. M., Zappitelli, M., Ronco, C., Goldstein, S. L., & Mottes, T. A. (2021). Quality improvement goals for pediatric acute kidney injury: Pediatric applications of the 22nd Acute Disease Quality Initiative (ADQI) conference. *Pediatric Nephrology, 36*(4), 733–746. https://doi.org/10.1007/s00467-020-04828-5

Shapiro-Mendoza, C. K., Palusci, V. J., Hoffman, B., Batra, E., Yester, M., & Corey, T. S. (2021). Half century since SIDS: A reappraisal of terminology. *Pediatrics, 148*(4). https://doi.org/10.1542/peds.2021-053746

Silbert-Flagg, J. & Pillitteri, A. (2018). *Maternal and child health nursing: Care of the childbearing and childrearing family* (8th ed.). Lippincott Williams & Wilkins.

Stanhope, M. & Lancaster, J. (2020). *Public health nursing: Population-centered health care in the community* (10th ed.). Elsevier.

Suni, E. (2021, November 22). *Teens and sleep: An overview of why teens face unique sleep challenges and tips to help them sleep better.* https://www.sleepfoundation.org/teens-and-sleep

Taketomo, C. K., Hodding, J. H., & Kraus, D. M. (2021). *Pediatric & neonatal dosage handbook: An extensive resource for clinicians treating pediatric and neonatal patients* (28th ed.). Wolters Kluwer.

Tanaka, K., Adams, B., Aris, A. M., Fujita, N., Ogawa, M., Ortiz, S., Vallee, M., & Greenbaum, L. A. (2020). The long-acting C5 inhibitor, ravulizumab, is efficacious and safe in pediatric patients with atypical hemolytic uremic syndrome previously treated with eculizumab. *Pediatric Nephrology, 36*(4), 1033–1033. https://doi.org/10.1007/s00467-020-04874-z

Tieder, J. S., Bonkowsky, J. L., Etzel, R. A., Franklin, W. H., Gremse, D. A., Herman, B., Katz, E. S., Krilov, L. R., Merritt, J. L., Norlin, C., Percelay, J., Sapien, R. E., Shiffman, R. N., & Smith, M. B. H. (2016). Brief resolved unexplained event (formerly apparent life-threatening events) and evaluation of lower-risk infants. *Pediatrics, 137*(5). https://doi.org/10.1542/peds.2016-0590

U.S. Preventive Services Task Force. (2018). Screening for adolescent idiopathic scoliosis: Recommendation statement. *American Family Physician, 97*(10). https://www.aafp.org/afp/2018/0515/od1.html

Vallerand, A. H. & Sanoski, C. A. (2021). *Davis's drug guide for nurses* (17th ed). F.A. Davis.

Velez, M. L., Jordan, C. J., & Jansson, L. M. (2021). Reconceptualizing non-pharmacologic approaches to neonatal abstinence syndrome (NAS) and neonatal opioid withdrawal syndrome (NOWS): A theoretical and evidence-based approach. *Neurotoxicology and Teratology, 88*. https://doi.org/10.1016/j.ntt.2021.107020

World Health Organization. (2022). *Breastfeeding.* https://www.who.int/health-topics/breastfeeding#tab=tab_2

Yuen, H. & Becker, W. (25, July 2021). *Iron toxicity.* StatPearls.

Basic Concept

STUDENT NAME _____

CONCEPT_____   REVIEW MODULE CHAPTER_____

Related Content

(E.G., DELEGATION, LEVELS OF PREVENTION, ADVANCE DIRECTIVES)

Underlying Principles

Nursing Interventions

WHO? WHEN? WHY? HOW?

STUDENT NAME _____

PROCEDURE NAME _____ REVIEW MODULE CHAPTER_____

Description of Procedure

Indications

Interpretation of Findings

Potential Complications

CONSIDERATIONS

Nursing Interventions (pre, intra, post)

Client Education

Nursing Interventions

STUDENT NAME _____

DEVELOPMENTAL STAGE _____ REVIEW MODULE CHAPTER_____

EXPECTED GROWTH AND DEVELOPMENT

Physical Development	Cognitive Development	Psychosocial Development	Age-Appropriate Activities

Health Promotion

Immunizations	Health Screening	Nutrition	Injury Prevention

STUDENT NAME _____

MEDICATION _____   REVIEW MODULE CHAPTER_____

CATEGORY CLASS_____

PURPOSE OF MEDICATION

Expected Pharmacological Action

Therapeutic Use

Complications

Medication Administration

Contraindications/Precautions

Nursing Interventions

Interactions

Client Education

Evaluation of Medication Effectiveness

ACTIVE LEARNING TEMPLATE: *Nursing Skill*

STUDENT NAME _____

SKILL NAME_____ REVIEW MODULE CHAPTER_____

Description of Skill

Indications

CONSIDERATIONS

Nursing Interventions (pre, intra, post)

Outcomes/Evaluation

Client Education

Potential Complications

Nursing Interventions

ACTIVE LEARNING TEMPLATE: *System Disorder*

STUDENT NAME _____

DISORDER/DISEASE PROCESS _____ REVIEW MODULE CHAPTER_____

Alterations in Health (Diagnosis)	Pathophysiology Related to Client Problem	Health Promotion and Disease Prevention

ASSESSMENT

Risk Factors

Expected Findings

Laboratory Tests

Diagnostic Procedures

SAFETY CONSIDERATIONS

PATIENT-CENTERED CARE

Nursing Care

Medications

Client Education

Therapeutic Procedures

Interprofessional Care

Complications

Therapeutic Procedure

STUDENT NAME _____

PROCEDURE NAME _____ REVIEW MODULE CHAPTER_____

Description of Procedure

Indications

CONSIDERATIONS

Nursing Interventions (pre, intra, post)

Outcomes/Evaluation

Client Education

Potential Complications

Nursing Interventions

Concept Analysis

STUDENT NAME _____

CONCEPT ANALYSIS_____

Defining Characteristics

Antecedents

(WHAT MUST OCCUR/BE IN PLACE FOR
CONCEPT TO EXIST/FUNCTION PROPERLY)

Negative Consequences

(RESULTS FROM IMPAIRED ANTECEDENT —
COMPLETE WITH FACULTY ASSISTANCE)

Related Concepts

(REVIEW LIST OF CONCEPTS AND IDENTIFY, WHICH
CAN BE AFFECTED BY THE STATUS OF THIS CONCEPT
— COMPLETE WITH FACULTY ASSISTANCE)

Exemplars